Working for Health

University Centre Barnsley

Telephone: 01226 | 644281

University of
HUDDERSFIELD

UniversityCentre
Barnsley

Open University Course: Working for Health (K203)

This Reader forms part of the Open University course *Working for Health* (K203), a 60 points second level undergraduate course. It is an optional course for the BA/BSc (Open) and the BA/BSc in Health and Social Care, as well as being a core course for the Diploma in Health and Social Welfare.

The chapters in this book have been designed as a source for students during their study of K203. The collection of readings has been chosen to challenge preconceptions and to evoke a critical understanding of health issues. Opinions expressed in the Reader are not necessarily those of the Course Team or of The Open University.

If you are interested in studying this course or working towards a related degree or diploma please write to the Information Officer, School of Health and Social Welfare, The Open University, Walton Hall, Milton Keynes, MK7 6AA, UK. Details can also be reviewed on our web page http://www.open.ac.uk

Working for Health

Edited by
Tom Heller, Rosemary Muston,
Moyra Sidell and Cathy Lloyd
at the Open University

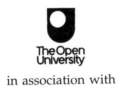

The Open
University

in association with

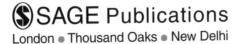

SAGE Publications
London ● Thousand Oaks ● New Delhi

SAGE Publications Ltd
1 Oliver's Yard
55 City Road
London EC1Y 1SP

SAGE Publications Inc
2455 Teller Road
Thousand Oaks
California 91320

SAGE Publications India Pvt. Ltd
B-42 Panchsheel Enclave
PO Box 4109
New Delhi 110 017

British Library Cataloguing in Publication data
A catalogue record for this book is available from the British Library

ISBN-10 0-7619-6997-7   ISBN-13 978-0-7619-6997-6
ISBN-10 0-7619-6998-5 (pbk)   ISBN-13 978-0-7619-6998-3 (pbk)

Printed on paper from sustainable sources

Typeset by Photoprint Ltd., Torquay, Devon
Printed and bound in Great Britain by
Cromwell Press Limited, Trowbridge, Wiltshire

Contents

Acknowledgements

The authors and publishers wish to thank the following for permission to use copyright material.

Chapter 1: HarperCollins Publishers for 'The past, the present and the future' from *A Medical History of Humanity from Antiquity to the Present* by Roy Porter, 1999.

Chapter 2: *The Lancet* for Robert Downie and Jane Macnaughton (1998) 'Images of Health', *The Lancet*, 351: 823–825.

Chapter 3: Macmillan Press Ltd for 'From clinical gaze to regime of total health' by David Armstrong from A. Beattie, M. Gott, L. Jones and M. Sidell (eds) (1993) *Health and Wellbeing: A Reader* (pp. 55–67).

Chapter 4: Royal College of Physicians for Douglas Black (1998) 'The limitations of evidence', *Journal of the Royal College of Physicians of London*, 32 (1): 23–26.

Chapter 5: University of California Press for 'Postmodernism and Illness' from *Illness and Culture in the Postmodern Age* by David Morris, 1998.

Chapter 6: The Royal Society of Medicine Press for John Bunker (1997), 'Ivan Illich and the pursuit of health', *Journal of Health Services Research and Policy*, 2 (1): 56–59.

Chapter 7: Routledge for 'A Social View of Health and Disease' by Michael Marmot from *Health and Social Organization* edited by D. Blane, E. Brunner and R. Wilkinson (1996) (pp. 42–67).

Chapter 8: Health Development Agency for Richard Wilkinson 'Social status, inequality and health' from *Inequalities in Health, HEA Seminars 1999* (pp. 33–46).

Chapter 10: Baywood Publishing Company Inc. for Lesley Doyal 'The politics of women's health: setting a global agenda', *International Journal of Health Services*, 26 (1): 47–65.

Chapter 11: Reproduced by permission of Oxford University Press Australia from *The New Public Health; An Australian Perspective*, by Fran Baum (ed.), OUP, 1998 © Oxford University Press, www.oup.com.au

Chapter 12: Lippincott Williams and Wilkins for Anthony J. McMichael (1999) 'From Hazard to Habitat: Rethinking Environment and Health', *Epidemiology and Society*, 10 (4).

Chapter 13: *The Lancet* for Gill Walt (1998) 'Globalisation of International Health', *The Lancet*, 351: 434–437.

Chapter 16: Comedia for 'The Health and Social Impact of Participation in the Arts' from *Use or Ornament?*, Francois Matarasso, 1997.

Chapter 17: The Royal Society of Medicine Press for Janet Butler (1993) 'Prevention may be more expensive than cure', *Journal of the Royal Society of Medicine*, 86: 341–344.

Chapter 18: BMJ Publishing Group for Raj Bhopal (1997) 'Is research into ethnicity and health racist, unsound, or important science', *British Medical Journal*, 314: 1751.

Chapter 19: Sage Publications Ltd for 'My body is my art' by Kathy Davis from *Embodied practices: Feminist perspectives on the body*, Kathy Davis (ed.), 1997.

Chapter 21: American College of Physicians for Donald Berwick (1996) 'Quality Comes Home', *Annals of International Medicine*, 125 (10): 839–843.

Chapter 23: BMJ Publishing Group for Julie Taylor, Nick Spencer and Norma Baldwin (2000) 'Social, economic and political context of parents', *Arch Dis Child* 113–120.

Chapter 26: Open University Press for 'Understanding chronic illness' from Moyra Sidell, *Health in old age: Myth, mystery and management* (pp. 57–69), 1995.

Chapter 27: Blackwell Science Ltd for Christine Webb 'Caring, curing and coping', *Journal of Advanced Nursing*, 23: 960–968.

Chapter 28: Jocalyn Lawler for 'Sexuality, the body and nursing' from Jocalyn Lawler, *Behind the screens: Nursing, somology and the problem of the body*, pp. 195–213, 1991.

Chapter 30: Bailliere Tindall for Mavis Kirkham 'Stories and Childbirth' from *Reflections on Midwifery* by Mavis Kirkham and Elizabeth Perkins, pp. 183–201, 1997.

Chapter 31: Findhorn Press for 'Research in holistic medicine' by Mike Fitter from *Medical Marriage* edited by Cornelia Featherstone, 1998.

Chapter 34: BMJ Publishing Group for Wolfgang Sadee (1999) 'Pharmacogenomics', *British Medical Journal*, 319: 1294.

Chapter 35: BMJ Publishing Group for Gunther Eysenback, Eun Ryoung Sa and Thomas Diepgen (1999) 'Towards the Millennium of cybermedicine', *British Medical Journal*, 319: 1294.

Chapter 37: BMJ Publishing Group for 'Future health scenarios and public policy' by Michael Peckham from *Clinical Futures* edited by Marshall Marinker and Michael Peckham, 1998.

Preface

Many disciplines have a contribution to make in the search for meaning and understanding of health and health issues. No single aspect of study, or any individual, can lay claim to having the answers to the questions that surround human health. This is an individual matter, *'What does your health mean to you'*, and also an intensely communal concern, *'What features in society tend to make it more, or less, healthy?'* 'Working for Health', the title of this collection, is intended to convey some of the dynamic nature of this search, and the importance of the effort that is required to get to grips with these apparently simple questions. Trying to understand the nature of health will require sightings and insights from many different vantage points. Mariners can plot their position while at sea from a couple of fixed points, but our task in defining health may be more complex and many more attempts at illuminating our subject are required. For the meaning of health is elusive, and can be transient, and there may be few fixed points from which to take our bearings.

The collection of writings that make up this book have been chosen to guide us in the search for meaning or meanings surrounding the subject of health. The editors and authors come from many of the disciplines which have traditionally laid claim to knowledge about health. Historians, sociologists, public health specialists, statisticians, economists, ethicists, psychologists, as well as doctors and nurses from a variety of specialities, have put down their markers in the papers you will find in this volume. Their attempts to discuss the meaning of health are all incomplete as individual items. Sometimes their views may even be contradictory or worryingly disparate, but together the collection is intended to contribute to the totality of the debate, and to stimulate you to continue your own search for meaning and understanding in this intensely interesting subject area.

In general terms the volume is intended to dispel the notion that any one academic or professional discipline has all the answers, but confirms that each one does have an important contribution to make to the whole. In the past it could be considered that doctors attempted to colonize this subject area and exert excessive power in the attempt to promulgate their world view. The 'medical model' ruled the waves, and all those who would challenge it were variously insulted, assaulted or marginalized. In attempting to introduce some balance into these debates, the editors have given space to critics of the medical model, but have also retained

Sir Douglas Black is a past President of the Royal College of Physicians and could be expected to hold the medical line against attack from other disciplines. But from within its uppermost ranks he looks at 'The Limitations of Evidence' (Chapter 4) and uses an eclectic approach to examine one of its current bastions, the concept of 'evidence based medicine' (EBM), on which much of the moral high ground of current medical practice is based. He puts forward an irresistible case for balance between the 'science' and the 'art' of medical practice and gives his opinion that 'the unstructured search for evidence may only lead to confusion'. David Morris (Chapter 5: 'Postmodern Illness') almost 'clinically' dissects the nature of illness and disease, while giving a clear exposition of the theory and methods of postmodernism. The contribution of postmodernism to the debate about health, illness and the nature of the medical task is explored. If postmodernism allows us to recognize the social construction of concepts such as health and illness from pluralistic building blocks taken from science, multiculturalism and many disparate disciplines, then all this can also be taken apart, destabilized and deconstructed using the same analyses. The result, for people wanting to understand, or even operate within, the previously apparently stable medical world, is 'something close to intellectual chaos: the controlled experiment from hell and "normal science" run amok'. In the final paper in this section John P. Bunker (Chapter 6: 'Ivan Illich and the Pursuit of Health') takes something of a defensive stance on behalf of the medical establishment. While charting some of the attacks on the medical model during his own career and the way that they have been repulsed, he argues for a separation of the social and medical determinants of health. He is keen that the 'baby' of medical treatment is not thrown away with the 'bath water' of social determinism. 'Social reform is not a substitute for health care, as the current social activists would have it. Rather, our social environment is a second, but quite separate, determinant of health and well-being.'

Preface

Many disciplines have a contribution to make in the search for meaning and understanding of health and health issues. No single aspect of study, or any individual, can lay claim to having the answers to the questions that surround human health. This is an individual matter, *'What does your health mean to you'*, and also an intensely communal concern, *'What features in society tend to make it more, or less, healthy?'* 'Working for Health', the title of this collection, is intended to convey some of the dynamic nature of this search, and the importance of the effort that is required to get to grips with these apparently simple questions. Trying to understand the nature of health will require sightings and insights from many different vantage points. Mariners can plot their position while at sea from a couple of fixed points, but our task in defining health may be more complex and many more attempts at illuminating our subject are required. For the meaning of health is elusive, and can be transient, and there may be few fixed points from which to take our bearings.

The collection of writings that make up this book have been chosen to guide us in the search for meaning or meanings surrounding the subject of health. The editors and authors come from many of the disciplines which have traditionally laid claim to knowledge about health. Historians, sociologists, public health specialists, statisticians, economists, ethicists, psychologists, as well as doctors and nurses from a variety of specialities, have put down their markers in the papers you will find in this volume. Their attempts to discuss the meaning of health are all incomplete as individual items. Sometimes their views may even be contradictory or worryingly disparate, but together the collection is intended to contribute to the totality of the debate, and to stimulate you to continue your own search for meaning and understanding in this intensely interesting subject area.

In general terms the volume is intended to dispel the notion that any one academic or professional discipline has all the answers, but confirms that each one does have an important contribution to make to the whole. In the past it could be considered that doctors attempted to colonize this subject area and exert excessive power in the attempt to promulgate their world view. The 'medical model' ruled the waves, and all those who would challenge it were variously insulted, assaulted or marginalized. In attempting to introduce some balance into these debates, the editors have given space to critics of the medical model, but have also retained the arguments of commentators who recognize the continuing contribution that medicine can make to the 'health' of any society.

The papers in this collection have been organized into six parts:

Theory and Ideology
Social Patterns of Health
Public Health Issues
The Human Side of Health
Caring and Curing
Looking to the Future

The division of the Reader into these parts reflects the editors' hope that the collection will help readers to travel from understanding theory towards more practical considerations of 'what needs to be done' about various contemporary health issues. The collection represents journeys from theory to practice, and also from a global scale, discussing grand theoretical sweeps and universal or international issues, to quite intimate and personal explorations of the meaning and understanding of health for individuals. The aim is to provide a collection that will be of interest and assistance to people with a general interest in health issues, to users of health services, to service providers and professionals, and to academics and those interested in the theory that underpins health care practice.

As editors we hope that we have provided you with a refreshing and stimulating collection. You will not find all these readings comfortable, because we have not shied away from controversy or complexity. We have chosen those readings which have helped us personally and collectively, in our own search to understand health-related issues, and which illustrate clearly exactly those subject areas that have been difficult for us to grasp. We will have succeeded in our task if, through this selection, you also are helped to understand some of the range of difficulties and complexities that surround this fascinating and challenging subject area.

PART I

THEORY AND IDEOLOGY

Part 1 of this collection provides insights into the nature of some of the challenges to the dominant medical model and positions the contribution of various disciplines within the debate that attempts to delineate the nature of health. This selection may not make comfortable reading for members of the medical or other caring professions, or indeed for people seeking simple statements or easy definitions regarding the nature of health or illness. Using historical and cultural insights, the six contributors have variously set about dismantling many preconceived notions about health and illness.

Roy Porter (Chapter 1: 'The Past, the Present and the Future') takes a broad historical canter through several centuries of medical 'science' and, while acknowledging the contribution that biomedical interventions have made, opines that medicine is really a 'downstream activity' engaging in 'Band-Aid salvage' which therefore has little or nothing to do with health. He concludes that in the current climate, 'medicine will have to redefine its limits even as it extends its capacities'.

Robin Downie and Jane Macnaughton (Chapter 2: 'Images of Health') examine a rich swathe of literature and the visual arts, searching for representations or images of health, but with little immediate success. For them health seems to be either represented and defined by its absence (the presence of disease or illness), or by other proxies of positive health, such as happiness or vigour. They ask the question, if you remove images of illness, what is left? They extrapolate from their own difficulties in trying to find satisfactory images for health to the quest of the entire medical profession; 'The protean nature of health explains why doctors, perhaps rightly, concentrate on trying to minimize sickness rather than on promoting positive health.' This explanation, however, does not satisfy David Armstrong (Chapter 3: 'From Clinical Gaze to Regime of Total Health'), who looks in much more detail at the historical dimensions of power and the ordering and reordering of the medical endeavour through historical ages. His view of the 'extended medical gaze' analyses the way that the medical sphere of influence has been extended from considering only the body and its functions, to considering the space between bodies (relationships, psychosocial space, etc.), and more recently transforming itself into the 'new public health', enveloping all of society and from which no one seemingly can escape.

Sir Douglas Black is a past President of the Royal College of Physicians and could be expected to hold the medical line against attack from other disciplines. But from within its uppermost ranks he looks at 'The Limitations of Evidence' (Chapter 4) and uses an eclectic approach to examine one of its current bastions, the concept of 'evidence based medicine' (EBM), on which much of the moral high ground of current medical practice is based. He puts forward an irresistible case for balance between the 'science' and the 'art' of medical practice and gives his opinion that 'the unstructured search for evidence may only lead to confusion'. David Morris (Chapter 5: 'Postmodern Illness') almost 'clinically' dissects the nature of illness and disease, while giving a clear exposition of the theory and methods of postmodernism. The contribution of postmodernism to the debate about health, illness and the nature of the medical task is explored. If postmodernism allows us to recognize the social construction of concepts such as health and illness from pluralistic building blocks taken from science, multiculturalism and many disparate disciplines, then all this can also be taken apart, destabilized and deconstructed using the same analyses. The result, for people wanting to understand, or even operate within, the previously apparently stable medical world, is 'something close to intellectual chaos: the controlled experiment from hell and "normal science" run amok'. In the final paper in this section John P. Bunker (Chapter 6: 'Ivan Illich and the Pursuit of Health') takes something of a defensive stance on behalf of the medical establishment. While charting some of the attacks on the medical model during his own career and the way that they have been repulsed, he argues for a separation of the social and medical determinants of health. He is keen that the 'baby' of medical treatment is not thrown away with the 'bath water' of social determinism. 'Social reform is not a substitute for health care, as the current social activists would have it. Rather, our social environment is a second, but quite separate, determinant of health and well-being.'

1
The Past, the Present and the Future

Roy Porter

At the close of the twentieth century, new horizons are visible, but so are new problems. Westerners are now living longer. But longevity means more time for illness, and implies that greater effort and resources will need to be devoted to keeping well – all the more so as it will increasingly fall to individuals to ensure (and insure) their passage through the longer journey. In a more health- and beauty-conscious culture, keeping up appearances will also become more costly and energy-consuming.

We live in an age of science, but science has not eliminated fantasies about health: the stigmas of sickness, the moral meanings of medicine continue. Previous centuries wove stories around leprosy, plague, tuberculosis and so on, thereby creating terror, guilt and stigma. But the modern age created similar taboos about cancer ('the big C') as untreatable, fatal and psychogenic, the product of the so-called 'cancer personality', the self that eats itself away through frustration and repressed anger. Therapy was hindered and suffering multiplied. Mythologies have now grown up around AIDS. In important respects, science itself has been the vehicle for the proliferation of health fantasies.

Moreover, despite all the advances, medical self-confidence has been shaken on several occasions during the past century: in 1918–19, when an influenza pandemic of unprecedented virulence swept the world, killing over 25 million people, and in medicine's powerlessness against AIDS. Other deadly viral diseases loom, such as the Marburg virus and Ebola fever. The recent discovery that the cattle disease Bovine Spongiform Encephalopathy (BSE) is probably, through infected beef, a source of Creutzfeldt-Jakob Disease (CJD) has sparked fears respecting other pathogens introduced into the food chain by ignorance, carelessness and greed. Such 'new diseases' are not unlucky accidents but part of the political and economic system the West pursues – relentless growth and often destructive development. They are also what the Darwinian struggle for survival predicts will never cease. Earlier optimism about magic bullets and a pill for every ill now seems symptomatic

First published in R. Porter, *A Medical History of Humanity from Antiquity to the Present*. London: Fontana, 1999, pp. 710–18.

of a shallow high-tech, quick-fix vision of the world, born of the laboratory and expecting the world to be as controllable as a laboratory.

From the Olympian view, how does medicine's historical balance-sheet stand? Hard to assess. Let us take the most tragic medical disaster: women dying in childbirth. Throughout the Western world, medicalized childbirth has finally, within the last half century, become safe for mother and child, with a less than one-in-10,000 risk of maternal mortality. In 1930 an Englishwoman going into labour had a one in 250 chance of not surviving, and a dozen women a day died of childbirth just a century ago (it is now down to one a week). In the worst Victorian maternity hospitals, between 9 and 10 per cent of women entering might leave in a coffin. The graph was even grimmer in the American south. Rank and riches afforded no insurance policy; nor were things unambiguously getting better over the years. Maternal mortality – the outcome of sepsis (puerperal fever), haemorrhage or toxaemia (eclampsia) – maintained its tragic plateau from mid Victorian times until the 1930s, and, as Semmelweis found in nineteenth-century Vienna, the peaks were sometimes quite Andean.

Was this carnage inevitable? Of course, some women died because they were famished, and others through septic abortions. Until the drugs revolution (sulpha drugs in the 1930s and antibiotics from the 1940s), there was not much that medicine could do to check lethal infections. But the majority of deaths could have been prevented by better obstetrics. In Britain, home deliveries were performed by low-status midwives who had little training, or by GPs whose obstetrical education had been perfunctory. It was not until 1902 that midwives had to be registered. In the United States, deliveries were increasingly performed in hospitals, by a high-intervention factory system which relied on sedation, forceps and Caesareans. In both countries, careless and cavalier practices inflated infection rates, long after the Listerian antiseptic revolution could have made labour far safer. Obstetrics was a Cinderella service; male practitioners did not accord mothers and babies much attention.

Things were different in some countries. Scandinavia and the Netherlands were safer places to have a baby. Why? Because their maternity services hinged upon highly qualified domiciliary midwives. Training equipped them to deal with all but the most exacting emergency cases; they were less trigger-happy with forceps and drugs; and delivery by midwife avoided the lethal cross-infections picked up in the germ-infested hospital or carried by the jack-of-all-trades family practitioner, rushing from infectious cases to women in labour. In short, the safest form of childbirth was traditionally away from hospital and from the doctors' clutches.

Why didn't all nations follow the Dutch or Danish leads? It wasn't because doctors elsewhere did not know the perils facing pregnant women. Pioneers like Semmelweis had already pointed the accusing finger at the profession and its slapdash habits, and many sincere

physicians agonized over the slaughter of the innocents. But gut preju-
dices and professional *esprit de corps* prevailed. Did not hospitals provide
the best that science could offer? And how *could* mere midwives provide safer deliveries than top physicians? – midwives, according to one
American physician, were 'filthy and ignorant and not far removed from
the jungles'. Medicine likes to think it is the most 'beneficent' profession,
but it is deeds not words that count.

We should certainly not hanker after some mythic golden age when
women gave birth naturally, painlessly and safely: the most appalling
Western maternal death rate today is among the Faith Assembly religious
sect in Indiana, who reject orthodox medicine and practise home births;
their perinatal mortality is 92 times greater than in Indiana as a whole.
Ignorance may be as lethal as complacency.

Much light is shed on the enigmatic role played by medicine in the
modern world by developments over smoking and health. By 1951, it
had been determined, in a large sample of hospital patients, that the
great majority of lung cancer sufferers were cigarette smokers. In 1956,
the results of a five-year study of the smoking habits of 40,000 medical
practitioners were published. Lung cancer deaths among doctors who
were heavy cigarette smokers (25 or more a day) were over 20 times
higher than among non-smokers. The study unleashed the criticism that
it did not identify the cause of lung cancer.

The psychologist Hans Eysenck (1916–97) offered a counter-study
exonerating cigarettes and claiming a statistical connection between
personality types and proneness to lung cancer. Nevertheless, by 1962
the Royal College of Physicians declared that smoking 'causes' lung cancer and, two years later, the US Surgeon-General's Advisory Committee
took the same line. In 1964 the Surgeon-General found that death from
cancer for men who smoked was 70 per cent higher than for non-
smokers. In 1979 another report from the Surgeon-General announced
that the main risk from smoking was not cancer but heart disease.
Doctors took the findings to heart: the numbers of British doctors who
smoked fell by 50 per cent between 1951 and 1964, a decline much
steeper than in the general population. Further links between smoking
and other serious diseases became clear – bronchitis, circulatory and
cardiovascular disorders.

But politicians were used to the stupendous tax revenues from cigarette
sales, and tobacco companies made large political donations and ran
forceful political lobbies. Change came slowly. Britain banned television
advertising of cigarettes in 1965 and in 1971 secured an agreement from
the industry that all cigarette packets would carry a government health
warning; in the US, too, health warnings were introduced on cigarette
packs. Restrictions on smoking in public places and at work multiplied,
particularly since the appearance of data indicting passive smoking. Yet,
in the early 1990s, 50 million Americans (nearly a quarter of the entire

population, including children) were still regular smokers, and federal experts put the death rate from smoking-related diseases at 1,000 a day. Among certain sectors of the population, notably young women, cigarette smoking was conspicuously increasing (smoking allegedly creates a powerful personal aura and is believed to aid slimming).

We now know that tobacco companies were long aware of the health risks of their products, thanks to experiments conducted by their own medical scientists but kept secret. Documentation shows that they deliberately targeted children and artificially raised the nicotine content of their cigarettes so as to increase addiction. In March 1997 the Liggett Group (the smallest of the five big US tobacco companies and the makers of Chesterfield cigarettes) announced a settlement with 22 American states in which it admitted that smoking was addictive, and caused heart disease, cancer and lung-related illnesses. The company agreed to provide evidence of meetings between the industry and lawyers which would prove tobacco firms had long known of the dangers of nicotine yet had continued to target cigarettes at underage smokers.

What has been the role of medicine in this vast health tragedy, costly in lives, costly in resources? Ironically, tobacco was introduced and promoted, around 1600, as a medicine, and long recommended by doctors for calming the nerves. Clinicians were astonishingly slow to sense the dangers; that was the work of statisticians and epidemiologists, once again revealing the divisions within medicine. Despite changes in the political climate – in the United Kingdom, the new Labour government announced in May 1997 its intention to ban all cigarette advertising – the likelihood is that a product known to cause the deaths of one third of a million people a year in the US alone will remain energetically promoted on the open market – because it is profitable to producers and governments, and popular with sectors of the public. Meanwhile, smoking is increasing in many of the poorer parts of the world – in China, cigarette consumption increased from 500 billion in 1978 to 1,700 billion in 1992. Africa shows a similar picture; much of the global increase is the result of hard-selling campaigns by Western multinationals.

Blame for all this can hardly be laid at medicine's door, but the facts indicate how little medicine weighs in the balance of health. With stupendous expense of human skill and money – smoking-related diseases cost the NHS £610 million a year – modern medicine has developed the capacity, through late-stage crisis management, to bestow a few extra months or years of life on some smokers who would otherwise have died of cardiovascular or lung conditions. The blessing to the individual may be inestimable (or it may simply mean a bad death), but that hardly registers on the global balance-sheet. The contribution of prolonging some smokers' lives is rather slight: most who have been diagnosed and treated do not live more than five years. Common sense suggests that the money spent on these forms of cardiology and oncology would be more

wisely spent on anti-smoking campaigns, and in research into other diseases.

We have invested disproportionately in a form of medicine ('Band Aid' salvage) whose benefits often come late, which buy a little time, and which are easily nullified by external, countervailing factors. Curative, interventionist medicine has played a modest part in shaping wider morbidity and mortality patterns within the community, but in terms of its professed aims – the greatest health of the greatest number – the Olympian verdict must be that much medicine has been off target.

Until the last 150 years, the role of clinical medicine in the improvement of health was tiny. Whether populations grew or shrank, were robust or suffered 'the thousand natural shocks that flesh is heir to', had little to do with medicine, despite its best efforts. That has changed, though not in simple or predictable ways. In the form of contraceptive pills, medical research is today responsible for capping some populations, while, in the form of rehydration kits and measures against infantile diarrhoea, it raises others. Medicine's role in the future of *Homo sapiens* on this planet is unforeseeable, because the Darwinian evolutionary battle between mankind and microbes is itself unpredictable. It is unlikely that medicine will play a role as important as politics, economics or disease.

Its standing is now highly contested. Never has it achieved so much or attracted such great suspicion. The breakthroughs of the last 50 years have saved more lives than those of any epoch since medicine began. Lewis Thomas (1913–93) wrote that when he began his career in the 1930s

> the major threats to human life were tuberculosis, tetanus, syphilis, rheumatic fever, pneumonia, meningitis, polio, and septicemia of all sorts. These things worried us then the way cancer, heart disease and stroke worry us today. The big problems of the 1930s and 1940s have literally vanished.

Medicine played a large part in that transformation. In 1940, penicillin was just being tried out on mice; within a decade it had saved millions of lives. The 1950s extended the 'first pharmacological revolution' on to a broad front: it produced, in psychotropics like chlorpromazine, the first effective medications for mental illnesses; other drug breakthroughs, notably steroids such as cortisone, made it feasible to capitalize on the growing understanding of the immune system. Immunosuppressants opened brave new world possibilities for transplant surgery. With bypass operations and heart transplants beginning in 1967, surgery seemed to know no bounds.

Technology and science contributed electron microscopes, endoscopes, keyhole surgery, CAT and PETT scans, Magnetic Resonance Imaging, lasers, tracers, ultrasound. Genetic screening and engineering have made great headway; gene replacement therapy beckons. Such advances have come from the vast investment in and endowment of medicine. In several European Union countries, more than 10 per cent of GNP now goes on health; in the US, the figure is touching 15 per cent.

But if medicine is expanding almost beyond the bounds of imagination, the euphoria of the age of penicillin or the 'pill' has turned to anxiety. Today's headlines are much more likely to be of fears about a new cholera epidemic sweeping South America or plague in India, the cloning of sheep today and maybe humans tomorrow. For all medicine's successes, who would deny a certain malaise? The atmosphere is one of hollow conquest. The age of infectious disease gave way to the age of chronic disorders. Longer life means more time to be ill, and medicine is more open to criticism.

Drugs have sometimes been disasters; iatrogenic illness has grown; research on afflictions like cancer, schizophrenia, diabetes, Alzheimer's and other degenerative diseases creeps at a snail's pace: doubts remain about the very subject of psychiatry. In Britain, the NHS was allowed to disintegrate in the 1980s and became a political football; in the US, insurance and litigation scandals dog the profession. In rich countries, the needy still get a poor medical deal. In the Third World, malaria and many other tropical diseases continue to spread, while diphtheria and tuberculosis, once believed routed, are resurgent in eastern and central Europe and in other industrialized nations. Not least, the AIDS pandemic has destroyed any naive faith that disease itself was *hors de combat*. The fact that AIDS remains without a cure reminds us that panaceas cannot be made to order.

Misgivings may be variously evaluated: do we call partial progress success or failure? Are shortcomings to be blamed on physicians or on politicians? But they are not the heart of the matter: medicine is arguably going through a far more fundamental crisis, the price of progress and its attendant inflated expectations. It is losing its way, or having to redefine its goals. In the *British Medical Journal* in 1949, Lord Horder (1871–1955) posed the question, 'Whither Medicine?', and returned the answer direct: 'Why, whither else but straight ahead'. Today, no thinking person within or outside medicine knows where 'straight ahead' is.

For centuries, the medical enterprise was too feeble to attract radical critiques. From Cato to Chekhov, medicine had its mockers; yet most who could, called the doctor when sick. People did not have high expectations, and when the doctor typically achieved little, they did not blame him much. Medicine was a profession, but it carried little prestige or power. All bowed before death.

In the twentieth century, medicine grew, conquering and commanding. It now costs the earth and, as its publicity has mushroomed, it has provoked a crescendo of criticism. Historians, social scientists, political analysts and the public converge to pose searching questions. From the 1950s, sociology put medicine under the microscope – and sometimes on the couch. One school of sociologists mounted assaults on professional dominance. Another contended that the categories of medicine – the very notions of health and sickness, as well as specific diagnosed disorders, like hysteria – were social labels, often involving stigma, victim-blaming, scapegoating and the designation of deviance with respect to class, race and gender. Nor was this critique the ritual chanting of trendy Lefties. At mid-century, the doyen of conservative American sociologists, Talcott Parsons (1902–79), drew attention to what he called 'the sick role', a notion reducing the estate of medicine to social ritual. Sociologists now regularly characterize it as a means of social control, reproducing social norms, exercising social power. Once medicine proved effective, the scourge of pestilence was forgotten, and the physician no longer had to be thanked and could be disparaged as a Figure of authority, a tool of patriarchy or a stooge of the state.

In another key respect, medicine has become the prisoner of its success. Having conquered many grave diseases and provided relief from suffering, its mandate has become muddled. What are its aims? Where is it to stop? Is its prime duty to keep people alive as long as possible, willy-nilly, whatever the circumstances? Is its charge to *make* people lead healthy lives? Or is it but a service industry, on tap to fulfil whatever fantasies its clients may frame for their bodies, be they cosmetic surgery and designer bodies or the longing of post-menopausal women to have babies? In *Gulliver's Travels* (1726), Jonathan Swift exposed, through his portrait of the wretched Struldbrugs, the follies of hankering after immortality. It may be that medicine has to learn that lesson all over again.

Many of these quandaries can be resolved in a particular case with common decency, goodwill and a sensible ethics committee. But in the wider world, who can decide the direction medicine should now take? In the rich world, it has accomplished its basic targets as understood by Hippocrates, William Harvey or Lord Horder – who will decide its new missions?

The irony is that the healthier Western society becomes, the more medicine it craves – indeed, it regards maximum access as a right and duty. Especially in free market America, immense pressures are created – by the medical profession, by medi-business, the media, by the high-pressure advertising of pharmaceutical companies, and dutiful (or susceptible) individuals – to expand the diagnosis of treatable illnesses. Scares are created. People are bamboozled into lab tests, often of dubious reliability. Thanks to diagnostic creep or leap, ever more disorders are revealed. Extensive and expensive treatments are then urged, and the physician who chooses not to treat may expose him/herself to mal-practice accusations. Anxieties and interventions spiral upwards like a space-shot off course.

The root of the trouble is structural. It is endemic to a system in which an expanding medical establishment, faced with a healthier population, is driven to medicalizing normal events like menopause, converting risks into diseases, and treating trivial complaints with fancy procedures. Doctors and 'consumers' are becoming locked within a fantasy that *everyone* has *something* wrong with them, everyone and everything can be cured.

Medical consumerism – like all sorts of consumerism, but more menacingly – is designed to be unsatisfying. The law of diminishing returns necessarily applies. Extending life becomes feasible, but it may be a life exposed to degrading neglect as resources grow overstretched and politics turn mean. What an ignominious destiny if the future of medicine turns into bestowing meagre increments of unenjoyed life!

The close of my history thus suggests that medicine's finest hour is the dawn of its dilemmas. For centuries medicine was impotent and thus unproblematic. From the Greeks to the First World War, its tasks were simple: to grapple with lethal diseases and gross disabilities, to ensure live births and manage pain. It performed these as best it could but with meagre success. Today, with 'mission accomplished', its triumphs are dissolving in disorientation. Medicine has led to inflated expectations, which the public eagerly swallowed. Yet as those expectations become unlimited, they are unfulfillable: medicine will have to redefine its limits even as it extends its capacities.

2

Images of Health

Robin Downie and Jane Macnaughton

Images of disease, illness, bereavement and death are common in literature, but images of health are more difficult to find, the reason being that health does not have a clear identity of its own. The experiences of disease and illness are intense and have a certain duration. Thus, they can become objects of attention in their own right and easily generate a rich variety of images. Being healthy, on the other hand, might just be a way of saying that we are not ill or diseased. If so, the lack of literature on health is not surprising, because there is nothing to write about. Medical practice seems to support this view of health, in that when treatment restores us to health it is really just removing disease or illness. Even if we say that there is more to health than just the absence of something, that it refers to some biological balance or equilibrium, we still do not have a concept that is likely to be a focus for a writer's attention. For when we are in this state of bodily equilibrium – when we are healthy – we do not notice our health but concentrate on other matters. Health is, as it were, transparent, whereas illness and disease are opaque. Health, therefore, easily escapes the attention of writers because in one sense it lacks the identity of illness or disease.

The 1946 World Health Organization (WHO) definition of health offers another sense of health: 'Health is a state of complete physical, mental and social well-being, and not just the absence of disease and infirmity' (WHO, 1946). This definition has, of course, been much criticized, but the problem for the purposes of this discussion is that it does not give health a clear identity, any more than do the 'absence of disease' or the 'equilibrium' views of health. For what has come to be known as 'positive health' is a concept in perpetual disguise. It is conceptually impossible to distinguish positive health from other states such as well-being, happiness, exhilaration, fitness or vigour. In other words, we shall not find many images of health unless we look for them under other descriptions or in other guises. But these other guises tell us a great deal about health, just as we can learn a great deal about someone by noting the clothes they wear. It is therefore on some of the many guises of health

First published in *The Lancet*, 351 (1998): 823–5.

that we shall concentrate, and also on the conceptual company that health keeps, such as beauty and youth.

In whatever guise it appears, health is regarded as a value, for it frequently appears in lists alongside other values, as in phrases such as 'healthy, wealthy, and wise'. The following anonymous verse about the four-leaf clover is typical:

> One leaf for fame, one for wealth
> One for a faithful lover,
> And one leaf to bring glorious health,
> Are all in a four-leaf clover. (Downie, 1994: 186)

But the health that is thought to be valuable or worth having, however varied its images, is usually more than the absence of disease or infirmity. As the Spanish-born Latin epigrammatist Martial (AD 40–104) stated, 'Non est vivere, sed valere est' (life's not just being alive but being well) (Martial, 1972). But there is a huge variation of opinion about what this 'being well' consists of. The only thing that seems to be agreed upon by writers is that there is no single state that is being well.

The same emphasis on the variable nature of states of health can be found in the writer/philosopher Nietzsche (1844–1900):

> For there is no health as such, and all attempts to define anything that way have been miserable failures. Even the determination of what health means for your body depends on your goal, your horizon, your energies, your drives, your errors, and above all on the ideals and phantasms of your soul. Thus there are innumerable healths of the body; and . . . the more we put aside the dogma of the 'equality of men', the more must the concept of a normal health, along with a normal diet and the normal course of an illness, be abandoned by our physicians. Only then would the time have come to reflect on the health and sicknesses of the soul, and to find the peculiar virtue of each man in the health of his soul: in one person's case this health could, of course, look like the opposite of health in another person. (Nietzche, 1967)

In the case of Richard Wagner (1813–83), his 'normal' state is one of 'exultation', as a letter to August Roeckel dated 26 January 1854, shows:

Exultation as health

In order to become a radically healthy human being, I went two years ago to a Hydropathic establishment; I was prepared to give up Art and everything if I could once more become a child of Nature. But, my good friends, I was obliged to laugh at my own naiveté when I found myself almost going mad. None of us will reach the promised land – we shall all die in the wilderness. Intellect is, as someone has said, a sort of disease; it is incurable. In the present conditions of life, Nature only admits of abnormalities. At the best we can only hope to be martyrs; to refuse this vocation is to put oneself in opposition to the possibilities of life. For myself, I can no longer exist except as an artist; since I cannot encompass love and life, all else repels me, or only interests me in so

far as it has a bearing on Art. The result is a life of torment, but it is the only life. Moreover, some strange experiences have come to me through my works. When I think of the pain and discomfort which are now my chronic condition, I cannot but feel that my nerves are completely shattered: but marvellous to relate, on occasion, and under a happy stimulus, these nerves do wonders for me; a clearness of insight comes to me, and I experience a receptive and creative activity such as I have never known before. After this, can I say that my nerves are shattered? Certainly not. But I must admit that the normal condition of my temperament – as it has been developed through circumstances – is a state of exultation, whereas calm and repose is its abnormal condition. The fact is, it is only when I am 'beside myself' that I become my real self, and feel well and happy . . . (Wagner, 1965: 290)

On the other hand, the quiet life of honest toil is much promoted in literature as the life of true health and well-being. Oliver Goldsmith (1730–74) writes in 'The Deserted Village':

A time there was, ere England's grief began,
When even rood of ground maintained its man;
For him light labour spread her wholesome store,
Just gave what life required, but gave no more;
His best companions, innocence and health;
And his best riches, ignorance of wealth. (Goldsmith, 1869)

But literature has its health cynics, such as James Thurber (1894–1961): 'Early to rise and early to bed makes a male healthy and wealthy and dead' (Thurber, 1939).

More typically, images of health are presented in terms of youth and vigour and beauty. Tolstoy (1828–1910) in his masterpiece *War and Peace* uses images of youth, vigour and health as metaphors for moral goodness. In Book 1 we are introduced to the young people of the Rostov family and in particular to the eldest son, Nicholas, who is described as: 'short with curly hair and an open expression. Dark hairs were already showing on his upper lip, and his whole face expressed impetuosity and enthusiasm' (Tolstoy, 1922).

Later, when he joins the army to campaign against Napoleon, we are again struck by his appearance: 'Rostov in his cadet uniform, with a jerk to his horse rode up to the porch, swung his leg over the saddle with a supple youthful movement, stood for a moment in the stirrup as if loath to part from his horse, and at last sprang down and called to his orderly' (ibid.). His sister, Natasha, is similarly portrayed as bursting with good humour and vitality: 'She . . . glanced at her younger brother, who was screwing up his eyes and shaking with suppressed laughter, unable to control herself any longer, she jumped up and rushed from the room as fast as her nimble little feet would carry her'. These attractive portraits follow immediately on from the opening scenes of the novel which take place at a soirée attended by the great and the good of St Petersburg society. These characters are portrayed as older, false and manipulative. The contrast is striking.

There seems to be widespread agreement from the time of Plato (1970: 404–12) to the present that diet and exercise (rather than healthcare or doctors) are the determinants of health. John Dryden (1631–1700) is an example of this tradition:

> Better to hunt in fields, for health unbought,
> Than fee the doctor for a nauseous draught.
> The wise, for cure, on exercise depend;
> God never made his work, for man to mend (in Dryden, 1956: line 92)

Some writers distinguish between physical and mental health. Maimonides (1135–1204), for example, writes of the two perfections of man: 'man has two perfections: a first perfection, which is the perfection of the body, and an ultimate perfection, which is the perfection of the soul. The first perfection consists in being healthy and in the very best bodily state. His ultimate perfection is to become rational in actuality' (1963). But not everyone agrees that the well-being of the mind or soul consists of the exercise of rationality. George Herbert (1593–1633) sees it as virtue:

> Only a sweet and virtuous soul,
> Like seasoned timber never gives;
> But though the whole world turn to coal,
> Then chiefly lives. (Herbert, 1972)

Others see mental health (and indeed physical health) as a balance of elements: 'Whatever dies was not mixed equally' (Donne, 1970). John Donne (1572–1631) is here writing of love, but he is using an idea of health that goes back to the Greeks. Indeed, the notion of mental health as expressed through a 'balanced personality' is still current in psychiatry. But others again see mental health as an extreme. For example, William Blake (1757–1827) in *The Marriage of Heaven and Hell* (Blake, 1951) represents some aspects of this point of view: 'Energy is Eternal Delight' or 'The road of excess leads to the palace of wisdom'.

It is noteworthy that there is a tradition that sees our mortal life as highly unsatisfactory. Bodily health, which maintains that life, is correspondingly described paradoxically as a kind of sickness. Shakespeare's disillusioned Timon of Athens is a good example: 'My long sickness / Of health and living now begins to mend, / And nothing brings me all things' (V, i, in Shakespeare, 1993).

Again when Socrates (469–399 BC) drinks the hemlock, which is his punishment for speaking the truth, Plato (428–348 BC) reports in the *Phaedo* that Socrates asks for a sacrifice to be made to Asclepius (Plato, 1951: 118). The point here is that he wishes to give thanks to the demigod of health for his recovery from the long sickness of life.

Our brief survey shows that the imagery of health is richer than at first it seems. But it has emerged that health is a multifaceted concept and cannot be pinned down in a single definition. The protean nature of health explains why doctors, perhaps rightly, concentrate on trying to minimize sickness rather than on promoting positive health.

REFERENCES

Blake, W. (1951) 'The marriage of heaven and hell', in *Selected Poems by William Blake*. Oxford: World's Classics.

Donne, J. (1970) 'The good morrow', in A. Allison et al. (eds), *The Norton Anthology of Poetry*, 3rd edn. New York and London: Norton.

Downie, R.S. (ed.) (1994) *The Healing Arts: an Oxford Illustrated Anthology*. Oxford: Oxford University Press.

Dryden, J. (1956) 'Epistle to my honoured kinsman John Driden', in J. Kinsley (ed.), *Collected Works*. Oxford: Oxford University Press.

Goldsmith, O. (1869) *The Deserted Village*, ed. J. Mason. London: Macmillan.

Herbert, G. (1972) 'Virtue', in *The New Oxford Book of English Verse*. Oxford: Oxford University Press.

Maimonides (1963) *The Guide of the Perplexed*, trans. S. Pines. Chicago: University of Chicago Press.

Martial (Marcus Valerius Martialus) (1972) *Epigrammata*, Book 6, no.70, in P. Porter (ed.), *After Martial*. Oxford: Oxford University Press.

Nietzsche, F.W. (1967) *The Joyful Science*. New York: Vintage Books.

Plato (1951) *Phaedo*. New York: Library of Liberal Arts.

Plato (1970) *Republic*, trans. B. Jowett. London: Sphere Books.

Shakespeare, W. (1993) 'Timon of Athens', in S. Wells et al. (eds), *The Oxford Shakespeare*. Oxford: Oxford University Press.

Thurber, J. (1939) 'The shrike and the chipmunks', *The New Yorker*, 29 April.

Tolstoy, L. (1922) *War and Peace*, trans. L. Maude and A. Maude, ed. H. Gifford. Oxford: Oxford University Press.

Wagner, R. (1965) *The Musicians' World: Letters of the Great Composers*, ed. H. Gal. London: Thames & Hudson.

World Health Organization (1946) *Constitution*. New York: WHO.

3

From Clinical Gaze to Regime of
Total Health

David Armstrong

In histories of medicine the late eighteenth century stands out as a particularly fertile period in that it gave birth to the modern system of clinical pathological medicine. This remarkable achievement is usually presented in terms of discovery: certainly there were political and social struggles surrounding the emergence of this new medicine, but in the end we are left with the clear image of the triumph of truth as medical scientists uncovered the diseases previously hidden within the human body.

At the heart of this new framework for understanding the nature of illness lay the notion of the pathological lesion. Prior to the end of the eighteenth century illness was perceived as moving between bodies and environments (as in humoral medicine) without ever stopping to become analysable. However, with the dissection of the corpse and concomitant developments in clinical technique, specific anatomical lesions were identified inside the body: these seemed to account for the outward appearances of illness – the so-called clinico-pathological correlation. Thus, for example, pain and tenderness on the 'outside' were seen to signify the existence of inflammation in internal tissues beyond immediate vision. These discoveries ushered in the hospital as a place in which bodies could be examined with proper rigour, the post-mortem as the event in which the true nature of disease was finally revealed, and the many facets of clinical method which still underpin medical practice today.

THE CLINICAL GAZE

Although conventional histories of medicine acclaim the late eighteenth-century discoveries of clinical pathology, it is still possible to pursue a less arrogant and self-centred analysis of Western medical history.

First published in A. Beattie, M. Gott, L. Jones and M. Sidell (eds), *Health and Wellbeing: a Reader*. London: Macmillan in association with The Open University, 1993, pp. 55–67.

intent on dominating and controlling others. In this model the extended gaze would be a dangerous force to be resisted, as several critics of medicine have advocated.[1] However, according to Foucault's notion of disciplinary power, surveillance is a productive rather than repressive force.

The extended medical gaze does not repress the liberty of the individual, but rather creates it. It is only through the extended gaze – within medicine and other agencies – that the psychological and social characteristics of wholeness and identity come to exist for those inert corporeal masses which the clinical gaze had fashioned throughout the nineteenth century. It is ironic that having had their subjectivity fabricated those same subjects insist that subjectivity is an invariate and universal component of human life; but it is also a subtle device through which the operation of this productive power is concealed.

DISCIPLINING BODIES

Although the major changes in medical surveillance during the twentieth century would seem to embrace the psychosocial space between bodies, this does not mean that the physical body itself has continued as a passive recipient of observation, as in the nineteenth century. In part through developments in the educational field, but increasingly through our preoccupation with the notion of 'health behaviour', the movement of bodies has become a major focus for twentieth-century disciplinary techniques (this section draws on Armstrong, 1988).

Early in the twentieth century it would have been impossible to conceptualize the notion of health behaviour. Indeed while the problem of behaviour was to achieve some limited recognition in 'behaviourism', most of the new discipline of psychology was concerned with the subject of human 'conduct' which was held to be the 'highest type of behaviour'. The term 'behaviour' itself was reserved to describe 'certain peculiarities which are only found in the movement of living things' (McDougall, 1908).

The shift from a world of instincts, conduct and habits to one of attitudes and behaviour can be traced through the attempts to discipline and manipulate the body of the child in the elementary schools earlier this century, a strategy which produced the great alliance between physical education and hygiene. Universal primary education had the task of managing and transforming the body of the child and to accomplish this goal the new schools at first simply borrowed the same techniques which had evolved in the army to transform raw recruits into disciplined soldiers. Drill routines, 'marching, counter-marching, diagonal marching, changing ranks and so on', were initially popular, other hand, some sociologists have explicitly rejected survey techniques on the grounds that they objectify respondents and have turned instead to methodologies which, they hold, more clearly respect or enhance patient subjectivity. Within the last two decades proponents of inter-action analysis, participant observations, ethnomethodology, and other more naturalistic methods have been critical of the dehumanizing aspects of medicine and of sociology itself; and yet the effect of their stance is to have strengthened the power of gaze of the new medicine to the essentially subjective.

Thus, at the same moment as patients entered medical discourse as subjects, they appeared in a parallel discourse in the human sciences; indeed, the changes in medical discourse often took precedence. This is not to argue that the human sciences have simply been the handmaidens of medicine: their frequent alliances, points of contact and shared con-cerns do not reflect a relationship of domination but of a common object, namely, the body and its relationships, and a common effect, the sub-jectivity of that same body. The human sciences have thus produced an often independent but parallel gaze to the body and within this inde-pendence have forged a new 'regime of truth'. This knowledge has increasingly been concerned with the subjectivity of experience and has often sought to conceal its recent invention through the notion of alienation which presents subjectivity as the immanent human condition that the human sciences have succeeded in 'liberating'.

Over the last two decades there has been an historical project in the human sciences and parts of medicine which has concerned itself with the identification of a distant disappearance of 'a sense of wholeness, inviolability and ethical judgement' through forces of repression and domination – which then enables claim to be made for the parallel rediscovery and reappearance of the sick man (Jewson, 1976). In effect, the recent social origins of the sick man are blurred as a historical discourse on alienation provides him with a political credo, a universal status and a plausible history; an invention is translated into a language of liberation, a positive power which creates is concealed in the identi-fication of a repressive power which is lifted. As Foucault points out, we continue to 'describe the effects of power in negative terms: it "excludes", it "represses", it "censors", it "abstracts", it "masks", it "conceals". In fact, power produces; it produces reality; it produces domains of objects and rituals of truth. The individual and the knowl-edge that may be gained of him belong to this production' (Foucault, 1977).

It is all too easy to see the changes accompanying the extended medical gaze in terms of a pernicious movement to constrain the lives of free citizens; indeed it cannot be coincidence that *Brave New World* and *Nineteen Eighty-Four* were written as these surveillance opportunities were deployed throughout the population. Yet this is to see surveillance as the instrument of a sovereign power, of a calculating centre which is sought to monitor everyone's ability to cope with interactions and feelings.

The fabrication of this psychosocial space surrounding all bodies can also be discerned in the techniques which doctors have deployed to 'interrogate' the patient (Armstrong, 1984; see also Armstrong, 1983b). Nineteenth-century manuals on clinical method only described how to examine the body and made perfunctory reference to the patient's 'history'. However, in the early years of the twentieth century there was a growing interest in what the patient might say. At first it was a question of provoking the pathological lesion to speech – achieved through the patient's history. Then it was recognized that the patient's words might not exactly speak for the pathological lesion as had previously been assumed: doctors were therefore advised on the use of certain techniques, such as avoidance of leading questions, to prevent the patient speaking of symptoms which could mislead the search for the lesion. By the late inter-war years these strange words which patients often spoke were no longer construed as the background 'noise' which might prevent the clinical truth from emerging clearly; instead the words represented the patient's affective state, and accordingly doctors were advised to seek out the patient's fears, feelings and anxieties as a legitimate part of medical 'case-taking'.

The increasing emphasis on monitoring the patient's mental functioning as part of the normal medical interview has continued. Nowadays doctors are taught the importance of affect and cognitions in the patient's story and the possible interrelationship of organic lesion and mental state. For example, it is now reported that most appendicitis is preceded by significant negative life events and that the psychological effect of these often lasts beyond the surgical operation to remove the offending appendix (Creed, 1981). Thus even surgery, the great bastion of the clinical gaze, is coming to extend its gaze from the body's interior to the psychological states and social relationships of that body. Why else have psychology and sociology, both of which emerged as distinct and autonomous disciplines in the twentieth century, become essential components of the medical curriculum?

Sociology made its principal contribution to post-war medicine when its mastery of survey techniques made it of value to an extended medical gaze intent on exploring the surveillance possibilities of this newly discovered technology. Sociologists, in close alliance with medicine, opened up areas of the health experiences of 'ordinary' people through surveys of health attitudes, of illness behaviour, of drug taking and of symptom prevalence.

More recently, as the medical gaze has focused on individual idiosyncrasies, personal meanings and subjectivity, sociology too has turned its attention to fresh possibilities. On the one hand, various survey techniques have been made more sophisticated so that they might take into consideration, bring out or measure individual meanings; on the

So too the increasing concern with contagion of more minor illnesses. Around the end of the first decade of the century it was recognized that schoolchildren might spread infection between themselves through contact. Schools therefore deployed a regime of surveillance which stressed less the significance of sanitation and more the importance of personal hygiene. Children with infectious diseases, from measles to the common cold, were required to remain at home for specified periods to prevent the spread of illness throughout the school and thereafter the community.

Under the nineteenth-century system of public health the natural environment was the potential source of ill health. Under the new hygiene the natural environment was not of itself dangerous, but merely acted as a reservoir. The danger now arose from people and their point of contact. In one form venereal disease existed within the body as a specific identifiable infection: but from the early twentieth century it was also construed as existing in the space mapped by intimate relationships. As the traditional techniques of clinical method could not interrogate this new space of illness new procedures had to be developed. The epidemiological gaze therefore began to shift from the environment to the mode of transmission between people and to the ramifications of social relationships. Preventive medicine was no longer restricted to environmental questions and sanitation but became concerned with the minutiae of social life. Might not health, Newman argued, be promoted 'by maintaining a clean mouth and clear breathing, and by abstinence from spitting, sneezing, coughing and shouting at each other?' (Newman, 1920).

Together, these various measures outlined an organizational structure which could both survey and constantly monitor the whole community. Hence, also, the emphasis on close scrutiny of details of patients' contacts and relationships, and the creation of a thorough record of family networks, friends and acquaintances through which to co-ordinate home visits, checks and follow-ups. In addition, this social surveillance raised the consciousness of health matters in the community thus observed and, on the one hand, enabled the intrusion of surveillance to be more easily justified, and, on the other hand, made the potential patient a part of the surveillance machinery.

A PSYCHOSOCIAL SPACE

The space between bodies that emerged early in the twentieth century was a physical space which micro-organisms could cross; but, more important, it was also a 'social-psychological' space in which could crystallize those attributes of bodies which are now referred to as identity. A powerful illustration of the emergence of this new space was the 'discovery' of the neuroses less than a century ago (Armstrong, 1980). Whereas nineteenth-century psychiatry had only been concerned with separating the mad from the sane, twentieth-century mental health has it, asks Foucault, that the school, the hospital, the prison, the barracks and the workshop have so much in common?

The clinical gaze of medicine was one of the new techniques through which bodies were analysed. It is apparent, as Foucault observed, that late eighteenth-century medicine began to perceive a body which had a new anatomy. Every time medicine had cause to deploy its new techniques and treat an illness, it drew the anatomical outline of a docile body. At first the procedure was unsure and the outline hazy but with time and with refinement the shape became more clear. As the nineteenth century progressed each and every consultation of the new pathological medicine functioned to imprint, by its sheer repetition, the reality of a specific anatomy.

AN EXTENDED MEDICAL GAZE

During the twentieth century the diagram of power has been rearranged (this section draws on Armstrong, 1983a). The clinical gaze, which for over a century had analysed the microscopic detail of the individual body, began to move to the undifferentiated space between bodies. Indeed, it is possible to discern in the early years of the century the beginning of a new framework for understanding illness. This emergence can be traced through various extensions to the dominant clinical gaze. First, the locus of illness can be seen to have begun to shift from within the body to a space which might be described as between bodies. Secondly, it is possible to map a series of new techniques which have developed to interrogate this new space of illness. And thirdly, the actual impact of these new approaches on the shape and character of the body can be identified as a new political anatomy emerges.

The main change in the nature of the clinical gaze during the twentieth century can be summarized as the extension of surveillance from the interior of the body to its exterior points of contact: disease has become increasingly located in the spaces between people, in the interstices of relationships, in the social body itself. In this new conceptualization pathology is not seen as an essentially static phenomenon to be localized to a specific point – as construed by the great historic breakthrough of the eighteenth-century clinic – but as a movement through the social body, appearing only intermittently. This new model of illness can be seen in the 'reconstruction' of certain established diseases such as tuberculosis and venereal diseases, and in the invention of several new forms of pathology.

Tuberculosis, which had, until the closing decades of the nineteenth century, been primarily a disease of individual bodies and of environmental neglect, became a disease of contact and social space. Equally the early twentieth-century concern with venereal disease and contact tracing illustrated the mapping of a social domain for the locus of illness.

Instead of seeing the period until the end of the eighteenth century as essentially one of darkness to be illuminated by the new truths of the dissecting room and post-mortem, we can view the latter developments as simply one more construction or perception about the nature of illness. Central to this new perception, as Michel Foucault argued in *The Birth of the Clinic* (1973), was the fabrication of the body by means of the 'anatomical atlas': the anatomical atlas directs attention to certain structures, certain similarities, certain systems, and not others, and in so doing forms a set of rules for reading the body and for making it intelligible. In this sense the reality of the body is only established by the observing eye that reads it. The atlas enables the anatomy student, when faced with the undifferentiated amorphous mass of the body, to see certain things and ignore others. In effect, what the student sees is not the atlas as a representation of the body but the body as a representation of the atlas.

The atlas is therefore a means of interpreting the body, of seeing its form and nature and establishing its reality. The modern body of the patient, which has become the unquestioned object of clinical practice, is a product of the exercise of those same clinical techniques. The clinical gaze, encompassing all the techniques, languages and assumptions of modern medicine, establishes by its authority and penetration an observable and analysable space in which is crystallized that apparently solid figure of the discrete human body.

MECHANISMS OF POWER

The analysis of the way the body is seen, described and constructed, Foucault suggests, might be called 'political anatomy' (Foucault, 1977). It is political because the changes in the way the body is described are not the consequences of some random effects or progressive enlightenment but are based on certain mechanisms of power which, since the eighteenth century, have pervaded the body and continue to hold it in their grasp. From that time the body has been the point on which and from which power has been exercised.

In eighteenth-century European society the body became treated 'as something docile that could be subject, used, transformed and improved'. The body became surrounded and invested with various techniques of detail which analysed, monitored and fabricated it. These various techniques all involved surveillance: bodies had to be inspected to judge their status, they had to be analysed to identify their deficits and they had to be monitored to evaluate their functioning. The importance of surveillance is illustrated in particular in the various techniques of examination that emerged to prominence in the eighteenth century such as the clinical examination in the hospital, the inspection in the prison, the test in the school and the military inspection in the barracks. Why is later being replaced by more 'carefully graduated and scientifically calculated' movements (Atkins, 1904: 151).

The disciplining of bodily movement in both army and school was gradually widened from the rigidity of drill to the more generalized techniques of physical training and physical education. The individual body could be trained, particularly through repetitive actions – so inculcating 'habits' – to achieve some goal such as fitness and efficiency. Training took control over the general physical development of the child, ensuring that full physical capacity was achieved, and it also had a 'corrective effect', remedying or adjusting 'any obvious defects or incorrect attitude or action of the body, or any of its parts' (Board of Education, 1909).

But it was not only the drill sergeant and the teacher who trained the child's body but also the child itself; training could equally well, and undoubtedly more efficiently and permanently, be achieved through education. Pure training only worked at the level of habit forming: 'the child unconsciously acquires habits of discipline and order, and learns to respond cheerfully and promptly to the word of command' (ibid.). Yet the more valuable aim was to instil the word of command into the child so it could function as its own drill master. Posture, fitness and efficiency were the initial objectives but with the gradual extension of the techniques through which the body was manipulated – physical culture, sports, gymnastics, dance, exercise and athletics – the goal widened towards a regime of total health.

Movement of the body had its effects on the mind: exercises could inculcate habits and, moreover, it seemed that the discipline of movement could focus the mind on the task in hand, eliminating stray thoughts – perhaps of a sexual nature – and build up 'character'. But equally, movement in some way reflected mental functioning. For example, it was claimed that there was a very close relationship between intelligence and success in athletics, and mental problems might be expressed in poor movement co-ordination just as true character could be read from the sports field, the gymnasium, the athletics ground and the dance school (Campbell, 1940: 351). Such strategies were, of course, largely limited to development of the child; but where education left off, medicine had techniques to pick up the management of behaviour throughout adult life.

THE ACTIVE PATIENT

Clinical medicine from the late eighteenth century involved an interaction between clinician and pathological lesion. The patient, as a person, had only existed within this dyad as a repository or, at most, as a rather unreliable translator for the lesion. In effect, the patient was no more than a passive physical object.

In the new public health of the twentieth century, however, which stressed the importance of both the physical and the social relationship between bodies, the individual was constituted as a more active physical and social being. Personal hygiene addressed this individual because it required commitment to certain activities, particularly those involving the sanitization of body interfaces such as skin, mouth, ears, teeth, bowels, etc., to prevent the transmission of disease from one person to another. In effect the object of the new personal hygiene was not the organic lesion but some activities of its potential host.

The reconstruction of patient identity through the new public health towards a more active and acting object was only one part of this transformation in medicine. The other component of the new personal hygiene was the recruitment of the patient to the medical enterprise. In the nineteenth century the public health official alone could monitor and control the dangers of natural environment. The new hygiene however could not rely on these officials as its agents of surveillance; instead it demanded involvement of 'patients' themselves. If human bodies were to be monitored and sanitized medicine required the active co-operation of those same bodies; patients had to be enlisted to practise their own hygienic regime; patients had to become agents of medicine, their own self-practitioners.

Thus the two related features of the new public health were forged early in the twentieth century. On the one hand the patient as a person became the object of medical attention, particularly in his or her own actions. On the other hand patients were also the subjects of medicine in the sense that they were recruited to monitor their own bodies. Since then, these two (and often confused) facets of patient identity have been explored, developed and reinforced. The active body of the patient required study, guidance and control if illness was to be avoided and health achieved. The malleable subjective mind of the patient in its turn demanded education and training if it was successfully to monitor and bring under some control its otherwise capricious body.

Early in the twentieth century the patient as actor was recognized in regimes of personal hygiene and in concerns for patient 'defaulters' from treatment, particularly from that of venereal disease. And by the middle of the century health education was firmly established as an essential part of the public health programme. 'Health authorities', wrote Derry-berry in 1945, 'are becoming increasingly aware that many diseases are uncontrollable without the active participation of the people themselves' (1945: 1401). Whereas a few decades earlier the community was involved in public health only when their electoral or political support was required, now people had to be involved from the very beginning of any programme because they themselves were the agents of health practice.

Opportunities for applying these new strategies emerged with the preventive health programmes of the immediate post-war years, particularly those relating to polio vaccination, community X-ray programmes for TB, and the new multi-phasic screening programmes. What were the public's attitudes towards vaccination? What factors precluded their involvement? How was participation and non-participation to be explained? Whereas during the early part of the century human behaviour had been seen as governed by instinct, that is from a fixed biological point, during the late 1950s public health discovered beliefs as the mainspring of human action. The theories of Rosenstock et al. of 1959 of why people failed to seek polio vaccination had become, by 1965, the basis for a more generalized model of health beliefs and focus on patient activity (Rosenstock, 1965: 94).

One of the effects of the recruitment of the patient as an integral component of health management was the change in the status and nature of 'patient' identity. The boundary between healthy person and patient became problematic. In the past the transition from person-status to patient-status had been marked by 'coming under the doctor'. In the new regime, which made the patient both an object of medicine and a lay health practitioner, patienthood began to lose its old meaning. This shift was marked by the extension of patient status (or at least potential status) as everyone came under medical/health surveillance through gradual recruitment to the medical enterprise. Post-war surveys of population morbidity and symptom prevalence confirmed that a rigid distinction between health and illness was meaningless: everyone had health problems, everyone was 'at risk'; health care merely touched the tip of the morbidity iceberg (Last, 1963). In addition the now problematic boundary between person and patient was subjected to a close analysis in the new subject of 'illness behaviour' which attempted to explain how and why patients chose to consult a doctor.

Illness behaviour, a term invented by Mechanic in 1960 (Mechanic and Volkart, 1960: 86), has often been challenged as being too restricted, as failing to encapsulate the wider concerns of health behaviour. Yet illness behaviour was not only an explanation of certain health-related activities but also part of the post-war fascination with the weakening person–patient boundary. The concept of illness behaviour showed that the transition between health and illness, between person and patient, was not predicated on an absolute and biological difference, but was underpinned by the notion of a person as his or her own health practitioner making judgements and decisions on the nature and limits of health and illness.

The patient was inseparable from the person because all persons had become patients, and with it changed their identity. Until the post-war years behaviour had been relatively unchangeable, set by heredity and repetitive patterning. In the post-war years behaviour became contingent: social psychologists, for example, discovered attitudes with

Newman, G. (1920) q...
Rosenstock, I.M. (1965) 'Why people use health services', *Millbank Memorial Fund Quarterly*, 44: 94.

medicine of Sydenham and Ryle. External research-based clinical evidence is derived in part from 'the basic sciences of medicine', but 'especially from patient centred clinical research into the accuracy and precision of diagnostic tests (including the clinical examination), the power of prognostic markers, and the efficacy and safety of therapeutic, rehabilitative and preventative regimens'. Although these types of relevant evidence range far beyond that derived from randomized trials and meta-analyses, Sackett allots a special place to that type of evidence as being 'so much more likely to inform us, and so much less likely to mislead us' than the 'non-experimental approaches', which in his view 'routinely lead to false-positive conclusions about efficacy'. Indeed, he regards evidence derived from the systematic review of several controlled trials as the 'gold standard' for judging whether a treatment does more good than harm. This is the message first proclaimed by Archie Cochrane (1972), whom to know was to love, but whose manifold gifts did not include inerrancy.

Sackett's description of what is meant by EBM is framed in terms of individual patient care; but the principle of using best available evidence is also relevant to 'group decisions' on the provision of services, in which 'the overriding objective . . . is that of maximising the total cost-utility in that group'. Both in individual medicine and in public health medicine, clinical judgements have to be modulated to an appropriate extent by considerations of ethics and of health economics (Gillon and Lloyd, 1994; Williams, 1997).

COMMENT ON EBM

There can surely be no difficulty in accepting the general proposition that medical practice and the provision of health care should be based on the best available evidence, or in welcoming the complementarity accorded by Sackett to 'individual clinical expertise' and 'external clinical evidence from systematic research'. Any movement which encourages self-scrutiny and self-criticism has to be a good thing, so long as it stops short of aborting that modicum of self-confidence which enables us to live and practise, while aware of the strong element of uncertainty that is inescapable in all branches of health care. However, since criticism is the acid that etches medical systems into better shape, I would raise one particular concern – the primacy given to 'RCT evidence' – and two more general ones: the validity and applicability of 'group evidence', and the extent to which the 'EBM principle' can be applied to the totality of medical practice.

Relative value of RCT evidence

The development of the randomized controlled trial (RCT) by Bradford Hill and Richard Doll is both theoretically and practically a milestone in medical history. It was a brilliant response to the increasing problems set by the proliferation of agents that are highly effective but also potentially hazardous from their side effects; it has in many clinical contexts provided sound information not only on which drug to use but also on how much of it to give. These are immense gains, but to the extent that Cochrane and Sackett imply a primacy over other sources of therapeutic evidence, I think they take a step too far, and one that would perhaps take them beyond Doll and Hill themselves.

The quality of evidence should be assessed not by the method by which it is obtained but by its strength or weakness. RCTs can produce evidence of great strength (and have often done so) when a clinical situation is: common, so that the trial can be carried out in one centre; easily defined, so that inclusion and exclusion are simple; and has little variation between patients. Whilst there are ways of organizing multi-centre trials that largely preserve their validity (at some cost in increased complexity), the most important derogation to the strength of RCT evidence stems from patient variation and imperfect clinical taxonomy. When there are many variables with an effect on outcome, as in coronary thrombosis, or when an apparently simple label conceals taxonomic complexity, as in the nephrotic syndrome (Black et al., 1970), then the results of RCTs tend to be inconclusive or conflicting, though probably still stronger as evidence than the results of unsystematized clinical observation of the effects of therapy.

There are other risks in the 'systematic review of several controlled trials', commended 'especially' by Sackett (1996) in comparison with the single trial. It is true that the influence of one trial, idiosyncratic for whatever reason, may be 'diluted out' by numerous others. But as against that, occult variations in procedure, such as may lie hidden even in a single multi-centre trial, must be almost inevitable in a group of trials subjected to meta-analysis. While trials can be scrutinized for gross errors of methodology, and excluded if such are found, less obvious but still material differences in procedure may not be apparent to a scrutiny diffused over a number of protocols. Another problem, particular to the aggregation of trials, is the systematic bias that arises from the reluctance of authors to report, and of editors to accept for publication, trials with a 'negative' result, which may be just as relevant as a 'positive' trial in forming a true picture (Grahame-Smith, 1995).

In summary, a well-conducted RCT on a clearly defined issue can yield evidence of a probability approaching certainty, and certainly greater than that derived from unstructured clinical scrutiny of the same issue. However, there remain issues of clinical importance whose complexity makes them, for the present, 'insoluble' by the RCT route, and whose solution must await further resolution by conventional clinical or patho-logical analysis. There is not here a hierarchy of methodological esteem, merely an order of difficulty, and the RCT must not take 'gold standard' precedence over all other methods of clinical investigation.

Validity and the applicability of 'group evidence'

In this section I use 'group evidence' as a shorter equivalent of Sackett's 'best available external clinical evidence from systematic research'. Evidence relevant to clinical decision-making is derived from many sources: the basic medical sciences; the social sciences; the science of the 'seats and causes' of disease; the observed natural history of disease; epidemiology; the skills of diagnosis, of which speaking with the patient is paramount; and the range of possible therapies, graded for practicability and efficacy. From such a variety of sources, it is likely that the evidence will be variable in validity and relevance, as well as being potentially overwhelming by its very extent. It is all the more important that the search should at least start in the right place, by that characterization of the actual problem that we call diagnosis. The old-fashioned danger of being sent to the wrong specialist has its informatic equivalent of being entered in the wrong algorithm, and undergoing a series of tests appropriate to someone else.

Accurate definition of the actual problem does not remove the entire risk in applying the evidence derived from group studies to the problems of an individual. Leaving aside possible flaws in the evidence itself, its applicability depends on the individual being conformable to the group in all relevant aspects. And 'relevant aspects' may be legion, for example in the risk factors relevant to outcome in coronary arterial disease.

Pragmatic limits of EBM

Even to think of disparaging an evidential approach must be the cardinal sin of an academic physician. My backsliding had an unlikely venue in the course of a meeting convened to give advice on the permanent vegetative state; the definition and management of this are not free from the form of uncertainty to which the term 'grey area' is commonly applied. During the discussion of these matters, we were told that 'all advice coming from the Department of Health must be evidence-based'. That was certainly a boldly stated ideal but in that context, and in many others, it scarcely corresponds to reality, unless one stretches 'evidence' to include the whole area in which we are guided by that elusive quality, common sense. Wrestling with the mechanisms, other than strict logic, by which the mind can attain certitude, Newman (1870) invoked an 'Illative Sense', which appears to be a faculty of correct reasoning from facts presented to us in apparently random fashion. Of course, in practical medicine our concern is rarely with certitude, but almost always with a degree of probability sufficient to justify the action that we propose to recommend; but in recognizing that degree of probability, I suggest that we are more commonly persuaded by a balance of likelihoods than we are driven forward by the iron laws of evidence.

The relative frequency of 'evidence-based' and 'more-broadly-based' decisions is a matter of speculation, but it is important to recognize that many of the situations with which medicine is concerned lie outside the realm of 'scientific medicine'. Even within clinical medicine, the majority of acute situations are self-limited, irrespective of treatment, and that has been an impartial bulwark both to historical and to complementary medicine. At the other extreme, there are illnesses that inevitably lead to death or incapacity. But there are also, happily, a minority of situations in which scientific medicine makes all the difference between a cure and disaster, and this minority grows steadily larger. In our legitimate concentration on those areas in which the treatment given is critical, we must keep in mind that they are still, however important, only a small part of the whole province of medicine, and that we have a 'duty of care' as well as a 'duty of cure'. EBM can contribute to the discharge of both of these, but it is far from being the only player on the field. Although I am no great lover of the taxonomy that distinguishes the 'science' from the 'art' of medicine (believing them to be interwoven activities), the point that I am trying to make has been better put in those terms by Robert Platt (1972), a great clinician who taught me a great deal: 'However far the science of medicine and surgery advances, the art of medicine will remain: the art of first identifying the patient's problem (which is something more than merely diagnosing his disease) and the art of applying the science to the needs of the individual patient'. If that is a sound critique for the practice of clinical medicine, how much more does it apply to the more general application of medical knowledge and skills which we designate as 'public health medicine'? Perhaps it is there above all that the fruits of existing evidence must first be critically examined, and then supplemented by insights derived from imaginative reasoning.

CONCLUSION

My intention in this chapter is not to disparage evidence-based medicine, but to deprecate any attempt to equate it with the whole of medicine. I recognize that no such attempt is being made by responsible advocates (Sackett, 1996), but a prophet is not in control of disciples who might deny the value of medical thought and experience in situations in which a categorical evidence base is still lacking. To deny that we must use evidence to the farthest extent that it can take us would be to be guilty of obscurantism and of 'anti-science' – charges which I may perhaps be fortunate to escape, if indeed I do. What I seek to emphasize is the importance of the prior intellectual analysis of the problem, be it clinical or organizational, in such a way as to define the type of evidence that is going to be relevant. An unstructured search for evidence may only lead to confusion. Of course, intellectual analysis is fallible, and the search for relevant evidence may have to change direction, but at all stages the search has to be planned, and not random.

When all relevant evidence has been gathered, and with its help the problem is 'understood', the transition from knowledge to action may indeed be assisted by evidence derived from comparable situations, and such must be sought. However, comparability is not identity, and treatment or planning needs continued intellectual review, including the planned search for retrospective evidence, without which plausible errors can lead to preventable disasters for individuals or groups.

REFERENCES

Black, D.A.K., Rose, G.A. and Brewer, D.B. (1970) 'Controlled trial of prednisone in adults with the nephrotic syndrome', *British Medical Journal*, 3: 421–6.

Cochrane, A.L. (1972) *Effectiveness and Efficiency: Random Reflections on Health Services*. London: Nuffield Provincial Hospitals Trust.

Gillon, R. and Lloyd, A. (1994) *Principles of Health Care Ethics*. Chichester: John Wiley & Sons.

Grahame-Smith, D. (1995) 'Evidence based medicine: Socratic dissent', *British Medical Journal*, 310: 1126–7.

Harris, H. (1981) 'Rationality in science', in A.F. Heath (ed), *Scientific Evolution*. Oxford: Oxford University Press.

Kuhn, T.S. (1970) *The Structure of Scientific Revolutions*, 2nd edn. Chicago: University of Chicago Press.

Medawar, P.B. (1984) *Pluto's Republic*. Oxford: Oxford University Press.

Newman, J.H. (1870) *An Essay in Aid of a Grammar of Assent*. London: Longmans Green & Co.

Platt, R. (1972) *Private and Controversial*. London: Cassell & Co.

Polanyi, M. (1956) 'Passion and controversy in science', *Lancet*, 270: 921–5.

Popper, K.R. (1959) *The Logic of Scientific Discovery*. London: Routledge & Kegan Paul.

Popper, K.R. (1963) *Conjectures and Refutations*. London: Routledge & Kegan Paul.

Sackett, D.L. (1996) 'The doctor's (ethical and economic) dilemma'. OHE annual lecture. London: Office of Health Economics.

Sackett, D.L., Rosenberg, W.N.C., Gray, J.A.M., Haynes, R.B. and Richardson, W.S. (1996) 'Evidence based medicine: what it is and what it isn't', *British Medical Journal*, 312: 71–2.

Williams, A. (1997) *Being Reasonable about the Economics of Health*. Cheltenham: Edward Elgar Publishing.

5

Postmodern Illness

David Morris

POSTMODERNISM UNDEFINED

The upstart term *postmodern* makes many people edgy. It has been so overused as to mean almost anything. Some employ it as a sign of intellectual power, as if it contained a secret erudite meaning, and the urge to dump such a troublesome term is hard to resist. As two American sociologists write, 'Postmodernism is everywhere. It has become the hip, the in, the trendy catchword of the late 1980s. There is even a "Postmodern Hour" on MTV' (Goldman and Papson, 1994: 224). The spell of the postmodern extends well beyond the 1980s, so the main issue is how to understand a concept that will not go away. Some analysts prefer to rush in with a definition, but it is folly to provide a firm definition for something still in flux, a flux that encompasses the definer. A more useful approach is to accept some degree of indefiniteness, with the irritation it inspires, as intrinsic to postmodernism. After all, the postmodern world almost reinvented uncertainty – in quantum physics and cross-dressing, for example – and such a shifting quarry is bound to resist a perfect definition. Instead of seeking to capture it whole, we will do better to examine some of the postmodern fragments that have helped to reshape the contemporary experience of illness, and meanwhile we can validly employ postmodern in its most restricted sense to denote the unfinished period that commences (roughly) with the second half of the twentieth century.

Does postmodernism represent a decisive break with the past – or an extension and development of modernist programmes? In some fields (architecture, for example) differences between postmodern and modern are obvious, but elsewhere the relationship is much harder to sort out. Even cultural trends that analysts agree to call postmodern are divided by disagreement and conflict. In short, there is not one postmodernism, monolithic and homogeneous, but a dialogue of postmodern voices.

First published in D. Morris, *Illness and Culture in the Postmodern Age*. Berkeley: University of California Press, 1998.

Postmodernism is self-consciously pluralistic and multicultural, a free-wheeling consortium of heterogeneous parts, where underlying consistencies are often less visible than the outward play of difference.

Postmodernism in its copious variety cannot be captured in slogans about the failures of Enlightenment rationality, about the loss of foundations, or about a linguistic turn in philosophy. It is equally hard to pin down as it applies to illness. Arthur W. Frank, in an extremely valuable analysis, argues that '[t]he *postmodern* experience of illness begins when ill people recognize that more is involved in their experiences than the medical story can tell' (Frank, 1996: 6). In Frank's version, modern and postmodern denote two distinct, successive styles of living with illness: a modern style that accepts the authorized medico-scientific narrative and a postmodern style in which patients reclaim power as creators and narrators of their own distinctive stories. There are, however, other equally important styles, features and themes in the postmodern transformation of illness.

Postmodernism – to offer another fragmentary description in lieu of a definition – indicates a world that we recognize as inescapably 'constructed'. It is constructed not so much with cement and steel, like the modernist skyscraper, as with images and representations. Its main power tools are television, cinema and the computer screen. The endless images they generate have grown so potent that representations sometimes take on an independent life and supplant whatever they supposedly depict or refer to. The modernist real world – a bold new venture built with the products of mills, factories and machine shops – dissolves into the computer-simulated postmodern universe of visual images. This simulated postmodern world is a place where life often seems less real (less sharp and full) than its representations on TV and where increasingly – as when a talking cartoon dog sells life insurance – there is nothing outside the image: an unprecedented state of affairs that sociologist Jean Baudrillard describes through his coinage *hyperreal*. 'The real,' as he puts it somewhat cryptically, 'is no longer real' (Baudrillard, 1988: 172).

The postmodern world is a place where 90 per cent of teenagers across the globe recognize the Chicago Bulls. The Chicago Bulls, in turn, are far more than the players on a Midwestern professional basketball team. The name, like the team, is a commodity marketed relentlessly on television, whence it escapes into popular culture and is appropriated by groups as diverse as urban gangs and high-fashion models, who return the image for circulation bearing ever new layers of constructed meaning or implication. Postmodernism in this familiar sense evokes the franchised, *déjà vu*, simulated reality where shopping malls in Pittsburgh and Los Angeles contain identical stores, where a Las Vegas casino reproduces the skyline of New York City, where the latest Hollywood action film opens simultaneously in Mozambique and Munich. It is the world of consumer capitalism, late-night talk shows, soundbite politics, satellite weather reports, gay pride marches, e-mail, and virtual libraries (which contain no books), to name a few post-war innovations. The attendant changes in our sensibilities and understanding have had a significant impact on the experience of illness.

DESTABILIZING DISEASE AND ILLNESS

What doctors mean by *disease* and *illness* is not exactly what patients mean. Contemporary medical textbooks define 'disease' as an objectively verified disorder or bodily functions or systems, characterized by a recognizable cause and by an identifiable group of signs and symptoms. 'Illness', by contrast, is used inside medicine to indicate the patient's subjective experience, which may or may not indicate the presence of disease. For example, tests show that many patients with chronic low back pain suffer from lumbar disk disease, but so do 70 per cent of people without low back pain. Lumbar disk disease, then, sometimes produces the chronic illness we call low back pain, but many people have the disease without the illness. At this level of analysis, the distinction between disease and illness is useful in preventing confusion. The two concepts have now become so encrusted with additional layers of meaning, however, that they prove not so much useful tools as awkward and antiquated carriers of what are now highly questionable assumptions.

The main assumption underlying the traditional distinction between disease and illness is that knowledge falls into two broad categories, objective and subjective. Every medical student in the United States memorizes the distinction on arrival in medical school. Moreover, in its respect for scientific rigour, medicine gives greatest value to knowledge that can be verified as objective. Thus disease as objective and illness as subjective are categories that convey a powerfully divided sense of worth. What the patient reports is subjective (and untrustworthy), what the lab reports is objective (and true). Numbers are objective (and serious), stories are subjective (and trivial). Doctors are the authorities on disease, while patients remain the more or less unreliable narrators of their own unruly illnesses. The distribution of power within the traditional doctor/patient couple is tellingly one-sided. One knows, the other feels; one prescribes, the other complies; one is paid, the other pays. Although this sharp division has begun to blur under the pressure of postmodern innovations such as the ubiquitous malpractice suit, the old conceptual infrastructure that sustained it is still, confusingly, in place. The distinction between disease and illness, in any case, is not as innocent as it looks.

Perhaps the traditional differences in the understanding of disease and illness are merely a reflection of the truism – which has far-reaching and mostly ignored implications – that doctors and patients view the world from different perspectives. For the patient, illness is always a lived experience, while a patient's report of illness indicates to doctors the likelihood of a medical problem requiring biological explanations of disease. This inescapable degree of separation between doctor and patient must not, however, be interpreted as confirming a rigid split between objective and subjective knowledge. The split between objective and subjective knowledge, while based in common sense, is far from clear. So-called objective statistics and lab reports are meaningful only so far as fallible human beings produce and interpret them, and interpreters differ. As happens too often, accidents occur, tests may be improperly conducted, or doctors receive faulty data. Although doctors like to regard themselves as objective, the objectivity of medicine is a myth fostered as much by patients as by doctors. In practice, as doctors know, anomalies pop up to complicate every norm. Diagnosis and treatment often go forward in the absence of conclusive facts. 'Lesions and signs do not always match,' Kathryn Montgomery Hunter writes, 'nor do signs and test results. Even lesions and test results sometimes may not correspond' (1991: 18). Objectivity remains a valued goal, but the daily practice of medicine is shot through with subjective decision-making and ambiguous data.

Similar ambiguities undermine the traditional distinction between disease and illness. The recent lively academic discussion concerning definitions of disease, talk that seldom penetrates into the clinic, most often leaves room for non-biological, extraphysiological and social circumstances. Borderline cases and changing social attitudes push back the limits of even roomy definitions. We now view alcoholism as a disease, for example, but it is often next to impossible to diagnose individual heavy drinkers with an objectively verified disorder. Is drug addiction a disease? What about chronic pain? Doctors in one clinic will offer a diagnosis of reflex sympathetic dystrophy – continuous post-trauma burning pain in a limb or extremity without significant nerve damage or observable lesions – while doctors in another clinic think the category is a sham. The ambiguous status of Gulf War syndrome (a multisymptomatic affliction of American troops who served in the 1991 war in Iraq) concerns institutional politics as much as science. Patients who suffer from an unverified illness are no less sick than patients whose disease matches the textbook. Sometimes they are worse: not only ill but also frustrated, disabled, worried, out of work, and out of hope. The traditional biomedical distinction between disease and illness, seemingly clear and reasonable, fits imperfectly in a world that is often opaque and irrational, where the logical and the biological often fail to coincide. Its most unfortunate side effect lies in forcing us to employ a language whose assumptions implicitly validate the medical profession and devalue the patient.

The term *postmodern illness* implies a shift, incomplete and ongoing, in which the patient, no longer merely a bundle of symptoms reported by an unreliable, subjective ego, emerges at moments as a valued participant in the medical process of diagnosis and treatment. In this shift 'disease' and 'illness' also undergo change. While continuing to convey their traditional biomedical meanings, they increasingly carry as a tacit subtext an awareness of how these artificial distinctions limit understanding and create unnecessary, harmful distance between patients and doctors. We are coming to see that disease and illness are not oppositions rooted in the nature of things, like fire and ice, but socially constructed categories with somewhat porous and imperfect application to the array of maladies, disorders, syndromes and conditions – some quite new and mysterious – that patients today ask doctors to care for. A study of postmodern illness needs to acknowledge and explore the changes that destabilize traditional medical usage in ways commensurate with the changing postmodern world.

Postmodern illness, as I use the phrase, encompasses both the patient's experience and whatever biological condition initiates or accompanies it. In effect, it conflates two concepts that medicine normally prefers to keep separate. The traditional division between disease and illness, however, while it makes good sense to a scientist tracking the AIDS virus under an electron microscope, simply cannot stand up to the complication of postmodern ailments and understandings. From a postmodern point of view, AIDS is never simply about the science of a microbe. People infected with the human immunodeficiency virus (HIV) live within cultures that directly affect their health: cultures marked in the developed world, for example, by homophobia, government funding, gay rights activists, research grants, racism, pharmaceutical companies, addicts and blood transfusions. Outside the lab, microbes follow the terrain of cultural geopolitics. Life-extending multiple drug therapies available to a US citizen in San Diego are unavailable – because they cost too much – to a patient in Port au Prince or Kinshasa. HIV was not simply discovered, like a comet, but slowly put together as a legitimate diagnosis through a process of social consensus that included debate among international laboratories, sometimes stormy annual conferences, peer-reviewed journals, grant proposals, and the exclusion of contrary views deemed extreme, incorrect or merely annoying. From a postmodern perspective, doctors and medical researchers are never wholly objective, despite even heroic efforts to achieve verifiable results, much as patients are never wholly subjective, despite evidence that we know the world as filtered through our individual egos. What underlies these changed assumptions, assumptions that destabilize a traditional biomedical reading of disease and illness, is a new understanding of culture.

THE CULTURE OF ILLNESS

The language we are learning to speak in the postmodern country of the ill gives a prominent place to the idea of culture. An awareness that both doctor and patient stand within a cultural context is what modifies both the objectivity valued in medicine and the subjectivity native to the patient's experience. Objective judgement, after all, is finally a cultural artefact, not everywhere defined or valued equally – sometimes this is not even possible, as in the inherently uncertain realm of subatomic physics. Similarly, the sick person is not a mere subjective monad locked within an individual ego, an untrustworthy prisoner of consciousness, but, like physicians, an actor within a widely shared, intersubjective culture. Culture, of course, is always a pluralized concept: the social basis of health differs widely across groups, nations and continents. Yet, no matter how rich or plural the possible diversity, a shared, inter-subjective culture is what creates the behaviour that sociologist Talcott Parsons identified as 'the sick role': a way of being (when we are ill) assigned to us usually without our knowledge (Parsons, 1951, 1958 and 1978). Illnesses, in the manner of sick roles, differ across time and space. Despite presumably identical processes of cell biology, the experience of cancer – including such transpersonal measures as incidence and mortality rates – is different on an impoverished reservation in Montana than inside the Beverly Hills compounds of the rich and famous. Western nations sharing many basic cultural similarities – England, France, Germany and the United States – reveal distinctive variations in the medical treatment they offer and in how they understand health and sickness. Illness, in short, is never wholly personal, subjective and idiosyncratic, nor is disease wholly objective, factual and universal, but both take on their specific, malleable, historical shapes through the mediations of culture. William James, the modernist father of post-modern pragmatist philosophy and the only major American philosopher with a degree in medicine, put it this way: '[h]uman motives sharpen all our questions, human satisfactions lurk in all our answers, all our formulas have a human twist' (1975: 117).

The rediscovery of culture might be called a precondition of post-modern thought. Although postmodernism takes almost as doctrine the rejection of claims that knowledge can be grounded in anything like an absolute, essentialist, universal or (God help us) metaphysical basis for thought, a belief in the importance of culture is as close to providing a foundation as postmodernism is ever likely to come. Beyond disputes about the definition of culture, countless issues are open to debate, including such chicken-and-egg controversies as whether culture is the source of all representations or rather the product of representations. It seems clear that cultural texts and contexts maintain an interaction complex enough to justify Stephen Greenblatt's concept of a 'poetics of culture' (1989). No one, despite the inevitable arguments, can doubt the within which they work – as Medawar (1984) pithily puts it: 'the history of science bores most scientists stiff. A great many highly creative scientists. . . take it quite for granted, though they are usually too polite or too ashamed to say so, that an interest in the history of science is a sign of failing or of unawakened powers'. Happily, a flawed framework does not prevent all accretion of knowledge through observation. The Greeks could add to physical science within a framework torn between Leucippus' atoms in a void and the four elements of Empedocles; somewhat sadly, the invention of gunpowder did not have to await either the theory of phlogiston or the discovery of oxygen.

Those who seek to advance medical science, or to practise competent medicine, are doubtless quite as likely to be detached from the evolution and validity of their basic assumptions as those in other branches of science or professional activity. So far as effectiveness of medical practice is concerned, this may not in earlier times have greatly mattered; over many centuries, the faithful followers of Galen adhered to a framework of the four humours, without any specific baleful effect on what they did or failed to do. But in that respect, things have changed. In many illnesses there are great benefits from giving the right treatment, and corresponding dangers from giving the wrong treatment or even from omitting treatment, which in days gone by was often the right thing to do. The sheer power and specificity of the drugs now available, the frequency of side effects, and the multiplicity of indications for their employment, demand the utmost responsibility in their use, a responsibility whose recognition has fostered the discipline of clinical pharmacology, an essential component of undergraduate and postgraduate medical education.

A more recent manifestation of this proper concern for the best possible deployment of remedies may be seen in the advocacy of 'evidence-based medicine' (EBM) (Sackett et al., 1996). In his 1996 Office of Health Economics Lecture, Professor David Sackett had an opportunity to describe EBM in a less formal and more extended way than would be appropriate in a journal article. For example, he is able to say: 'I'm a student of neither ethics nor health economics, and my knowledge in these areas is mundane'. But he seems to me to have the root of the matter when he says: 'although I've drawn salaries from universities, governments, and now from the NHS, I've always considered my real employers (i.e. those with the highest call on my loyalty) to be my patients, my students, and the junior doctors on my clinical teams'.

Sackett defines EBM as 'the conscientious, explicit and judicious use of current best evidence in making decisions about the care of individual patients'. This involves 'integrating individual clinical expertise with the best available external clinical evidence from systematic research'. Individual clinical expertise derives from the care of patients and from accumulated personal knowledge of the natural history of disease – the medicine of Sydenham and Ryle. External research-based clinical evidence is derived in part from 'the basic sciences of medicine', but 'especially from patient centred clinical research into the accuracy and precision of diagnostic tests (including the clinical examination), the power of prognostic markers, and the efficacy and safety of therapeutic, rehabilitative and preventative regimens'. Although these types of relevant evidence range far beyond that derived from randomized trials and meta-analyses, Sackett allots a special place to that type of evidence as being 'so much more likely to inform us, and so much less likely to mislead us' than the 'non-experimental approaches', which in his view 'routinely lead to false-positive conclusions about efficacy'. Indeed, he regards evidence derived from the systematic review of several controlled trials as the 'gold standard' for judging whether a treatment does more good than harm. This is the message first proclaimed by Archie Cochrane (1972), whom to know was to love, but whose manifold gifts did not include inerrancy.

Sackett's description of what is meant by EBM is framed in terms of individual patient care; but the principle of using best available evidence is also relevant to 'group decisions' on the provision of services, in which 'the overriding objective . . . is that of maximising the total cost-utility in that group'. Both in individual medicine and in public health medicine, clinical judgements have to be modulated to an appropriate extent by considerations of ethics and of health economics (Gillon and Lloyd, 1994; Williams, 1997).

COMMENT ON EBM

There can surely be no difficulty in accepting the general proposition that medical practice and the provision of health care should be based on the best available evidence, or in welcoming the complementarity accorded by Sackett to 'individual clinical expertise' and 'external clinical evidence from systematic research'. Any movement which encourages self-scrutiny and self-criticism has to be a good thing, so long as it stops short of aborting that modicum of self-confidence which enables us to live and practise, while aware of the strong element of uncertainty that is inescapable in all branches of health care. However, since criticism is the acid that etches medical systems into better shape, I would raise one particular concern – the primacy given to 'RCT evidence' – and two more general ones: the validity and applicability of 'group evidence', and the extent to which the 'EBM principle' can be applied to the totality of medical practice.

Relative value of RCT evidence

The development of the randomized controlled trial (RCT) by Bradford Hill and Richard Doll is both theoretically and practically a milestone in impact of culture on everyday life. It shapes us like the force of gravity. In fact, the postmodern era has so vastly extended the domain of culture that it now includes the realm traditionally considered its opposite: nature. You cannot hike into the remotest uninhabited widerness today without inhaling particles of human civilization. The concept of wilderness is itself a cultural construction, of course. Even wild nature in all its sheer materiality – from floods to mud slides – now reveals the shaping or meddling hand of humankind.

Culture, in its tamer versions, usually takes the tangible shapes created by various interrelated symbol systems, systems that are also cultural creations, like the codes governing Parisian fashion or the choreographed moves of kung fu. Scholars have noted that postmodern culture achieves a certain uniqueness by placing closely together elements borrowed from widely disparate symbol systems, like the Pachelbel D-Minor Canon played behind a television ad for luxury cars. Postmodern culture typically leaps across space and time when, for example, an Anasazi pot is displayed in a Victorian hotel refurbished in contemporary Denver. Its eclectic, rootless style is international, postcolonial, affluent, underwritten by a late-capitalist consumer economy that transforms local markets into connections in a global network. As Jean-François Lyotard observes, 'one listens to reggae, watches a western, eats McDonald's food for lunch and local cuisine for dinner, wears Paris perfume in Tokyo and "retro" clothes in Hong Kong' (1984: 76). Not all, however, is affluence and jet-set travel. In contrast to the modernist focus on Europe, postmodernism engages the voices of far-flung and often oppressed groups, from women in the developing world to Chinese political dissidents. African-Americans, for example, infuse postmodern culture with fragments of contemporary black experience, such as the persona of the risk-taking, high-flying, impromptu performer: Michael Jordan hanging above the rim, Martin Luther King Jr. marching toward the police lines, the latest hip-hop artist testing the edge. Electronic technologies, meanwhile, connect people and data formerly dispersed and isolated across the globe. Participants in an Internet support group for cancer patients illustrate just one more way in which postmodern culture has changed the experience of illness.

An awareness of the role that culture plays in the experience of illness unavoidably invokes questions and texts lying far outside the ordinary range of medical knowledge. We must explore, for example, not only laboratory data and epidemiological research but also novels, television programmes, films, advertising, bodybuilders and obscenity laws. The disparate texts and activities that represent the domain of culture cannot be off-limits to a study of postmodern illness. The result, from a biomedical point of view, is something close to intellectual chaos: the controlled experiment from hell and 'normal science' run amok. From a postmodern point of view, however, it is only by opening the clinic and research laboratory to an increasing number of messy cultural variables that medicine, which is scientific but not strictly speaking a science, will begin to understand what most patients already know or strongly suspect about the changed arena of contemporary illness.

REFERENCES

Baudrillard, J. (1988) 'Simulacra and simulations' (1981) reprinted in M. Poster (ed.), *Selected Writings*. New York: Polity Press.

Frank, A.W. (1996) *The Wounded Storyteller: Body, Illness, and Ethics*. Chicago: University of Chicago Press.

Goldman, R. and Papson, S. (1994) 'The postmodernism that failed', in D.R. Dickens and A. Fontana (eds), *Postmodernism and Social Inquiry*. New York: Guilford Press.

Greenblatt, S. (1989) 'Towards a poetics of culture', in H.A. Veeser (ed.), *The New Historicism*. New York: Routledge. pp. 1–14.

Hunter K.M. (1991) *Doctors' Stories: The Narrative Structure of Medical Knowledge*. Princeton: Princeton University Press.

James, W. (1975) *Pragmatism* (1907), ed. F. Bowers and I.K. Skrupskelis. Cambridge, MA: Harvard University Press.

Lyotard, J.-F. (1984) *The Postmodern Condition: A Report on Knowledge* (1979), trans. G. Bennington and B. Massumi. Minneapolis: University of Minnesota Press.

Parsons, T. (1951) *The Social System*. New York: The Free Press.

Parsons, T. (1958) 'Definitions of health and illness in the light of American values and social structure', in E. Gartly Jaco (ed.), *Patients, Physicians, and Illness: A Sourcebook in Behavioral Science and Health*. New York: The Free Press. pp. 121–44.

Parsons, T. (1978) *Action Theory and the Human Condition*. New York: The Free Press.

6

Ivan Illich and the Pursuit of Health

John P. Bunker

'Why are some people healthy and others not?' ask two new books (Evans et al., 1994; Amick et al., 1995). The answers their authors give differ dramatically. While both are in strong agreement on the importance to health of inheritance, lifestyle and the social and physical environment, they differ in how much credit, if any, to give to medical care. It is ironic that today, when medicine's substantial and growing benefits to health are well established, medicine is subject to its greatest attacks since the beginning of the nineteenth century.

When my class graduated from medical school in the middle of the century the benefits of medicine and surgery were unquestioned by us. The Dean had said at Commencement, 'Gentlemen, half of what you are taught as medical students will in ten years have been shown to be wrong, and the trouble is, none of your teachers knows which half.' But new and more effective treatments were being introduced every month and the potential for preventing and curing illness appeared to have no limits. It never occurred to us, as we entered practice, that there were problems ahead.

ONSET OF DOUBTS

My own doubts were raised only when, 20 years later, I spent a year of sabbatical study in London. I became impressed by how similar medical and surgical practice was in the UK and the USA and yet, in many ways, how very different. I found, for example, that patients in the UK were half as likely, on average, to undergo surgery in a given year as were patients in the USA (Bunker, 1970). Life expectancy at that time was slightly greater in the UK, so more surgery in the USA did not mean their surgeons were saving more lives. Perhaps the quality of life was better served by surgery in the USA, but there were no data to demonstrate it and we still don't know. In the absence of evidence to the

First published in the *Journal of Health Services Research and Policy*, 2 (1), January 1997: 56–9.

contrary, the higher rates of surgery in the USA were interpreted as unnecessary surgery by some observers.

That was in 1970. The medical profession in both countries had begun to worry about the possible harm that medicine and surgery might incur, while the benefits of medicine were largely taken for granted. The British medical epidemiologist, Thomas McKeown, sharing these doubts, attempted to measure the role of medicine in furthering health and concluded that it was a very small one (McKeown, 1976). McKeown attributed the dramatic increase in life expectancy over the previous 100 years primarily to nutritional, environmental and behavioural factors, but he conceded that the evidence was only circumstantial. He believed that he had shown that medical care was not responsible and concluded that social and environmental factors must have been the cause. (In a second edition he acknowledged that 'it is not possible to estimate with any precision the contribution which therapeutic and other advances have made to the decline of the multiple non-infective causes of death which together were associated [at that time] with about a quarter of the reduction of mortality: McKeown, 1979.)

ILLICH'S ATTACK ON MEDICINE

The doubts concerning medicine were seized upon by the Austrian theologian, Ivan Illich, who was at that time engaged in a literary crusade against technology and the many ways in which he believed the public good was being harmed. In his 1975 book, *Medical Nemesis: the Expropriation of Health*, Illich argued that medical care did more harm than good, citing the by then substantial critical literature, much of it written by doctors themselves. At the time I considered it an ill-informed and irresponsible attack on the medical profession, but in retrospect we had only ourselves to blame: we had been so preoccupied with the problems of medical care that we failed to put them in the context of the good that medicine did and that we believed could be taken for granted. Attempting to make the case for medicine, two of its leaders, for example, could only suggest that 'what the doctor does is something that is extraordinarily difficult to analyze and measure' (McDermott, 1978) and that 'although most clinicians do not doubt that there has been substantial improvement in the treatment of disease during the past few decades, it is difficult to assess the dimensions' (Beeson, 1980).

Looking back today I realize that I misunderstood what Illich was up to. I had read *Deschooling Society*, in which he attacked the educational system for serving to indoctrinate the young in the overproduction of goods to satisfy the consumer society. Much the same theme reappears towards the end of *Medical Nemesis* (1975) in which he wrote that 'like school education and motor transportation, clinical care is the result of a

capital-intensive commodity production'. But he did not limit his accusa-
tion to one of over-treatment, an argument that I and others had already
made. His real argument was that medical care enslaves rather than
frees, and that 'medical nemesis is the experience of people who are
largely deprived of any autonomous ability to cope with nature, neigh-
bors, and dreams, and are technically maintained within environmental,
social, and symbolic systems'.

Illich wrote that 'better health care will depend, not on some new
therapeutic standard, but on the level of willingness and competence to
engage in self-care' and he defined self-care broadly as consisting of
'personal activities [that] are shaped and conditioned by the culture
in which the individual grows up: patterns of work and leisure, of
celebration and sleep, of production of food and drink, of family relations
and politics'. Illich has described this ideal state as an 'autonomous and
creative intercourse among persons, and the intercourse of persons with
their environment . . . individual freedom realized in personal interdependence and, as such, an intrinsic ethical ideal' (Illich, 1990). He
called this a state of conviviality, and his notion of its health enhance-
ment is remarkably consonant with current views of the impact of the
social environment on health (Patrick and Wickizer, 1995).

Illich's attack has been largely ignored by the medical profession
(though he states that there have been bulk orders of *Medical Nemesis*
from medical schools), and there is little if any evidence that it has
affected the continuing growth of the medical establishment. But it has
not been forgotten: *Medical Nemesis* was reprinted in 1990 by Penguin
and in 1995 by Marion Boyars. The latter, retitled *Limits to Medicine*,
includes a new preface, and in it Illich makes his purpose crystal clear: 'I
used medicine as a paradigm for any mega-technique that promises to
transform the *conditio humana*. I examined it as a model for any enterprise claiming, in effect, to abolish the need for the art of suffering by a
technically engineered pursuit of happiness' (Illich, 1995). (The preface,
taken from a 1994 lecture at a conference for nurses, also contains his
extraordinary and revealing statement that 'I am not a nurse and,
emphatically, I do not care about health'.)

SOCIAL DETERMINANTS OF HEALTH

Medical care today is a considerably less apposite model for Illich's
stated purpose. Not only has medicine continued to expand with new
and improved therapies, but the effects of the new therapies are now
routinely evaluated. While the benefits of medical care are substantial,
they account for only part of the large increase in life expectancy
experienced since the beginning of the century. Two books summarize
recently documented effects of the other, largely social, determinants of
health. *Why Are Some People Healthy and Others Not? The Determinants of*

Health of Populations (Evans et al., 1994) asks the right question, provides some of the answers, but gives little credit to medical care. The other, *Society and Health*, the product of a conference held in Boston in 1993, might also have neglected the role of medical care, had my associates and I not succeeded in convincing the conference organizers that medicine deserved a hearing (Amick et al., 1995).

A central message in each of these books, and one that has long been known, is that the health of the wealthy is better than that of the poor, the unemployed and the uneducated. There is also the important new message that will be familiar to many readers: it isn't just the poor who are sicker. There is a gradient of health evenly distributed across income, education and occupation levels. Individuals with middle income or high school diplomas die earlier and experience more frequent and more serious illness than those having completed a university degree or commanding a higher income. At every educational and income level, individuals with higher wages or more education are healthier. Top management lives longer and is healthier than middle management; white collar employees live longer than blue collar employees.

It may be taken for granted that poor people are apt to be less healthy. The mystery is why there should be such large differences in health among individuals and families who have resources and income more than adequate to provide all of the basic necessities of life. The large residual differences in health have something to do with our social lives, how many social contacts we have and whether we are part of one or more cohesive social groups. The better health of individuals with strong ties to family, friends and community has been widely documented: adults who live together live longer than those who live alone; members of churches or other social groups live longer than those who have few social contacts. The plausible role of biological pathways, leading from social disconnection to disease, has been extensively explored in a nine-year study of the residents of Alameda County, California (Berkman and Breslow, 1983). Smoking, alcohol intake and a sedentary lifestyle contributed to the ill health of individuals with fewer social contacts, but so, nearly equally, did marital status, contact with friends and relatives, and organizational membership – the social network within which individuals function.

Natural experiments on immigrants moving to the USA from countries with low rates of heart disease offer dramatic illustrations of the social network phenomenon. The incidence of heart disease in Japan is remarkably low, yet most Japanese moving to the USA have rapidly assumed the higher rate of heart disease of other Americans. But Japanese in the USA who retain the tight family structure traditional in Japan retain a relative immunity to heart disease. The prevalence of coronary heart disease in families adopting an American lifestyle has been reported to be three to five times greater than in those retaining a traditional Japanese culture, a difference that could not be accounted for by diet, smoking, or any of the other major risk factors for heart disease (Marmot and Syme, 1976).

Similar observations have been made in the Italians who emigrated in 1882 from the Italian town of Roseto to Pennsylvania, where they founded a town by the same name (Wolf and Bruhn, 1993). In the new Roseto they retained the relative freedom from coronary heart disease that they had enjoyed in Italy as long as they retained their traditional family-oriented social structure; but as they became assimilated into the surrounding American culture, where the individual, rather than the family and community, was considered to be the dominant social and economic unit, the incidence of coronary heart disease rose rapidly. Again, the deterioration in cardiac status could not be explained by the usual risk factors. Diet had actually improved and there was a marked fall in smoking. The Rosetans had become more sedentary but hardly enough to explain the large increase in heart disease.

THE PURSUIT OF HEALTH: WHICH PATH TO TAKE?

The differences in health between the well-to-do and the poor are large; a difference in life expectancy of five or six years, equivalent to a twofold difference in the likelihood of dying at almost every age. This is about the difference in life expectancy between pack-a-day smokers and non-smokers and similar in magnitude to my estimate of medicine's contribution to increases in life expectancy since 1900 (Bunker et al., 1995). Are estimates of life expectancy effects reliable enough to provide a basis for social or political action?

Documentation of the effectiveness of medical therapies, especially those recently introduced, is surprisingly strong, the result to a considerable extent of the need to justify the costs of treatment to governments and private insurance companies. A great deal is also known about the association between healthy and unhealthy lifestyle and longevity. How education, income and a variety of so-called social factors affect how long we live is much less clear. Income and education are almost certainly proxies for something else, perhaps control over one's personal and professional life (Syme, 1989), perhaps the social cohesion or sense of community (Patrick and Wickizer, 1995).

In the pursuit of health, how should we proceed? Writing in *Why Are Some People Healthy and Others Not?*, Evans and Stoddart suggest that 'perhaps Ivan Illich is right, and the health care system as a whole has a net negative impact on the health of the population it serves'. Other chapters suggest that funds 'might actually have a greater marginal effect on a nation's health status' if they were to be spent on other social needs and ask 'what can be done . . . to support the public objective of reduced resources to medical care for equivalent impacts on public health?' such as highway maintenance, education, police protection and

environmental clean-up (Evans et al., 1994). These are all highly important goods in their own right, of course, with urgent and valid demands
independent of their effects on health.

The association of social and economic status with health has been
known for many years. In the UK, the Black Report documented two-
and threefold differences in mortality across social classes (Townsend
and Davidson, 1982). Its publication in 1980 was met with a widespread
demand for social reform. The massive social restructuring that it would
have entailed was hardly welcomed by Margaret Thatcher's incoming
government and no action has yet been taken. Today there is a renewed
clamour for action, notably the King's Fund report that urges improvement in housing, lessening of poverty, reduction in smoking, and better
access to medical care (Benzeval et al., 1995).

Large-scale efforts at behavioural modification, encouraging the public
to adopt healthier lifestyles, have been largely unsuccessful (Carleton
et al., 1995; Davison et al., 1992). The public sees such programmes as
'victim blaming'. They resent being held responsible for poor health
when so many of the determinants of health (inheritance, the social and
physical environments, and the risks of occupation) are beyond their
control (Davison et al., 1992). Unhealthy personal habits have, if anything, increased during the century, as reflected in the loss of at least a
year in life expectancy to tobacco and alcohol-related diseases, AIDS and
violence (Bunker et al., 1995).

Efforts to coerce the public to adopt healthier personal habits having
failed, the prospects for improving the public's health by social or
environmental reform do not seem much brighter. It is not just that
governments are reluctant to make the enormous political changes that
would be required. More importantly, it is by no means clear what needs
to be done. Indeed, the social activists who urge that we invest less in
medical care and more in social programmes to improve health give very
little practical advice. The final chapter of *Why Are Some People Healthy
and Others Not?* calls for 'hygeia' rather than 'panakeia', public health
measures in preference to the panacea of the medical care system. Yet
'even where recognition [of social, economic and cultural factors] is now
emerging, there is little sense . . . of how best to reallocate scarce
resources so as to improve the health impact of public programs' (Evans
et al., 1994). Deploring 'our unwillingness to study social class', let alone
to take action, Leonard Syme at the University of California in Berkeley
suggests that 'we do not feel that anything can be done about it. Social
class is a product of vast historical, economic, and cultural forces,
and short of revolution, it is not something one targets for intervention. So we give up and instead urge people to lower their fat intake'
(Syme, 1994).

It is ultimately the public who decide whether to adopt a more healthy
lifestyle, whether to give up smoking, to drink in moderation, to take
more exercise, to lose weight. Successful or not, the needs and demands

for medical services will remain undiminished. (If, for example, a healthier lifestyle leads to additional years of life, the costs of medical care with advancing years will be, if anything, greater.)

It is the public, again, who will, or should, decide how much they wish to invest in medical care, the increasing benefits of which are now almost routinely measurable. Medical care costs more today primarily because it can do more, and the results of what it can do can be measured with increasing precision. Early in the century there were very large annual increases in life expectancy, to which medical care contributed relatively little. Life expectancy rose from about 45 years in 1900 to about 70 years in 1950, medicine contributing an estimated two of the 25 years of increase. Life expectancy rose by another seven years between 1950 and 1990, medicine now contributing nearly half of the continuing gain, together with an estimated five years' relief from the poor quality of life associated with chronic disease (Bunker, 1995).

The economist William Baumol has repeatedly explained that as industrial efficiency and productivity increase, time and resources become available for labour-intensive activities, notably medical care, education and the performing arts. It is simply a question of how we want to spend the resources and money that an increasingly productive economy will continue to make available (Baumol, 1989, 1995). Baumol's views, and the elementary economic theory of which he reminds us, have barely surfaced in the recent national health care debates, the focus of which has been on constraining costs. While there is strong resistance to increasing the investment of personal or public funds in health care, there is little prospect of its reduction.

If Illich's views on the practice of medicine are largely irrelevant today, as I believe they are, he may at least have done us a favour by forcing the medical profession to confront the problem of accountability. But be that as it may, his intuitive belief in the health-enhancing effects of friendship, social intercourse and personal interdependence, which he called con-viviality, now has strong evidentiary support. We do not yet fully understand how or why personal relations are so strongly associated with health, let alone how to improve health as a result. Social reform is not a substitute for health care, as the current social activists would have it. Rather, our social environment is a second, important but quite separate, determinant of health and well-being.

REFERENCES

Amick, B.C. III, Levine, S., Tarlov, A.R. and Walsh, D.C. (eds) (1995) *Society and Health*. New York: Oxford University Press.

Baumol, W.J. (1995) *Healthcare as a Handicraft Industry*. London: Office Health Economics.

Baumol, W.J., Blackman, S.A.B. and Wolff, E.N. (1989) *Productivity and American Leadership*. Cambridge, MA: MIT Press.

Beeson, P.B. (1980) 'Changes in medical therapy during the past half century', *Medicine*, 59: 79–99.

Benzeval, M., Judge, K. and Whitehead, M. (1995) *Tackling Inequalities in Health: an Agenda for Action*. London: King's Fund.

Berkman, L.F. and Breslow, L. (1983) *Health and Ways of Living: the Alameda County Study*. New York: Oxford University Press.

Bunker, J.P. (1970) 'Surgical manpower: a comparison of operations and surgeons in the United States and in England and Wales', *New England Journal of Medicine*, 282: 135–44.

Bunker, J.P. (1995) 'Medicine matters after all', *Journal of the Royal College of Physicians*, 29: 105–12.

Bunker, J.P., Frazier, H.S. and Mosteller, F. (1995) 'The role of medical care in determining health: creating an inventory of benefits', in B.C. Amick III, S. Levine, A.R. Tarlov, D.C. Walsh (eds), *Society and Health*. New York: Oxford University Press.

Carleton, R.A., Lasater, T.M., Assaf, A.R., Feldman, H.A., McKinlay, S. and the Pawtucket Heart Health Program Writing Group (1995) 'The Pawtucket heart health program: community changes in cardiovascular risk factors and projected disease risk', *American Journal of Public Health*, 85: 777–85.

Davison, C., Frankel, S. and Davey Smith, G. (1992) 'The limits of lifestyle: re-addressing "fatalism" in the popular culture of illness prevention', *Social Science and Medicine*, 6: 675–85.

Evans, R.G., Barer, M.L. and Marmor, T.R. (eds) (1994) *Why are Some People Healthy and Others Not? The Determinants of Health of Populations*. Hawthorne, NY: Aldine de Gruyter.

Illich, I. (1972) *Deschooling Society*. London: Marion Boyars.

Illich, I. (1975) *Medical Nemesis: the Expropriation of Health*. New York: Pantheon.

Illich, I. (1990) *Tools for Conviviality*. London: Marion Boyars.

Illich, I. (1995) *Limits to Medicine*. London: Marion Boyars.

McDermott, W. (1978) 'Medicine: the public good and one's own', *Perspectives in Biology and Medicine*, 21: 167–87.

McKeown, T. (1976) *The Role of Medicine: Dream, Mirage, or Nemesis?* London: Nuffield Provincial Hospitals Trust.

McKeown, T. (1979) *The Role of Medicine: Dream, Mirage, or Nemesis?* 2nd edn. Princeton, NJ: Princeton University Press.

Marmot, M.G. and Syme, S.L. (1976) 'Acculturation and coronary heart disease in Japanese-Americans', *Americal Journal of Epidemiology*, 104, 225–47.

Patrick, D.L. and Wickizer, T.M. (1995) 'Community and health', in B.C. Amick III, S. Levine, A.R. Tarlov, D.C. Walsh (eds), *Society and Health*. New York: Oxford University Press.

Syme, S.L. (1989) 'Control and health: a personal perspective', in A. Steptoe and A. Appels (eds), *Stress, Personal Control and Health*. Chichester: John Wiley.

Syme, S.L. (1994) 'The social environment and health. Health and wealth: proceedings of the American Academy of Arts and Sciences', *Daedalus, Journal of the American Academy of Arts and Sciences*, 123 (4): 79–86.

Townsend, P. and Davidson, N. (eds) (1982) *Inequalities in Health: the Black Report*. Harmondsworth: Penguin.

Wolf, S. and Bruhn, J.G. (1993) *The Power of Clan: the Influence of Human Relationships on Heart Disease*. New Brunswick, NJ: Transaction Publishers.

PART II

SOCIAL PATTERNS OF HEALTH

The second part of this book explores 'Social patterns of health' and examines the detailed evidence that has been gathered in an attempt to ascertain whether or not these patterns help us in our quest to understand the concept of 'health'. The bulk of the chapters in this reader reflect the views of the editors who tend towards favouring a broad, pluralistic, but largely social, model of health. Our health, as individuals, is inextricably linked to the health of the people around us, in our relationships, in our families, localities, communities and nations. The chapters in Part II attempt to lay out the ground rules for some of these encounters, and even to quantify some of the effects that these social phenomena have on the health of the people within these various structures.

Michael Marmot has spent a lifetime charting and researching the patterns and trends of disease (and by its absence, health) throughout the UK and while making international comparisons. His contribution to this collection (Chapter 7: 'A Social View of Health and Disease') summarizes and synthesizes conclusions that are the result of his and other people's research and analysis. The conclusions are irresistible: health and disease are socially patterned, and the magnitude of these patterns is convincingly illustrated throughout this chapter. Poor people have less money, but also less 'health' than those higher up the social scale. They die earlier of almost every measured cause of death, and this gradient continues right to the top of the social scale. Even those people who presumably have enough food, adequate housing and a certain amount of disposable income are 'less healthy' than those above them on the income scale, who have even more of these worldly goods and who live longer to enjoy them. Perhaps more significant is the finding that these social patterns are not fixed but have the ability to change over relatively short periods of time. While falling short of advocating massive social restructuring, Marmot does offer his opinion that, 'If the gradients vary there must be reasons why. Better understanding of the reasons may form the basis of action to alleviate them.'

Richard G. Wilkinson (Chapter 8: 'Social Status, Inequality and Health'), provides us with further clues to the aetiology of these health inequalities and also, by implication, further pointers to the social manipulation that would be necessary to eradicate these health inequalities from any society. His analysis leads to the conclusion that it is the *relative* differences within any society that lead to health inequalities. Societies which are relatively socially homogeneous, with smaller differentials between the richest and the poorest members of that society, are in general 'healthier' than those where wide disparities exist. About half of the measurable adverse health effects can be ascribed to this cause, while the other half seems to be connected with elements within society which can be labelled as 'social cohesion', or connected to the notion of 'social capital'. His research leads inevitably into conjecture about the sorts of social policy that would be required to minimize these adverse health effects: 'When thinking about policy in this field we should think about it on two levels. One is reducing the objective scale of inequality and the other is to make sure our institutions make people feel valued and appreciated.'

Stephen Morris (Chapter 9: 'Economics and Equity in the Distribution of Scarce Health Care Resources') considers the social distribution of health care resources within the context of an apparently chronic scarcity of money for universal, publicly funded health services. Not everything that could be done to improve people's health can be done, because we are continually told that there are not enough resources to go round. For this reason economics has become a necessary discipline to include in contemporary debates about health. This chapter looks at some of the principles that could, or should, underpin economic decision-making and considers the notions of equity, efficiency and equality. Morris's findings are stark, if unsurprising: the richer social classes and higher earners currently receive a greater proportion of health expenditure than the amount of illness in those groups would justify if principles of equity were applied accurately. Similarly there are certain geographical regions which receive greater financial resources for health care than their levels of illness would justify. Morris's chapter is a contribution to understanding the way that economic principles might illuminate the social policy initiatives required to work towards fairer distribution of scarce resources. The fact that resources are distributed in such a manifestly unequal fashion reflects something to do with power, rather than social justice.

Lesley Doyal (Chapter 10: 'The Politics of Women's Health: Setting a Global Agenda') explores power relationship with regard to gender inequalities throughout the world. Her claim that: 'At the heart of all feminist critiques of medicine is the recognition that women lack power in health care institutions. This limits their ability to determine medical priorities or to influence the allocation of scarce resources' is well supported by examples throughout her text. Most excitingly she charts many of the ways that women throughout the world are attempting to counter detrimental power situations, using health issues as a focus for their activities. International campaigning work by women to press for a variety of linked demands, such as humane medical care, reproductive self-determination and freedom from violence, is important at a policy level, but also at the level of the experience of each individual woman who approaches the health service or who is trying to keep herself 'healthy'. But much still needs to be done on all these counts: 'We have seen that women are continuing to challenge medicine in an attempt to get their needs for both physical and mental health care met more effectively. Though some progress can be identified much remains to be done.'

7

A Social View of Health and Disease

Michael Marmot

Health and disease are socially patterned. Rates of occurrence of disease states vary according to social and economic conditions, culture, and other environmental factors. This is true today, as it was during the major social and economic changes that came with industrialization. Not only do they vary, but the evidence suggests that variations in rates of occurrence of disease are actually determined by social and economic factors. It is the purpose of this chapter to demonstrate this variation and to present a framework for understanding its causes.

SOCIAL, ECONOMIC AND CULTURAL DIFFERENCES IN DISEASE WITHIN COUNTRIES

Our own exploration of this area began with the Whitehall study of British civil servants. Figure 7.1 shows mortality from a range of causes in the first Whitehall study. When we began this work, it seemed unlikely that social class differences would be as large in civil servants as they were in the country as a whole. These were all non-industrial civil servants in office-based jobs. At that time their jobs were stable, with high security of employment, and presumably free from chemical and physical industrial hazards. We were surprised, therefore, to discover that the nearly threefold difference in mortality between bottom and top grades of the civil service was larger than the difference between the top and bottom social classes in national mortality data (OPCS, 1978; Fox and Goldblatt, 1982). This presumably reflects the precise hierarchical classification of occupations within the civil service.

To investigate the causes of these social differentials, we launched a second study of civil servants, the Whitehall II study (Marmot et al., 1991; 1997; Pilgrim et al., 1992; Stansfeld and Marmot, 1992a, 1992b; Brunner et al., 1993; Marmot et al., 1993; North et al., 1993; Roberts et al., 1993; Stansfeld et al., 1993, 1995a). This later research showed that there were gradients in morbidity and health behaviour (smoking) in

First published in D. Blane, E. Brunner and R. Wilkinson (eds), *Health and Social Organization*. London: Routledge, 1996, pp. 42–67.

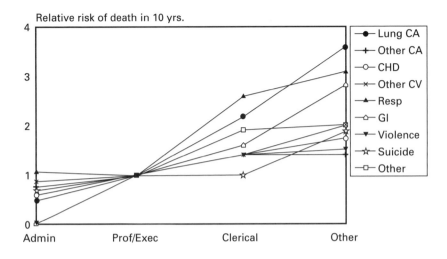

Figure 7.1 *Mortality by employment grade among British civil servants. CA cancer, CHD coronary heart disease, CV cardiovascular, Resp respiratory, GI general infection (Marmot et al., 1984a)*

Whitehall I and Whitehall II, in addition to the mortality gradients (Marmot et al., 1991). There is no suggestion that these gradients in morbidity were somehow due to the British civil service being atypical.

There are two points worth emphasizing from these data. First, there is a gradient in morbidity and mortality. Each group has worse health than the one above it in the hierarchy. The task for explanation here is not why is there a link between poverty and ill health but why is there a social gradient that runs across the whole of society. In the higher grades of the civil service there is no poverty, yet those who are near the top have worse health than those at the top, and the gradient continues all the way down.

This is not to imply that there is no longer a problem of poverty in wealthy countries. On the contrary, young black men in Harlem, in New York City, for example, have six times the US average mortality (McCord, 1990). Interestingly, although the relative risk of violent death was large, the greatest contributor to the absolute excess in mortality was cardiovascular disease. Income levels in Harlem are less than a third of the US average. The definition of poverty in wealthy countries has been much debated. One part of the debate has centred on whether poverty should be measured in absolute or in relative terms. The Rowntree Report on income and wealth in Britain produced both measures (Joseph Rowntree Foundation, 1995). As a relative measure, it reported the percentage of the population that had incomes below half the average, after allowing for housing costs. This fell to a low point of 7 per cent of the population in 1977 and rose to 24 per cent in 1990. In absolute terms, the bottom tenth of the distribution had a 17 per cent fall in real income between 1979 and 1991, the second bottom 10 per cent had no change. This contrasted with a 36 per cent rise in average incomes. However, only the top 30 per cent of the distribution had incomes rising as fast as the average (Joseph Rowntree Foundation, 1995).

We have, therefore, two types of problem to understand and address. First, the relation between inequality and ill health (Wilkinson, 1986): secondly, the relation between poverty and ill health (World Bank, 1993).

The second point arising from these Whitehall analyses is the generality of the findings across causes of morbidity and mortality. Specific diseases have specific causes. Cutting across these, there may be a predisposition to ill health that is related to position in the social hierarchy. There are similar gradients for various measures of morbidity and for the general measure of self-reported health. A particular demonstration of the general importance of environment in the patterning of disease comes from the study of migrants (Marmot et al., 1984b). In general, disease rates among migrants reflect influences from the country of origin and the country of destination. There are some genetic abnormalities such as thalassaemia or sickle cell disease. Apart from these, we observe a pattern of disease in migrants that resembles that of the old country in the early years after migration, and comes to resemble that of the new country with the progress of time. Men of Japanese ancestry living in the United States have rates of coronary heart disease intermediate between the low rates in Japan and the high rates in the United States (Syme et al., 1975). Japanese men in Hawaii have lower rates than those in California (Marmot et al., 1975).

There has been much debate as to the extent to which ethnic differences in disease can be attributed to socioeconomic factors. In the United States, for example, it appears that the bulk of the black/white differences in health can indeed be accounted for by social and economic factors (Pappas et al., 1993). Comparing ethnic groups is not the same as comparing migrants and non-migrants. The position of blacks in the United States may indeed be largely determined by socioeconomic circumstances. This appears not to be the case for migrants to England and Wales. Figure 7.2 examines mortality from ischaemic heart disease by country of birth and social class in England and Wales. The high mortality in immigrants from the Indian subcontinent and the low mortality in immigrants from the Caribbean persist within social classes and hence cannot easily be attributed to socioeconomic circumstances. Indeed, there is a suggestion that the social class pattern of mortality in the South Asian and Caribbean immigrants differs from the inverse relation between social class and mortality seen in the country as a whole (Marmot et al., 2000).

These migrant data illustrate an important point about the influence of social circumstances. Because social factors are more distant in the causal

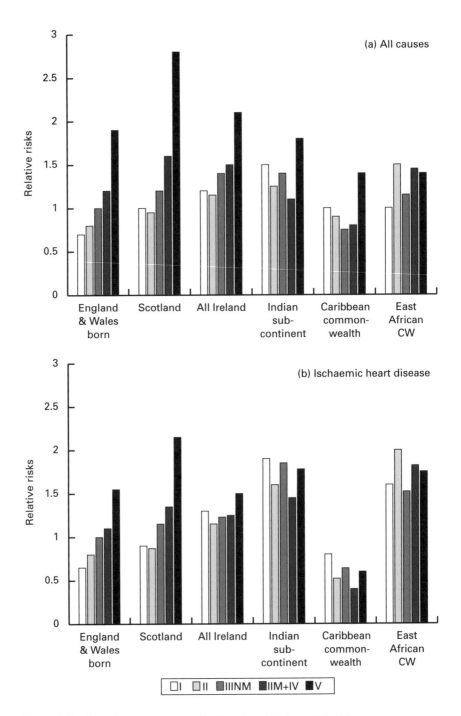

Figure 7.2 *Mortality by country of birth and social class, 1979–85.*
(a) All causes (Marmot et al., 1995b) (b) Ischaemic heart disease (Marmot
et al., 1995b)

chain than biological processes, their effects may be contingent on other circumstances. There is evidence, for example, that the social class distribution of heart disease changes with level of economic development (Marmot, 1992: 3). With the emergence of ischaemic heart disease as a major cause of death, it appears at first to be more common in higher socioeconomic groups. Subsequently, the social class distribution changes to the one more commonly seen now in industrialized countries, with higher rates in lower socioeconomic groups.

This changing social class pattern presumably means either that important causal factors have changed their social class distribution or that the relative importance of different factors has changed. For example, the social class distribution of smoking appears to have reversed. It now shows a clear social gradient, with high rates in low socioeconomic groups. Other things may not have changed their social class distribution. The disadvantage of low social position in terms of psychosocial factors related to inequality may not have changed. These psychosocial factors may not have led to an increased risk of ischaemic heart disease in the absence of important causes, such as high intake of saturated fat, smoking, sedentary lifestyle and obesity. This emphasizes the importance of studying the links between social, economic, cultural and other determinants of ill health.

MEASURES OF SOCIAL INFLUENCES ON HEALTH

In the United States, social position is usually referred to as socioeconomic status and is commonly measured as some combination of occupation, income and education. In Britain much of the evidence for the relation between social position and ill health has come from analyses using the Registrar-General's social classes (OPCS, 1978). This classification is based on grouping occupations into social classes. It has continued to be widely used for the pragmatic reason that it is a potent predictor of a wide range of health outcomes. It regularly attracts criticism because the basis of the grouping is unclear (Goldblatt, 1990). Goldthorpe has contrasted three different systems of measuring social stratification. The first is based on the prestige of occupations. The second is based on social status and is a measure of whether members of a social group are treated as equals. The third is social class. Goldthorpe's preference is for a measure of social class that locates individuals in households within the economic sphere (Erikson and Goldthorpe, 1992).

There are at least two reasons for wishing to be precise about social classification. The first relates to the pragmatic issue of better prediction, the second to understanding. The argument is that a measure that has a clear conceptual base and higher validity is more likely to convey meaning when attempting to interpret a correlation. This is desirable but maybe illusory. Education has appeal as a measure because it appears to

Table 7.1　*Rate ratios[a] for short and long spells of sickness absence by employment grade and level of education*

Measure	Men		Women	
	Short spells[b]	Long spells[c]	Short spells[b]	Long spells[c]
Employment grade				
Unified grades 1–6	1.0	1.0	1.0	1.0
Unified grade 7	1.96	2.03	1.51	1.11
Senior Executive Officer	2.30	2.25	2.09	1.08
Higher Executive Officer	3.04	3.27	3.13	2.13
Executive Officer	5.33	4.49	3.57	2.47
Clerical Officer/Office Support	6.85	6.33	4.04	3.76
Educational level (years)				
≤ 16	1.0	1.0	1.0	1.0
17–18	1.17	0.90	1.03	0.83
< 19	1.29	0.94	1.29	0.96

(a) Rate ratios for employment grade are adjusted for age and level of education and those for education are adjusted for age and grade. All rate ratios 95% CI.
(b) Seven days or less.
(c) Over seven days.

convey what it is about social position that may be causally related to increased risk. If education were then shown to be a stronger predictor than, say, occupational prestige, this could lead to the presumption that it is education, not factors related to occupation, that is more important in the causal chain leading to ill health. This may be an overinterpretation. If it were the case that education was measured more precisely than occupational prestige, that alone could account for its stronger predictive power.

Data from the Whitehall II study show that grade and education are independent predictors of sickness absence. Table 7.1 shows, however, that when both predictors are put into the same predictive model, grade emerges as the stronger independent predictor. This is contrary to most investigators' findings with measures of education and occupation. It may be that, in the Whitehall II study, factors related to occupation are more important in the aetiology of socioeconomic differences in health than are factors related to education. Before reaching this conclusion, however, we should consider the relative precision of measurement. In Whitehall II, grade of employment is a precise measure of hierarchical position, whereas our measure of education is relatively imprecise. This may be one of the relatively few examples where an occupation-based measure of class is more precise than a measure based on education. This may be at least part of the explanation of the greater predictive power of grade.

Townsend proposed measures of socioeconomic deprivation. He developed an index for classifying areas that combines household access to a car, housing tenure (whether a dwelling is owned, rented from the local

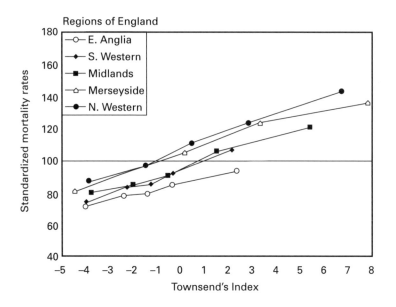

Figure 7.3   *All-cause mortality in regions of England by degree of deprivation divided into fifths (Eames et al., 1993)*

authority or privately rented), percentage unemployed and percentage living in crowded conditions (Townsend et al., 1988). Figure 7.3 contains analyses of mortality in small geographical areas (electoral wards) grouped according to scores on the Townsend index. It shows that the average mortality in each quintile of social deprivation is higher than in the quintile below it (Eames et al., 1993). One interpretation of this apparent gradient is that relative deprivation is an important predictor of mortality level. Alternatively, it is possible that there is a threshold of deprivation above which mortality is raised, and each quintile contains progressively greater proportions of deprived households.

SOCIAL PATTERNS OF DISEASE ARE NOT FIXED

One response to the demonstration of social variations in disease rates is that they exist everywhere and are therefore intrinsic to social organization. It is implied that, if social differentials in health are a consequence of the complex organization of society, there is little that can be done about them.

While it is true that social differentials in health have been observed widely, wherever they have been sought, the magnitude of the differentials, i.e. the slope of the gradient, is not fixed. It varies over time and place. Analyses confirm a widening differential in mortality between manual and non-manual groups for every region in Britain (Marmot and McDowall, 1986). Similarly, in Finland there has been a widening gap in mortality across social groups (Valkonen et al., 1990).

The data in Figure 7.3 show that the relation between social deprivation and mortality varies across regions within England. The slope of the relation appears to be somewhat shallower in East Anglia, for example. Further, at equivalent levels of deprivation on the Townsend score there are regional differences in mortality. This may result from the measures having different 'meaning' in different parts of the country. In other words, a given score may not indicate equal levels of deprivation in different geographical regions. These are, after all, indicators. A second interpretation is that the relation between deprivation and mortality actually varies in different geographical areas. There may be other factors determining geographical differences in mortality.

If socioeconomic gradients in health change over relatively short periods of time, and are different in different countries and geographical settings, such gradients need not be inevitable. If the gradients vary there must be reasons why. Better understanding of the reasons may form the basis of action to alleviate them.

SOCIAL DETERMINANTS OF INTERNATIONAL DIFFERENCES

Comparison of disease patterns on a global scale leads to the obvious conclusion that social, economic and cultural forces are primary in determining the major differences in infant mortality, life expectancy and disease patterns that exist around the world. When informed that life expectancy at birth in 1992 in Guinea-Bissau and Afghanistan is 43 years, whereas life expectancy in Japan is 78.6 years, we have little difficulty in speculating that this fact may be related to the economic fortunes of the different countries. In fact the real gross domestic product per capita (expressed in purchasing power parities) is $19,400 in Japan and $700–$750 in Guinea-Bissau and Afghanistan (United Nations Development Programme, 1994).

Although poverty, expressed as real income, is a major reason for these huge international differences in health status, there is no simple link between GDP and life expectancy. This is illustrated in Table 7.2, from the Human Development Report published by the United Nations Development Programme (1994). The report uses a Human Development Index which combines real GDP, life expectancy and education. It then ranks countries from 1 (Canada) to 173 (Guinea) on this index. Table 7.2 shows some exceptions to the link between income and life expectancy, for three groups of countries, within which the countries have similar levels of GNP. Guinea and Sri Lanka have similar levels of income per

Table 7.2   *Similar income, different Human Development Index, 1991–92*

Country	GNP per capita (US$)	HDP rank	Life expectancy (years)	Adult literacy (%)	Infant mortality (per 1,000 live births)
GNP per capita around $400 to $500					
Sri Lanka	500	90	71.2	89	24
Nicaragua	400	106	65.4	78	53
Pakistan	400	132	58.3	36	99
Guinea	500	173	43.9	27	135
GNP per capita around $1,000 to $1,100					
Ecuador	1,010	74	66.2	87	58
Jordan	1,060	98	67.3	82	37
El Salvador	1,090	112	65.2	75	46
Congo	1,040	123	51.7	59	83
GNP per capita around $2,300 to $2,600					
Chile	2,360	38	71.9	94	17
Malaysia	2,520	57	70.4	80	14
South Africa	2,540	93	62.2	80	53
Iraq	2,550	100	65.7	63	59

Human Development Index, a composite measure of life expectancy, education and income as purchasing power parities (United Nations Development Programme, 1994).

capita, but life expectancy in Guinea is 43.9 years and in Sri Lanka 71.2. As the table shows, within the income band, the higher the adult literacy rate the longer the life expectancy. There is a similar finding within each of the other two income bands.

The general conclusion from this example is that social factors are likely to exert a strong influence on life expectancy. Level of education is a powerful predictor in addition to income. Caldwell speculated that countries such as Sri Lanka which achieve long life expectancies in spite of low incomes have certain features in common. These include 'a substantial degree of female autonomy, a dedication to education, an open political system, a largely civilian society without a rigid class structure, a history of egalitarianism and radicalism, and of national consensus' (Caldwell, 1986). As a test of these notions, he showed that countries whose infant mortality was lower than would have been predicted from their GNP had a high female proportion at school.

Similarly, Hobcraft showed, in 25 developing countries, that mother's education shows a linear relation to survival chances (Hobcraft, 1993). Figure 7.4 shows the association between maternal education and child survival, adjusted for paternal occupation as well as paternal education and region. Similarly, the relation between paternal occupation and child survival is adjusted for the other variables. Adjustment attenuates the relation of father's occupation quite markedly. The odds ratio in the most favoured category is changed from 0.56 to 0.84. By contrast adjustment

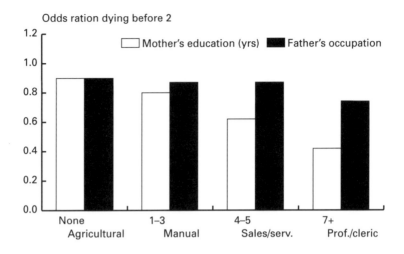

Figure 7.4   *Adjusted odds ratios of dying before 2 years of age, according to mother's education and father's occupation in 25 developing countries. Each parent's ratio is adjusted for the other's, plus father's education and region (Hobcraft, 1993)*

changes the odds ratio in the most favoured maternal education category only from 0.42 to 0.52. One interpretation of these data is that they support the direct causal link with mother's education. Possible explanations include: a shift in familial power structures permitting the educated woman to exert greater control over health choices; increased ability to manipulate the modern world; and a shift from fatalistic acceptance of health outcomes towards implementation of health knowledge (Hobcraft, 1993). There needs, however, to be a caveat. Maternal education may simply be a more precise and more quantitative ranking of social position than father's occupation and occupational status. Greater measurement precision alone could account for the 'better performance' of maternal education in multivariate models.

Up to a level of GNP of about $5,000 per capita, there is a tight relation between income and life expectancy (World Bank, 1993). Above that level of income the relation with life expectancy is shallow. Wilkinson shows that the relation is much tighter with income inequalities (Wilkinson, 1992).

The general point to emerge from Wilkinson's work is that social and economic influences on health are not confined to developing countries, nor are they encapsulated by measures of mean income alone. Similarly, the message from the work of Caldwell (1986), Hobcraft (1993) and the Human Development Report (United Nations Development Programme, 1994) suggests that other factors related to social organization are crucially important.

FRAMEWORK FOR EXPLAINING SOCIAL AND ECONOMIC DISEASE PATTERNS

The landmark Black Report posed four classes of explanation for inequalities in health: artefact, selection, culture and behaviour, and material conditions (Blane, 1985). Research since the Black Report makes it clear that the first two explanations are unlikely (Goldblatt, 1990; Power et al., 1991). Other factors are important (Marmot et al., 1995a).

Dahlgren and Whitehead have produced a general framework of the determinants of health, reproduced here as Figure 7.5. Much of research and policy to improve health focuses on biological factors in the inner-most circle, or individual lifestyle factors in circle 4. This is perhaps a natural extension, both of the clinical approach to disease and of the revolution in biological understanding. The first emphasizes the primacy of the individual patient; the second the molecular and biochemical basis of pathogenesis. Research into prevention has, to a large extent, focused on individual risk factors for disease. These, in general, have resided in the inner two circles, i.e. individual biological characteristics or lifestyle factors. Approaches to prevention have tended to follow this research by emphasizing the manipulation of individual risks.

Diet, smoking, alcohol, physical activity or risk-taking sexual and other behaviours as part of 'lifestyle' are of undoubted importance in the aetiology of the major causes of morbidity and mortality. We accept the importance of these lifestyle factors but then ask two types of

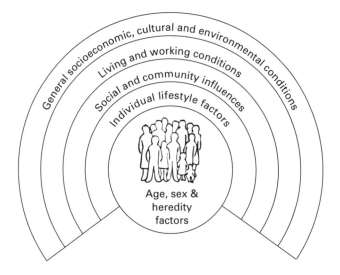

Figure 7.5   *Factors influencing health (Dahlgren and Whitehead, 1991)*

question. To what extent are they influenced by social, cultural and economic factors? Are there other psychosocial pathways that influence health?

POLICY IMPLICATIONS

A framework that emphasizes the social determinants of health has important implications for health policy. To a large extent in political discussion health policy is usually equivalent to policies for the organization and funding of medical services. All societies spend a large proportion of their resources on medical care. It is therefore appropriate to have vigorous debate and research as to the extent to which it is meeting society's needs. It is not appropriate for the health debate to stop there. The framework emphasized here suggests that policies for health should focus on the wider inputs to health. Such inputs are beyond the sphere of influence of health departments and need to involve a variety of agencies, departments and settings both public and private.

REFERENCES

Blane, D. (1985) 'An assessment of the Black Report's explanation of health inequalities', *Sociology of Health and Illness*, 7: 421–45.

Brunner, E.J., Marmot, M.G., White, I.R., O'Brien, J.R., Etherington, M.D., Slavin, B.M., Kearney, E.M. and Davey Smith, G. (1993) 'Gender and employment grade differences in blood cholesterol, apolipoproteins and haemostatic factors in the Whitehall II study', *Atherosclerosis*, 102: 195–207.

Caldwell, J.C. (1986) 'Routes to low mortality in poor countries', *Population and Development Review*, 2: 171–220.

Dahlgren, G. and Whitehead, M. (1991) 'Tackling inequalities: a review of policy initiatives', in M. Benzeval, K. Judge and M. Whitehead (eds), *Tackling Inequalities in Health: an Agenda for Action*. London: Kings Fund Institute.

Eames, M., Ben-Shlomo, Y. and Marmot, M.G. (1993) 'Social deprivation and premature mortality: regional comparison across England', *British Medical Journal*, 307: 1097–102.

Erikson, R. and Goldthorpe, J.H. (1992) *The Constant Flux*. Oxford: Clarendon.

Fox, A.J. and Goldblatt, P. (1982) *Socio-demographic Mortality Differentials*. OPCS Longitudinal Study 1. London: HMSO.

Goldblatt, P. (1990) 'Mortality and alternative social classifications', in P. Goldblatt (ed.), *Longitudinal Study: Mortality and Social Organisation*. London: HMSO.

Hobcraft, J. (1993) 'Women's education, child welfare and child survival: a review of the evidence', *Health Transition Review*, 3 (2): 159–75.

Joseph Rowntree Foundation (1995) *Inquiry into Income and Wealth*. York: Joseph Rowntree Foundation.

McCord, C. (1990) 'Excess mortality in Harlem', *New England Journal of Medicine*, 322: 173–7.

Marmot, M.G. (1992) 'Coronary heart disease: rise and fall of a modern epidemic', in M.G. Marmot and P. Elliott (eds), *Coronary Heart Disease Epidemiology.* Oxford: Oxford University Press.

Marmot, M.G. and McDowall, M.E. (1986) 'Mortality decline and widening social inequalities', *The Lancet*, 1: 274–6.

Marmot, M.G., Syme, S.L. and Kagan, A. (1975) 'Epidemiologic studies of CHD and stroke in Japanese men living in Japan, Hawaii and California: prevalence of coronary and hypertensive heart disease and associated risk factors', *American Journal of Epidemiology*, 102: 514–25.

Marmot, M.G., Adelstein, A.M. and Bulusu, L. (1984b) 'Lessons from the study of immigrant mortality', *The Lancet*, 1: 1455–8.

Marmot, M.G., Smith, G.D., Stansfeld. S., Patel, C., North, F., Head, J., White, I., Brunner, E. and Feeney, A. (1991) 'Health inequalities among British civil servants: the Whitehall II study', *The Lancet*, 337: 1387–93.

Marmot, M.G., North, F., Feeney, A. and Head, J. (1993) 'Alcohol consumption and sickness absence: from the Whitehall II study', *Addiction*, 88: 369–82.

Marmot, M.G., Bobak, M. and Davey Smith, G. (1995a) 'Explanations for social inequalities in health', in B. Amick, S. Levine, A. Tarlov and D. Walsh (eds), *Society and Health* Oxford: Oxford University Press. 172–210.

Marmot, M.G., Ryff, C.D., Bumpass, L., Shipley, M. and Marks, N. (1997) 'Explanations for social inequalities in health: next questions and converging evidence', *Social Science and Medicine*, 44: 901–90.

Marmot, M.G., Head, J.A. and Swerdlow, A.J. (2000) 'Socio-economic circumstances and trends in immigrant mortality'.

North, F., Syme, S.L., Feeney, A., Head, J., Shipley, M.J. and Marmot, M.G. (1993) 'Explaining socio-economic differences in sickness absence: the Whitehall II study', *British Medical Journal*, 306: 361–6.

Office of Population Censuses and Surveys (1978) *Occupational Mortality 1970–72.* London: HMSO.

Pappas, G., Queen, S., Hadden, W. and Fisher, G. (1993) 'The increasing disparity in mortality between socio-economic groups in the United States. 1960 and 1986', *New England Journal of Medicine*, 329: 103–9.

Pilgrim, J.A., Stansfeld, S.A. and Marmot, M.G. (1992) 'Low blood pressure, low mood?', *British Medical Journal*, 304: 75–8.

Power, C., Manor, O. and Fox, J. (1991) *Health and Class: the Early Years.* London: Chapman & Hall.

Roberts, R., Brunner, E., White, I. and Marmot, M. (1993) 'Gender differences in occupational mobility and structure of employment in the British civil service', *Social Science and Medicine*, 37: 1415–25.

Stansfeld, S.A. and Marmot, M.G. (1992a) 'Deriving a survey measure of social support: the reliability and validity of the Close Persons Questionnaire', *Social Science and Medicine*, 35: 1027–35.

Stansfeld, S.A. and Marmot, M.G. (1992b) 'Social class and minor psychiatric disorder in British civil servants: a validated screening survey using the General Health Questionnaire', *Psychological Medicine*, 22: 739–49.

Stansfeld, S.A., Davey Smith, G. and Marmot, M.G. (1993) 'Association between physical and psychological morbidity in the Whitehall II study', *Journal of Psychosomatic Research*, 37: 227–38.

Stansfeld, S.A., Feeney, A., Head, J., Canner, R., North, F. and Marmot, M.G. (1995) 'Sickness absence for psychiatric illness', *Social Science and Medicine*, 40: 189–97.

Syme, S.L., Marmot, M.G., Kagan, H. and Rhoads, G. (1975) 'Epidemiologic studies of CHD and stroke in Japanese men living in Japan, Hawaii and California', *American Journal of Epidemiology*, 102: 477–80.

Townsend, P., Phillimore, P. and Beattie, A. (1988) *Health and Deprivation: Inequality in the North*. London: Croom Helm.

United Nations Development Programme (1994) *Human Development Report 1994*. New York: Oxford University Press.

Valkonen, T., Martelin, T. and Rimpela, A. (1990) *Socio-economic Mortality Differences in Finland 1971–85*. Helsinki: Central Statistical Office in Finland.

Wilkinson, R.G. (1986) 'Socio-economic differences in mortality: interpreting the data on their size and trends', in R.G. Wilkinson (ed.), *Class and Health*. London: Tavistock.

Wilkinson, R.G. (1992) 'Income distribution and life expectancy', *British Medical Journal*, 304: 165–8.

World Bank (1993) *World Development Report 1993*. New York: Oxford University Press.

World Bank (1994) *World Development Report 1994*. New York: Oxford University Press.

8

Social Status, Inequality and Health

Richard G. Wilkinson

RELATIVE INCOME

The driving force behind health inequalities in developed societies is not absolute differences in living standards, but relative differences. Once countries have gone through the epidemiological transition, and the infectious diseases associated with absolute poverty have given way to the degenerative diseases as the main causes of death, further increases in the standard of living have only weak effects on average standards of health (Wilkinson, 1994, 1996). Whether you look at cross-sectional evidence or at changes over 20–30 years, no more than 10 or 15 per cent of the differences in life expectancy between developed countries are related to differences in their material living standards. One country's economy can grow twice as fast as another's for 25 years without necessarily having larger improvements in life expectancy.

Differnces in absolute income between developed societies have probably ceased to be powerful determinants of health. Perhaps advantages in some areas are offset by deteriorations – like the decline in exercise and the rise in obesity – in others. In contrast, however, *within* each country there are close relationships between health and individual income – or almost any other measures of social and economic circumstances. This is the relationship which we have come to know as the phenomenon of 'health inequalities'. This paradox is resolved if we accept that once we have reached the threshold standard of living marked by the epidemiological transition, then health is affected primarily by relative standards. Essentially, income differences within countries are closely related to differences in health because they map on to differences in social status, whereas income differences between countries have little significance for social status and so have little impact on health. What counts is not improving your absolute material circumstances regardless of others, but where you stand in relation to others.

First published in HEA seminars, *Inequalities in Health*, London: Health Education Authority, 1999, pp. 33–46.

INCOME DISTRIBUTION

The strong association between income distribution and population mortality rates confirms the importance to health of social relativities. Greater equality seems to be good for health. There are now some 20 different research reports to this effect – a proportion of which were 'independent' discoveries of the relationship in the sense that they came from people who appeared unaware of the rest of the literature. The hypothesis that greater equity is associated with better health has now been explicitly tested several times on data completely independent of the data used in all earlier reports (Kennedy et al., 1996). Most recently Lynch and colleagues reported that inequality is not merely predictive of mortality rates among the 50 states of the United States, but also among the 282 Standard Metropolitan Areas (Lynch et al., 1998).

SOCIAL COHESION

Before going into the likely mechanisms involved in this relationship, we should note that more egalitarian societies tend to be more socially cohesive than less egalitarian ones. In his well-known study of the strength of 'civic community' in the regions of Italy, Putnam notes that his index of people's involvement in local community life is highly correlated with income distribution ($r = 0.81$) – more equality, more cohesion (Putnam et al., 1993). On the basis of his surveys, and talking more about an egalitarian social ethos rather than about income inequality, Putnam said: 'Citizens in more civic regions, like their leaders, have a pervasive distaste for hierarchical authority patterns' (1993: 104); 'Political leaders in the civic regions are more enthusiastic supporters of political equality than their counterparts in less civic regions' (p. 102). His interviews with local political leaders and samples of local people led him to conclude that 'Equality is an essential feature of the civic community' (p. 105).

Qualitative evidence from a number of other examples also suggests that societies which are unusually egalitarian and unusually healthy tend to be highly cohesive. Life expectancy increased unusually rapidly in Britain during the decades which include the First and Second World Wars. The well-known sense of camaraderie was based partly on a sense of unity in the face of a common enemy but, on top of that, income distribution narrowed dramatically and the government pursued policies on taxes and subsidies designed to make the burden of war seem equally shared.

PSYCHOSOCIAL PATHWAYS

How then are mortality rates linked, if indeed they are, to relative income and greater equality, and to the increased social cohesion which seems to go with narrower income differences?

First, the epidemiology of health inequalities points increasingly to the power of psychosocial factors rather than to the direct effects of exposure to toxic aspects of the material environment. The work on sense of control, job insecurity, social relations, life events and childhood emotional precursors of poor health is impressive. To take just a few recent examples: observational studies have shown two-, three- and even fourfold differences in mortality associated with high and low levels of social integration (House et al., 1988; Berkman, 1995). Experiments have shown that when people are given nasal drops containing cold viruses, those with friendships in fewer areas of life are four times as likely to develop colds as people with friendships in more areas (Cohen et al., 1997). A study of atherosclerosis over a period of four years in almost 1,000 men found it built up faster among men who experienced a sense of hopelessness (Everson et al., 1997).

Not only are these big effects, but if we add to that the fact that larger proportions of the population are exposed to these psychosocial risk factors than to some of the harmful material exposures, we can see that their 'population attributable risk' makes them very powerful determinants of population health.

The power of psychosocial factors is now finding firmer foundations in the rapidly growing understanding of the physiological pathways through which they can affect physical health (Chrousos et al., 1995; Lovallo, 1997; Martin, 1997). At centre stage seems to be the concept of chronic stress.

As well as their direct health impact on neuroendocrine and immunologic function, psychosocial stresses will also increase exposure to behavioural risk factors. Part of our inability to stop smoking, to avoid our tendency to eat for comfort, or to indulge in a range of other health-damaging behaviours must be related to whether we feel in control of our lives and feel happy and successful. It is difficult to keep to resolutions about changing behaviour and living without props when we feel depressed and inadequate (Marsh and McKay, 1994; ASH, 1993; Skrabski and Kopp, 1996).

DIRECT EFFECTS OF SOCIAL STATUS

The sources of stress associated with low social status can be divided into two categories. The first includes things like unemployment, bad housing and financial insecurity, which are usually associated with low social status but are not inherent in it. The second includes forms of stress, such as feelings of inferiority or inadequacy, shame, humiliation, etc. which are closer to the essence of low social status. Our rather asocial understanding of human beings has meant that we got to grips with the health effects of the first category well before we recognized the second. But the work on the physiological effects of social status among non-human primates encourages us to place more emphasis on the second category.

Descended from species with strong social ranking systems which had fundamental implications for welfare and reproductive success, we are likely to be pre-programmed to be particularly attentive to issues of hierarchy and to experience them as having a particular psychic charge. The implications for access to resources and reproductive success would have selected individuals who found low social status aversive in itself. Similarly, part of the importance of friendship may be a reflection of the defensive importance of alliances, particularly in a social hierarchy. Maintaining good social relations has probably always been crucial to welfare. Unlike members of other species which may compete with us for food, our fellow human beings can be the most deadly source of competition – for food, clothes, housing, jobs and sexual partners. But if we get the relationships right, other members of our own species can also be the most important source of support, comfort, love, learning and socialization.

HOMICIDE

The distribution of homicide and violent crime provides an unexpectedly powerful indication of how directly stressful low social status can be and of how closely this may be related to the increased incidence of other causes of death lower down the social hierarchy. In order to explore what it was about social cohesion that seemed to be associated with narrower income differences and low mortality rates, Kawachi, Kennedy and I decided to look at how rates of different kinds of crime fitted into the relationship between income distribution and mortality among the 50 US states.

In the event, we found that violent crime, but not property crime, was much more common in the areas with high income inequality and high mortality rates (Wilkinson et al., 1998). The homicide rate was closely correlated with income inequality ($r = 0.74$) and with all non-homicide mortality ($r = 0.70$). Not only that, but the variance in homicide almost exactly fitted the covariance of income distribution and other causes of death. These relationships were confirmed by the correlations with other categories of violent crime.

The implication seems to be that the social milieu which produces homicide is also the social milieu which produces high death rates from other causes.

So what kind of social environment, linking income inequality to mortality, produces high homicide rates? Remarkably it seems to hinge directly on problems of social status. A brief glance at some of the literature on the causes of violence shows a very strong emphasis on people thinking that others do not respect them.

SOCIAL COMPARISON – DEPRESSION AND VIOLENCE

Social comparison is surely the medium through which issues of respect and inequality (or Adam Smith's 'regard') might be expected to have an impact on us. Oliver James (1997) uses the concept of social comparison to explain the main features of a growing social malaise common to many developed countries. A number of developed societies have seen a long-term increase in rates of depression, violence, suicide and drug use, particularly among young people (Rutter and Smith, 1995). The central concept evoked by James to explain these trends is not income distribution (which has only widened for part of the period since 1950 in which he is interested), but *social comparison*. He suggests that the last half-century has seen a dramatic increase in the frequency with which we make social comparisons. Children in primary school are ranked by test scores, people worry about whether they are fatter than the ideal, we compare our meagre abilities and achievements with those of the media personalities and stars, we worry about whether we are as interesting, intelligent, or as funny as our friends, and we not only compare our career progress and material success with others, but we facilitate the comparisons by adopting an extraordinarily one-dimensional view of what counts as career progress and success. In one field after another we rate ourselves against impossible standards, see our shortcomings and experience ourselves as failures. James suggests that the rise in depression and violence is a result of increasing stimuli to make invidious social comparisons. Clearly social comparison is close to the heart of what gives inequality its psychic charge.

Part of the burden of both depression and violence in society should perhaps be seen as alternative responses to low social status and invidious social comparisons – violence can be seen as a way of contesting inferiority while depression may represent an acceptance of it and of a sense of failure. (Given the different consequences of low social status for reproductive success in males and females in hierarchical species such as baboons, the fact that men are more likely to be violent and women more likely to be depressed may seem to make some evolutionary sense.) But even more important in the present context, is that both serve as indicators of the inherently stressful nature of low social status itself.

INCOME DISTRIBUTION, DIGNITY AND BELONGING

When thinking about policy in this field we should think about it on two levels. One is reducing the objective scale of inequality and the other is to make sure our institutions make people feel valued and appreciated. The correlations between measures of social cohesion and income distribution suggest that between a half and two-thirds of the regional or state differences in cohesion are ascribable to differences in income distribution alone. Reducing the objective extent of inequalities is therefore a first priority for anyone interested in health or social cohesion.

When thinking about how we can reduce the insecurities which make us prey to debilitating social comparisons it is useful to bear in mind that social hierarchy is not our only evolutionary legacy. On top of it is something rather different. The hunting and gathering societies which have dominated almost all of the last two million years of human evolution have been described as 'assertively egalitarian' (Woodburn, 1982). Surveys of the literature from over 100 anthropological accounts of some 24 recent hunter and gatherer societies spread over four continents have led to the conclusion that these societies were characterized by 'egalitarianism, cooperation and sharing on a scale unprecedented in primate evolution' (Erdal and Whiten, 1996: 140). 'They share food, not simply with kin or even just with those who reciprocate, but according to need even when food is scarce' (p. 142).

It is intriguing to note that 'equity theory', developed by social psychologists quite independently of any of this evolutionary or anthropological material, suggests that 'When individuals find themselves participating in inequitable relationships, they become distressed. The more inequitable the relationship, the more distressed individuals feel. . . . The exploiter's distress may be labelled "guilt", "shame", "dissonance", "empathy", "conditioned anxiety", or "fear of retaliation". The victim's distress may be labelled "anger", "shame", "humiliation" ' (Austin et al., 1976: 166). Like the counter-dominance view of primitive equity, equity theory rests on the explicit assumption that we are selfish but that members of a group develop equitable systems so that they can 'avoid continual warfare and maximise collective reward' (Walster et al., 1976: 2). As Walster and colleagues note, even as individuals people use a number of methods to try and restore equity. People who feel underpaid by their employer may respond by trying to re-establish equity by wasting time and not working, by doing things which make the employer work harder, or by damaging company equipment.

The psychological legacy from this egalitarian past is our concern for fairness which social psychologists have amply demonstrated and which we are all used to seeing even in very young children. Equity theory was developed as 'a general theory of social interaction' because of the evidence that we intuitively recognize that a sense of fairness and social justice is an almost indispensable component of human social relationships. Feelings of unfairness always create tension and division and can give rise to an extraordinarily charged sense of anguish and distress.

How does this help us define the kind of socially nurturing structures which we should be aiming at? In hunting and gathering societies it seems likely that personal welfare and security were associated with being included in the processes of sharing and material reciprocity which bound people into the social group. The best insurance policy was to be part of the sharing group and system of mutual aid. Perhaps what makes disrespect and low social status so psychically charged is that it signals that one is excluded from, or only marginal to, the sharing group. It contrasts with the sense of self-worth or self-validation which comes from knowing that one's contribution to a common project or to the welfare of others is valued and appreciated. Thus perhaps the greatest damage done by inequality in modern societies takes place when it denies people a sense of self-worth and cuts them off from a role and activity which they know is valued and respected by others. In short, perhaps inequality becomes damaging to health primarily when it becomes great enough to deny people a sense of belonging.

A SOCIAL AUDIT

If we are to reduce the health burden of low social status, we not only need to reduce the objective inequalities in incomes, power and status, but also to make a kind of social audit of how our institutions function in terms of providing people with a sense of value and self-worth. We must avoid practices and treatment which belittle, which stigmatize and humiliate people. Minimum wages and standards of living must be consistent with a sense of personal dignity. We need to think about the social implications of the school regime and teaching methods: whether there are opportunities for all children to feel good at something; whether those who are less good feel humiliated or ridiculed, whether some leave school with the fundamental sense of shame which comes with a failure to achieve basic literacy or numeracy skills. At work we need to ensure that people's contribution is valued and that they feel appreciated and respected as equal human beings, and that the social environment at work is not scarred by unnecessary marks of hierarchy and status distinctions. By giving people a sense of being valued members of their communities, workplaces and schools, family life is more likely to become mutually supportive rather than an arena in which people pass on the external stresses and humiliations to each other.

REFERENCES

ASH: Action on Smoking and Health (1993) *Her Share of Misfortune*. London: ASH.

Austin, W., Walster, E. and Utne, M.K. (1976) 'Equity and the law: the effect of a harmdoer's "suffering in the act" on liking and assigned punishment', in L. Berkowitz and E. Walster (eds), *Advances in Experimental Social Psychology*, vol 9: *Equity Theory: towards a General Theory of Social Interaction*. New York: Academic Press.

Berkman, L.F. (1995) 'The role of social relations in health promotion', *Psychosomatic Research*, 57: 245–54.

Chrousos, G.P., McCarty, R., Pacak, K., Cizza, G., Sternbery, E., Gold, P.W. and Kvetnansky, R. (eds) (1995) in *Stress: Basic Mechanisms and Clinical Implications*. Annals of the New York Academy of Sciences, vol. 771. New York Academy of Sciences.

Cohen, S., Doyle, W.J., Skoner, D.P., Rabin, B.S. and Gwaltney, J.M. (1997) 'Social ties and susceptibility to the common cold', *Journal of the American Medical Association*, 277: 1940–4.

Erdal, D. and Whiten, A. (1996) 'Egalitarianism and Machiavellian intelligence in human evolution', in P. Mellars and K. Gibson (eds), *Modelling the Early Human Mind*. McDonald Institute Monographs. Cambridge: McDonald Institute for Archaeological Research. pp. 139–60.

Everson, S., Kaplan, G., Goldberg, D.E., Salonen, R. and Salonen, J.T. (1997) 'Hopelessness and 4-year progression of carotid atherosclerosis', *Arteriosclerosis, Thrombosis, and Vascular Biology*, 17 (8): 1490–5.

House, J.S., Landis, K.R. and Umberson, D. (1988) 'Social relationships and health', *Science*, 241: 540–5.

James, O. (1997) *Britain on the Couch: a Treatment for the Low Serotonin Society*. London: Random House.

Kennedy, B.P., Kawachi, I. and Prothrow-Stith, D. (1996) 'Income distribution and mortality: cross sectional ecological study of the Robin Hood index in the United States', *British Medical Journal*, 312: 1004–7. See also: Kennedy, B.P., Kawachi, I. and Prothrow-Stith, D. (1996) 'Important correction. Income distribution and mortality: cross sectional ecological study of the Robin Hood index in the United States', *British Medical Journal*, 312: 1194.

Lovallo, W.R. (1997) *Stress and Health: Biological and Psychological Interactions*. London: Sage.

Lynch, J., Kaplan, G.A., Pamuk, E.R., Cohen, R.D., Heck, K.E., Balfour, J.L. and Yen, I.H. (1998) 'Income inequality and mortality in metropolitan areas of the United States', *American Journal of Public Health*, 88: 1074–80.

Marsh, A. and McKay, S. (1994) *Poor Smokers*. London: Policy Studies Institute.

Martin, P. (1997) *The Sickening Mind*. London: HarperCollins.

Putnam, R.D., Leonardi, R. and Nanetti, R.Y. (1993) *Making Democracy Work: Civic Traditions in Modern Italy*. Princeton, NJ: Princeton University Press.

Rutter, M. and Smith, D.J. (1995) *Psychosocial Disorders in Young People: Time Trends and their Causes*. Chichester: Wiley.

Skrabski, A. and Kopp, M.S. (1996) 'Health behaviour, psychiatric symptoms and psychosocial background factors', in J.-P. Dauwalder (ed.), *Psychology and Promotion of Health*. Zürich: Hogrefe & Huber.

Walster, E., Berscheid, E. and Walster, G.W. (1976) 'New directions in equity research', in L. Berkowitz and E. Walster (eds), *Advances in Experimental Social Psychology*, vol. 9: *Equity Theory: towards a General Theory of Social Interaction*. New York: Academic Press.

Wilkinson, R.G. (1994) 'The epidemiological transition: from material scarcity to social disadvantage?' *Daedalus* (journal of the American Academy of Arts and Sciences), 123 (4): 61–77.

Wilkinson, R.G. (1996) *Unhealthy Societies: the Afflictions of Inequality*. London: Routledge.

Wilkinson, R.G., Kawachi, I. and Kennedy, B. (1998) 'Mortality, the social environment, crime and violence', *Sociology of Health and Illness*, 20 (5): 578–97.

Woodburn, J. (1982) 'Egalitarian societies', *Man*, 17: 431–51.

9

Economics and Equity in the Distribution of Scarce Health Care Resources

Stephen Morris

THE EXISTENCE OF SCARCITY IN HEALTH CARE

The fundamental problem that economics attempts to address is that of scarce resources. In the context of health care by 'resources' we mean all the things that are used in the production of health care such as doctors, nurses, professions allied to medicine, medicines, hospital beds, X-ray machines and all the other things that are used to provide health care.

The basic economic problem of scarcity is exceptionally acute in the UK National Health Service (NHS). This is because the need and demand for health care in the UK exceed the resources available to the NHS. In 1998 total health care expenditure in the UK was £52,126 million (Office of Health Economics, 1998). While the amount of money spent on health care is clearly substantial, evidence does exist that health care resources are still in short supply. In the media there are frequently stories reporting a lack of health care resources of some kind and the effects of this on staff and patients, all of which seem to indicate significant underfunding in the NHS and the existence of scarcity. One statistic often used as evidence of scarce resources is the size of treatment waiting lists. The NHS hospital inpatient waiting list in England in recent years is shown in Figure 9.1. This shows, for example, that in 1996 there were as many as 500,000 patients waiting for an inpatient procedure. While this number may have fallen in recent years, clearly it is still very large.

PROBLEMS ARISING FROM SCARCITY IN HEALTH CARE

The existence of scarcity in the health care sector necessarily implies that choices are required in order that limited health care resources are used in a particular way. Because, for instance, there are not enough doctors and nurses, hospitals and hospital beds, the NHS is unable to provide all the health care that ideally we would like, and therefore we must choose between competing uses of resources. Examples of the types of difficult choices faced every day by health care professions because of the problem of scarcity are as follows:

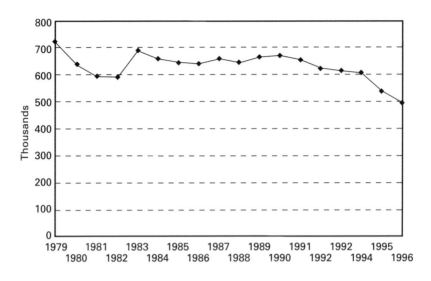

Figure 9.1   *NHS hospital inpaitent waiting lists for England (Office of Health Economics, 1998)*

(a)   Should treatment A be made available to patients? (For example, should Viagra be made available on the NHS?)
(b)   Should method B or method C be adopted for treating this patient? (For example, should simvastatin or fluvastatin be prescribed to patients with raised cholesterol levels?)
(c)   Should patient D be given treatment or patient E? (For example, which patient should receive a hip replacement immediately?)
(d)   Should condition F be treated or condition G? (For example, should tattoo removals be provided in preference to fertility treatment?)

These are examples of common questions raised concerning the allocation of resources. More generally, there are essentially three issues arising from the problem of scarcity in health care:

1   What health care interventions or treatments should be made available?
2   How should these treatments be provided?
3   Who should receive these treatments?

One fundamental question faced by health care decision-makers every day relates to issue 3 above ('Who should receive these treatments?'). Because of the problem of scarcity, individuals may not be able to obtain all the health care that ideally they would like. Therefore, it will be necessary to develop some method for dividing up these limited health care services among all individuals in society. Inevitably this will lead to some discussion of whether this division is a 'fair' one.

Another word for fairness is equity. While people would generally agree that the desire to achieve equity or fairness prevails within any society, what is meant by the word equity will differ between individuals. It is a subjective concept, so what one person thinks of as being a fair way of distributing scarce resources may be quite different from what another person thinks of as being fair.

EQUITY VERSUS EFFICIENCY

One notion commonly used in economics is that of efficiency. Efficiency is often incorrectly interpreted to mean 'cost-cutting'. It is commonly but wrongly argued that something is efficient if it is cheap and only because it is cheap (for example, this is an efficient way of treating patients because it is cheap). This is not what efficiency means. There are a number of possible definitions of efficiency but this is not one of them, as we shall see below. It is also commonly perceived that there is a trade-off between equity and efficiency – in simple terms, that it is not possible for something to be both efficient and fair.

The notion of efficiency is not universally helpful in dealing with the problem of scarcity because there may be many ways of distributing scarce health care resources that are equally efficient. The difficulty is in choosing between them. To choose between them requires some notion of equity or fairness, indicating how we should value the welfare of different members of society relative to each other. One obvious principle to follow could be that everyone should be treated equally. In other words, we may believe a fair allocation of resources to be one where everyone is treated the same. Another view might be that certain members of society should be treated more favourably than others. This raises the question of who those individuals should be.

We shall now discuss different equity principles that could be used to distribute scarce health care resources. We discuss only a few possibilities because the actual number of possibilities is unlimited. Deciding which principle we should adopt is a difficult issue faced by health care decision-makers every day. A key point to remember is that it is important that we have an equity goal that can be used to distribute health care resources. We shall discuss briefly the following notions of equity:

1   Utilitarianism
2   Equality
    2.1.   Equality of health
    2.2.   Equality of expenditure
    2.3.   Equality of use (for equal need)
    2.4.   Equality of access (for equal need)
3   Maximin
4   'Fair innings'

UTILITARIANISM

The basic principle behind utilitarianism is to act in such a manner as to maximize the utility or welfare of society. A policy of strict utilitarianism will ultimately seek to distribute health care so that the greatest good is achieved for the greatest number of individuals. In practical terms this may lead to a situation where relatively low-cost health care programmes which have the potential for benefiting large numbers of people would be provided in preference to high-cost health care programmes which have only a small health benefit for a limited number of individuals.

A policy of utilitarianism may lead to distributions of health care which are considered unsavoury by society because it will inevitably mean that some individuals in society (possibly the most sick) lose out in some way to maximize the welfare of the majority. That is, a few individuals may lose out for the good of the rest of society.

EQUALITY

As mentioned above, one potential principle to follow concerning the distribution of health care could be that everyone should be treated equally. This raises the obvious question, 'In what respect should everyone be treated equally?' We discuss four possibilities below.

Equality of health

Using this definition of equity, the distribution of health care is considered fair if it results in every individual obtaining the same level of health. This does not necessarily mean equality of health across all age and sex groups because this would be biologically impossible. However, within age and sex groups, equality of health means just that: equal or the same health for everyone.

Health is affected by a number of factors, such as diet, lifestyle, education and housing, and not just health care. Indeed, the actual effects of health care may often be quite limited. Therefore these other factors need to be included in any distribution of health care aiming to equalize health. Additionally, within age and gender groups equal health may not be possible because of the state of technology. Some illnesses are currently incurable, so a policy aimed at improving the health of some individuals to bring about equality of health would be unsuccessful.

Equality of expenditure

A distribution of health care that concentrates on equality of expenditure would be relatively easy to achieve, because at its most simple all it would require is that each individual receives the same distribution or quantity of health care.

The health status of individuals differs widely across society, and the incidence of ill health is higher for some individuals than others. Some individuals require more health care than others do. If health care is provided in such a way that expenditure on each individual is equal, then no recognition is given of the differences in the level of needs across society. This may result in a situation where certain health care resources are under-utilized, but where there is a need for them elsewhere.

Equality of use (for equal need)

Another possibility is equality of use. Because of the uneven distribution of illness and therefore the uneven need for health care across individuals in society it would not be sensible to give all individuals equal use of health care services. So this equity goal may be modified to become equal use for equal need. On a practical level this would mean that if two individuals have the same condition that requires the same treatment, then their use or consumption of health care services is the same.

This presupposes that individuals have the same attitudes to health and health care because uptake and compliance with health care services would be equal for individuals with the same health care needs. This ignores the fact that variations occur in preferences for both health and health care. The receipt of health care involves different levels of utility for different individuals (for example, some individuals have a greater fear of dentists than others), yet equal use for equal need as a definition of equity requires that such variations are not taken into account when distributing health care.

Equality of access (for equal need)

Equal access for equal need simply means that individuals are provided with the same opportunity to use needed health care services. This definition of equity has advantages over equality of use for equal need because it may legitimately lead to different patterns of health care utilization arising from different preferences of individuals towards health and health care. What is important is not that individuals with the same need for health care use the same health care services, but rather that they have the same opportunity to use (or the same access to) the same health care services.

In practical terms, equal access may be obtained if the costs incurred by two individuals using a particular health care service are valued the same. The costs involved include travel costs and time costs as well as monetary costs arising directly from health care. As with most possible definitions of equity, equality of access for equal need becomes difficult to achieve within the constraints imposed by scarce resources. Pursuit of equal access to health care for equal need would require, for example,

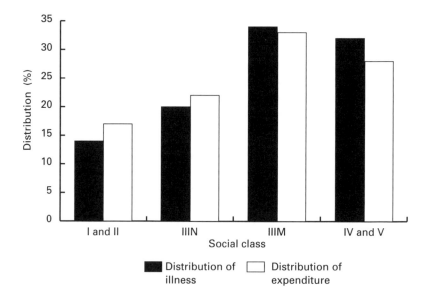

Figure 9.2 *Comparison of the distribution of illness and total health care expenditure by social class (adapted from LeGrand, 1978)*

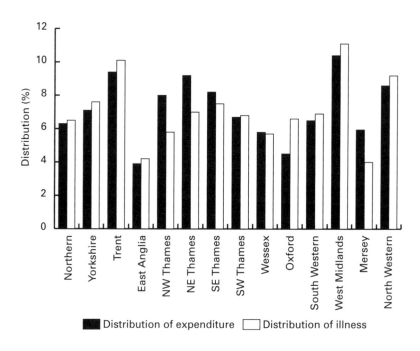

Figure 9.3 *Comparison of the distribution of illness and total health care expenditure by geographical region (Central Statistical Office, 1995; OPCS, 1994)*

expenditure. The figure offers a comparison of the distribution of total health care expenditure and illness in England, by geographical region. This shows considerable variation across geographical region not only of illness, but also of total health care expenditure. Furthermore, it suggests that the unequal distribution of health care expenditure cannot be wholly explained by geographical variation in illness, since there are differences between the proportion of expenditure which a region receives, and the proportion of illness incurred by that region. For example, North West Thames incurs approximately 5 per cent of all illness, yet receives approximately 8 per cent of total health care expenditure.

CONCLUSIONS

Health care professionals every day are faced with painful choices concerning which patients to treat and the best way to treat them, because of the problem of scarcity. One factor that will inevitably be considered when making these decisions is the notion of equity which, simply stated, asks: 'Is this a fair thing to do?' This raises the obvious question, 'What do we mean by equity or fairness?' Clearly this is something on which there may be considerable disagreement across individuals because what one individual thinks of as being fair (for example, 'I think *in vitro* fertilization programmes should be made readily available to everyone who wants them') may be completely different to what another individual thinks of as fair (for example, 'I think *in vitro* fertilization programmes should not be made readily available to everyone because I would rather the money was spent on treating cancer patients').

From a policy perspective what we mean by equity in the distribution of health care resources is a crucial question. It is important to specify precisely what is meant by equity in order to devise appropriate policies for pursuing equity goals. On the basis of the evidence that is available on the allocation of scarce health care resources in the NHS, there is an unequal distribution of health care across social classes, income groups and geographical regions. However, this cannot be accounted for by the distribution of illness, in which there is also considerable variation. Of course, whether or not this is fair depends on our own subjective point of view and this differs across individuals, across populations and across societies.

REFERENCES

Central Statistical Office (1995) *Regional Trends*. London: HMSO.

Le Grand, J. (1978) 'The distribution of public expenditure: the case of health care', *Economica*, 45: 125–42.

Office of Health Economics (1998) *Compendium of Health Statistics*, 10th edition. London: OHE.

OPCS: Office for Population Censuses and Surveys (1994) *General Household Survey 1993*. London: HMSO.

Wagstaff, A., Van Doorslaer, E. and Paci, P. (1991) 'Equity in the finance and delivery of health care: some tentative cross-country comparisons', in A. McGuire, P. Fenn and K. Mayhew (eds), *Providing Health Care: the Economics of Alternative Systems of Finance and Delivery*. Oxford: Oxford University Press.

10

The Politics of Women's Health: Setting a Global Agenda

Lesley Doyal

Health care was a major concern of second-wave feminists in North America, Australia, New Zealand and Europe. However, its political importance has now diminished in many of these countries, along with the decline of grassroots feminism itself. The centre of gravity of women's health politics has shifted to the Third World, where campaigns have become increasingly vigorous in the face of recession, structural adjustment policies and widespread environmental deterioration. Latin America in particular has a very powerful and growing tradition of women's health advocacy, and Asian organizations are also growing rapidly. Campaigners for women's health now represent a significant political reality in many parts of the world, and their voices have grown stronger over the past decade.

As well as spreading to many different countries, the practice of women's health politics is also becoming increasingly international (Kisekka, 1992; Tudiver, 1986). This is in part a response to the multinational nature of many threats to women's well-being – dangerous reproductive technologies for instance, as well as the export of environmental and occupational hazards. However, it also reflects the more general growth of international collaboration in women's politics that followed the 1975–85 UN Decade for the Advancement of Women.

Such activities are never easy since they bring together women with different material interests, desires, commitments, styles of working and frameworks of meaning. But whatever their circumstances, women have always directed their energies toward broadly the same ends. Reproductive self-determination, affordable, effective and humane medical care, satisfaction of basic needs, a safe workplace and physical security continue to be high on all feminist health agendas.

REPRODUCTIVE RIGHTS AND WRONGS

Reproductive rights issues are now central to women's health politics in most parts of the world (Garcia Moreno and Claro, 1994). Historically,

First published in the *International Journal of Health Services*, 26 (1), 1996: 47–65.

most initiatives have consisted of single issue campaigns for birth control. However, these are increasingly located within a broader framework that includes not just the right to prevent conception but also the right to sexual autonomy, to safe motherhood, and to a healthy environment for child rearing (Correa and Petchesky, 1994; Dixon-Mueller, 1993; Gerber Fried, 1990).

Most reproductive health campaigners work at the community level, empowering others through information, advice and care. Broader initiatives are also flourishing, however, as women identify and publicize the deficiencies of many family planning and abortion services, expose the hazards of some medical techniques, and fight for greater participation in reproductive research and development. In recent years many of these campaigning groups have begun to work together in regional and national alliances. The Latin American and Caribbean Women's Health Network co-ordinates many of the activities in that region, working in collaboration with Isis International. A similar network has recently been set up in South and South-East Asia. In Brazil, the National Feminist Network for Health and Reproductive Rights now has nearly 50 member organizations, and co-ordinating groups exist in Argentina, Chile and Colombia (Garcia Moreno and Claro, 1994). A variety of organizations are also working across north–south boundaries.

The volume of campaigning on reproductive issues and the growing links at both national and international levels testify to the vitality of this area of women's health politics. However, this should not be allowed to obscure the very varied interests of the many groups of women involved. Some are primarily concerned with increasing access to birth control. In much of Latin America, for instance, women have been drawn into political action by their inability to obtain safe and effective contraception and by the denial of abortion rights. In many Asian countries, on the other hand, women have been politicized by their experiences of coercive policies that gave them little right to refuse contraception or sterilization.

Significant differences are also evident in debates about strategy. Some women believe that working with government agencies – with 'the state' – or with international family planning organizations can never be an appropriate means to achieve reproductive rights. They argue that only marginal gains will be made and that these may be at the cost of legitimizing existing population policies (Garcia Moreno and Claro, 1994: 26). Others believe that fundamental change is impossible without entering the corridors of power either as workers or campaigners (Broom, 1993; Watson, 1990).

Today millions of women are still without effective means of contraception, and the fight to achieve this continues. It is now clear, however, that access alone is not enough. Women's health advocates have been highly critical of both the safety and the acceptability of many of the most commonly used methods and of the social inequalities embedded in many family planning services. Hence the emphasis in campaigning has now expanded to include not just availability but also safety and quality of care.

But whatever the availability and effectiveness of contraception, women will always need access to safe abortion, both as a back-up and sometimes as a preferred method of birth control. A recognition of this reality is manifest in continuing campaigns for its legalization. In Ireland, the struggle is still hard despite pressure to harmonize with the rest of Europe (Murphy-Lawless, 1993). In Brazil, women's groups managed to prevent the insertion of a foetal protection clause in the 1988 constitution, but the fight for decriminalization continues (Garcia Moreno and Claro, 1994). In Hungary, Romania and Poland women have fought to retain abortion rights threatened as the power of the Catholic Church is revitalized (Fuszara, 1993; Jankowska, 1993), while in former East Germany, campaigners have tried to maintain rights threatened by unification with the West (Funk, 1993). However, it is in the United States that one of the most vigorous campaigns has been fought – first to legalize abortion and then to maintain that gain (Gerber Fried, 1990).

Maternity continues to be a primary cause of morbidity and mortality for women in many parts of the world. Not surprisingly, those most at risk are least likely to have the resources to fight for change, and for generations these deaths were largely invisible. However, a number of international organizations campaigned during the 1980s to get maternal mortality on the agenda, and hundreds of women's groups have now taken up the cause. In 1988 delegates at the Fifth International Women and Health Meeting in Costa Rica launched the Campaign against Maternal Mortality and Morbidity. As part of the Campaign, 28 May was designated International Day of Action for Women's Health, and this has now become an annual focus of activity for many health groups, especially those outside the developed countries. Significantly, this day has also been adopted by WHO, marking an important link between women's health advocates working in very different environments.

Women in many Third World countries have used the campaign to call for access to effective and appropriate obstetric care tailored to meet the circumstances of their lives. For most, this means a close link between maternity services and primary health care as well as the use of traditional methods where appropriate. By this means they hope to get the benefits of modern obstetric techniques without losing what is valuable about culturally specific 'low technology' care (Jordan, 1986). In developed countries, too, maternity campaigners have called for appropriate care, but not surprisingly, the detail of their demands has been very different. Most are concerned not to increase levels of obstetric intervention, but to reduce them.

Some women living in rich countries do lack medical support. This is particularly evident in the United States, where lack of funding often leaves poor mothers deprived of the necessary services (Barbee and

Little, 1993; Ruzek, 1978). However, the major protagonists in the politics of pregnancy have been white middle-class women who can rely on a baseline of effective care for safe delivery but wish to prevent medical intervention exceeding what they regard as reasonable for the health of mother and child.

In Europe, North America and Australia, the consumer movement in maternity care reached its height during the late 1970s and early 1980s (Kitzinger, 1990; Shearer, 1989). Its major themes were increased choice for women and greater control over their own labour. Specific demands included a less clinical birthing environment, the limiting of high-technology interventions to genuine emergencies, and enhanced opportunities for the active participation of fathers. Campaigners pointed out that many of the new obstetric techniques were untested and that others had been shown to be harmful. They also emphasized the inadvisability of care policies that alienated mothers both from the birth process and sometimes from the baby itself.

The global campaign for reproductive rights is a complex and multi-faceted political reality. It takes many different forms but has the common thread of a belief in women's right to determine what happens to their own bodies. Not surprisingly, therefore, reproductive rights activists have often come into conflict with doctors and other health workers who continue to exert considerable control over important parts of their lives. Yet women do need some of what medicine has to offer. The next section explores this contradiction further through outlining the broader feminist critique of medicine.

CHALLENGING MEDICINE

The ease with which women can get health care varies dramatically. It is determined by their individual wealth or poverty and by the scope and cost of services in their local community. Some women are wealthy enough to ensure control over their own health care, but millions continue to experience the effects of professional domination and a denial of their right to participate in important decisions about their own lives (and deaths). As a result they have begun to challenge both the quantity and quality of care available to them and to question the basis upon which medicine itself is currently organized.

In the late 1960s and early 1970s women's health politics in the developed countries focused mainly on self-help and on women's capacity to take care of themselves and each other. Most of these local groups have now disappeared, along with the broader 'consciousness raising' groups characteristic of second-wave feminism. However, many women continue to be involved in more specialized health groups, some of which operate at a national level. The majority of these are mutual support and aid groups organized around the needs of people facing particular challenges. Some are mixed but many are women-only with a focus on gender-specific problems (Hatch and Kickbusch, 1983). As well as providing mutual support and information, many of these groups are also involved in campaigns to ensure that the needs of their members are met more effectively. In the United States the National Women's Health Network now has some 17,000 members, both individuals and organizations. They have worked hard for changes in the US health care system, and the combination of mutual aid and consumerist politics has often been a powerful one.

In some countries women have set up their own health centres. However, the viability of these initiatives has varied markedly, according to the social and economic context in which they have been developed. In Britain, for instance, very few services have been created outside the mainstream. This reflects in part the limited market for private care when it is available in the National Health Service without direct cost. But there is also a political reluctance to offer services that many women could not afford to buy.

All around the world, examples can be found of clinics offering women-centred care to fill gaps in official provision. These are important initiatives offering much-needed services as well as valuable examples of good practice. However, individual projects can never meet the universal need for high-quality health care. Hence women also continue to campaign for changes in the organization, funding and content of mainstream health services. They are seeking improved access and affordability, greater effectiveness in curing diseases or relieving symptoms, and more humanity in caring relationships.

Despite improved access to health services in many parts of the world, there are still major concerns about the effectiveness of much of the treatment available to women. Many are inappropriately diagnosed and treated by the doctors they consult. This is due in part to the lack of scientific evaluation of many medical procedures used on both sexes, but it is exacerbated by gender bias in medical decision-making. These distortions in the production and use of medical knowledge are now being challenged on a number of fronts (Rosser, 1992).

At the heart of all feminist critiques of medicine is the recognition that women lack power in health care institutions. This limits their ability to determine medical priorities or to influence the allocation of scarce resources. It also has a significant impact on their individual experiences as users of health services. It affects their capacity to play an active part in their own treatment and often leaves them feeling uncared for. In some countries, women's complaints about their treatment have led to changes in the education of doctors. However, there are few controls on the quality of the encounter between individual patients and the physicians and surgeons whose skills they need. In order to empower women within this relationship, some campaigners have attempted to

Such actions are often exhausting and terrifying, generating opposition not just from political opponents but from local people who believe that women should stay at home with their families. However, it is clear that they have been important not just in effecting social change but also in beginning to transform the women themselves. It is this potential for psychological and economic empowerment that makes campaigning for basic needs such an important element in the global politics of women's health.

PUTTING VIOLENCE ON THE POLITICAL AGENDA

Every day millions of women continue to be denied their right to physical security, as enshrined in the 1948 Declaration of Human Rights (Bunch and Carillo, 1990). Over the last two decades, campaigns have been waged in a number of countries to make this huge burden of violence visible (Davis, 1994; Dobash and Dobash, 1992; United Nations, 1989). A recent survey by the feminist network Isis documented nearly 400 separate groups fighting violence against women in Latin America alone (Heise, 1993). There have also been many international initiatives, reflecting the global nature of the problem. Largely as a result of pressure from Latin American and Caribbean women, 25 November has been designated International Day of Violence Against Women. Significant gains have been made in many parts of the world, but much remains to be done, especially in those countries where violence is increasing. Growing landlessness and poverty, greater militarism, and a shift toward fundamentalism in religious and social values have all been identified as factors in this intensification.

One of the earliest strategies to deal with the consequences of male violence was the organization of refuges for survivors. The first was set up in England in 1971, and the number there has now grown to over 100. Though the picture is constantly changing, recent estimates suggest that there are now more than 700 in the United States alone (United Nations, 1989: 77). Rape crisis centres, too, have proliferated, offering support and advice to women who have suffered sexual attacks. In Third World countries, both refuge and rape crisis centres spread rapidly during the 1980s. The first women's aid shelter in Malaysia was set up in 1981, and a network of services for female survivors of violence is now being created across Asia and Oceania and in some parts of Africa. In the former socialist states, too, organizations for abused women are beginning to appear for the first time (Siklova and Hradlikova, 1994).

Though the number of refuges is increasing, many are underfunded and dependent on volunteer labour. Only in a few countries has extensive lobbying led governments to take violence against women seriously. In Hong Kong, New Zealand, Japan, Brazil, Papua New Guinea and Malaysia, for instance, women's refuges now receive state funding. In

Australia in particular, the strength of the women's movement led to significant state support as early as 1975. Sexual assault centres and refuges receive funds from the government but are operated independently by women's groups, often affiliated to other voluntary organizations.

As well as providing services for abuse survivors, women have also been involved in campaigns to change those aspects of their social environment that continue to promote violence. Indian women, for instance, have attempted to change the legislation relating to sexual crimes (Gandhi and Shah, 1992 Chapter 3). The first demonstration against the existing rape laws was organized in Delhi on International Women's Day 1980. It was attended by 3,000 women, making it one of the first public affirmations of the need for an autonomous women's movement in India. Groups such as the Forum Against Oppression of Women have worked with other organizations to get changes in the laws relating to dowry death and *sati* (wife burning), and similar campaigns have been organized in Pakistan and in Bangladesh.

In some countries therapy programmes have been developed for persistent batterers, but their effectiveness has yet to be demonstrated. Elsewhere community education strategies have attempted to reach a wider population of both actually and potentially violent men, and those who could help to control them. These programmes have used a variety of strategies to alert the maximum number of people to the reality and unacceptability of violence against women. In Papua New Guinea an impressive campaign has been developed in collaboration with the National Council of Women. It has included village meetings throughout the country as well as direct action by local groups to protect and support battered women. Some success has been reported, with the issue of violence being widely debated. However, the threat to women everywhere remains very great.

CONCLUSION

Millions of women are now engaged both individually and collectively in the fight for better health. They have formulated goals, created strategies, and devised methods appropriate for their own circumstances. Campaigns have been both 'bottom up' and 'top down', and interventions have been made at local, regional and international levels. Women have worked for change both inside and outside medical institutions and formal organizations and have organized themselves in mixed as well as single-sex groups. Some would define themselves as feminist while others would not. No single movement has emerged but all share a common belief in women's right to health. If this goal is to be achieved, its realization must be a central concern not just in feminist politics but in wider campaigns for sustainable development, political freedom, and economic and social justice.

REFERENCES

Braidotti, R. et al. (1994) *Women, the Environment and Sustainable Development: Towards a Theoretical Synthesis*. London: Zed Books.

Broom, D. (1993) *Damned if We Do: Contradictions in Women's Health Care*. Sydney: Allen and Unwin.

Bunch, C. and Carillo, R. (1990) *Gender Violence: A Development and Human Rights Issue*. Dublin: Attic Press.

Barbee, E. and Little, M. (1993) 'Health, social class and African-American women', in S. James and A. Busia (eds), *Theorising Black Feminisms: The Visionary Pragmatism of Black Women*. London: Routledge.

Correa, S. and Petchesky, R. (1994) 'Reproductive and sexual rights: A feminist perspective', in G. Sen et al. (eds), *Population Policies Reconsidered: Health, Empowerment and Rights*. Boston, Mass.: Harvard University Press.

Dankelman, J. and Davidson, I. (1988) *Women and Environment in the Third World: Alliance for the Future*. London: Earthscan.

Davis, M. (1994) *Women and Violence: Realities and Responses Worldwide*. London: Zed Press.

Dixon-Mueller, R. (1993) *Population Policy and Women's Rights: Transforming Reproductive Choice*. Westport, Conn: Praeger.

Dobash, P. and Dobash, R. (1992) *Women, Violence and Social Change*. London: Routledge.

Funk, N. (1993) 'Abortion and German unification', in N. Funk and M. Mueller (eds), *Gender Politics and Post Communism: Reflections from Eastern Europe and the Former Soviet Union*. London: Routledge.

Fuszara, M. (1993) 'Abortion and the formation of the public sphere in Poland', in N. Funk and M. Mueller (eds), *Gender Politics and Post Communism: Reflections from Eastern Europe and the Former Soviet Union*. London: Routledge.

Gahlot, D. (1993) 'A spark of hope for slum dwellers', in Women's Feature Service (ed.), *The Power to Change: Women in the Third World Redefine their Environment*. London: Zed Press.

Gandhi, N. and Shah, S. (1992) *The Issues at Stake: Theory and Practice in the Contemporary Women's Movement*. New Delhi: Kali for Women.

Garcia Moreno, C. and Claro, A. (1994) 'Challenges from the women's health movement: women's rights versus population control', in G. Sen et al. (eds), *Population Policies Reconsidered: Health, Empowerment and Rights*. Cambridge, MA: Harvard University Press.

Gerber Fried, M. (ed.) (1990) *From Abortion to Reproductive Freedom: Transforming a Movement*. Boston: South End Press.

Hatch, S. and Kickbusch, I. (eds) (1983) *Self Help and Health in Europe*. Copenhagen: WHO.

Heise, L. (1993) 'Violence against women: The missing agenda', in M. Koblinsky et al. (eds), *The Health of Women: A Global Perspective*. Boulder, Col.: Westview Press.

Jain, S. (1991) 'Standing up for trees: Women's role in the Chipko movement', in S. Sontheimer (ed.), *Women and the Environment, a Reader: Crisis and Development in the Third World*. London: Earthscan.

Jankowska, H. (1993) 'The reproductive rights campaign in Poland', *Women's Studies International Forum*, 16 (3): 291–6.

Jordan, S. (1986) *Technology Transfer in Obstetrics: Theory and Practice in Developing Countries*, Working Paper 126. Department of Anthropology, Michigan State University.

Kisekka, M. (1992) 'Women's organized health struggles: the challenge to women's associations', in M. Kisekka (ed.), *Women's Health Issues in Nigeria*. Zaria, Nigeria: Tanaza Publishing.

Kitzinger, J. (1990) 'Strategies of the early childbirth movement: A case study of the National Childbirth Trust', in J. Garcia et al. (eds), *The Politics of Maternity Care Services for Childbearing Women in Twentieth Century Britain*. Oxford: Clarendon Press.

Moser, C. (1989) 'Gender planning in the third world', *World Dev*, 17: 11.

Moser, C. and Peake, L. (eds) (1987) *Women, Human Settlements and Housing*. London: Tavistock.

Murphy-Lawless, J. (1993) 'Fertility, bodies and politics: The Irish Case', *Reproductive Health Matters*, 2: 53–64.

Rodda, A. (1991) *Women and the Environment*. London: Zed Books.

Rosser, S. (1992) 'Re-visioning clinical research: Gender and the ethics of experimental design', in J. Holmes and L. Purdy (eds), *Feminist Perspectives in Medical Ethics*. Bloomington: Indiana University Press.

Ruzek, S. (1978) *Women's Health Movement: Feminist Alternatives to Medical Control*. New York: Praeger.

Shearer, H. (1989) 'Maternity patients' movements in the United States 1826–1985', in I. Chalmers et al. (eds), *Effective Care in Pregnancy and Childbirth*. Oxford: Clarendon Press

Shiva, V. (1989) *Staying Alive: Women, Ecology and Development*. London: Zed Books.

Sontheimer, S. (1991) *Women and the Environment, a Reader: Crisis and Development in the Third World*. London: Earthscan.

Siklova, J. and Hradlikova, J. (1994) 'Women and violence in post-communist Czechoslovakia', in M. Davis (ed.), *Women and Violence: Responses and Realities Worldwide*. London: Zed Press.

Tudiver, S. (1986) 'The strength of links: international women's health networks in the eighties', in K. McDonnell (ed.), *Adverse Effects: Women and the Pharmaceutical Industry*. Penang, Malaysia: International Organization of Consumer Unions.

United Nations. (1989) *Violence against Women in the Family*. Vienna: Centre for Social Development and Humanitarian Affairs.

Watson, S. (ed) (1990) *Playing the State*. London: Verso.

PART III

PUBLIC HEALTH ISSUES

This part explores many of the issues surrounding the development of the 'New Public Health' and some of the problems and opportunities that become apparent when health and health policy expands into almost all areas of living.

Fran Baum (Chapter 11: 'Healthy Public Policy') lays out the agenda for the 'New Public Health'. Explicitly the all-inclusive nature of the concept is outlined when 'Healthy public policy covers a broad range of activities in most sectors of society and aims to alter the socioeconomic and physical environments in which we live.' Under the banner of public health, every policy and every decision will henceforth be scrutinized for its potential to affect the health of those within its field of influence. Shrugging aside the possible criticism that the new advances might represent 'health imperialism', Baum details the overtly political nature of the task of healthy public policy. Health is firmly within the political arena where issues of power and influence are as important to analyse as health outcomes. The balance between individual and community rights and responsibilities is summed up: '– an effective new public health relies on policies that *do* [our emphasis] restrict the freedom of individuals, but which can be justified in terms of the gains in health status in the population as a whole'.

Anthony J. McMichael (Chapter 12: 'Rethinking Environment and Health') 'widens the gaze' of health policy makers and analysts when considering the effects of human-made toxic contaminants, mass urbanization and global climatic change. All these features, and many more, have the ability to fundamentally affect the health of the population of the world, mostly in an adverse way. The call for policy changes that could halt the catalogue of potential adverse health effects which follow the human manipulation of 'the stratosphere, the troposphere, the forests, the soils, the oceans and the world biotic repertoire', is not the plea of an isolated eco-freak, but a considered opinion drawn from a mass of epidemiological evidence. Most importantly, sustainability arguments are set out, and the case made that previous gains in health and increased life expectancy have almost certainly been derived from processes which have eroded the planet's 'natural capital'.

Attempting to come to grips with the increasingly global nature of health is the daunting task undertaken by Gill Walt (Chapter 13:

'Globalization of International Health'). There can be no doubt that recent changes in international relationships and structural reordering of nation states has had an effect on the health of all the world's population. But are these recent changes bringing about positive effects, or are they causing harm? and what organizational changes within health-related organizations might be required to maximize any of the potential benefits and reduce harm? Walt opens the debate on these issues and describes some of the ways that multinational organizations, such as the World Bank and the World Trade Organization, have become increasingly involved in global health issues. Broadly, she concludes that the effects of globalization have probably been to *increase* health inequalities, both within countries and between countries. Furthermore, international organizations will have to make substantial changes to the way they organize their activities to have any impact on these adverse health effects.

Measuring and attempting to quantify some of these effects at a number of levels is the subject of Alex Scott-Samuel's contribution (Chapter 14: 'Health Impact Assessment'). Scott-Samuel sets out the ways in which Health Impact Assessment (HIA) can be used to try to determine the health impact of any policy, programme or even small-scale projects. In undertaking this task he stresses the importance of stating the explicit values on which the assessment is made. These assessments are not value free, but reflect the values of those undertaking the work and those, presumably, of the commissioning agencies. 'HIA should openly declare its values – and social, material and environmental equity should feature strongly among them. This is because public policy impacts disproportionately on the already disadvantaged.' Similarly the *process* of undertaking HIA is important and he advocates the use of 'participatory methods which fully involve those affected by public policy at every stage of the assessment, and openness of all stages of the HIA process to public scrutiny'.

Linda Jones and Adrian Davis (Chapter 15: 'Young People, Transport and Environmental Risk: Perceptions and Responses') examine one specific area of public policy – transport – and in particular its impact on young people's health and well-being. These authors note that while parents manage risk by creating barriers to their children's independent mobility, the young people themselves deal with environmental risk (scary places, spaces and people) by 'constructing safety'. This research calls for health educators and policy-makers to respond to the needs of young people by 'creating safe places to go outside the home' and to help by transforming their 'local areas into safer more accessible environments'.

François Matarasso (Chapter 16: 'The Health and Social Impact of Participation in the Arts') examines the way in which arts initiatives have been used to address socioeconomic problems. He discusses the evaluation of the possible health outcomes of such projects. Exploring policy concerns at this apparently micro-level is important because, for each of us, health is such an individual feature of our lives. Matarasso sets about the task of evaluating the artistic and cultural inputs into the lives of individuals and communities. Particularly focusing on cultural work in deprived areas, he found that this sort of expressive input has helped people as individuals in their personal growth, that it has contributed to social cohesion, assisted in creative planning for deprived areas, brought about elements of real social change as part of a community develop-ment strategy and delivered real socioeconomic benefits for people and for whole communities.

Janet A. Butler (Chapter 17: 'Prevention May Be More Expensive Than Cure') looks at another shibboleth of public health policy and attempts to examine some of the complexity around the issues of preventing illness and maintaining health. All organized health care systems spend sig-nificantly more on treating illness than in maintaining the health of people under their care. This has led to the popular claim that, for example, the British National *Health* Service (NHS) is in fact an illness service. Butler examines some of the economic effects of switching resources from curative service towards prevention, and helps us con-sider some of the factors that should be taken into account when determining resource allocation policy within the health service. The final chapter in this part examines public health research policy as it relates to the study of ethnicity and health. Raj Bhopal (Chapter 18: 'Is Research into Ethnicity and Health Racist, Unsound, or Important Sci-ence?') takes a disparaging view of much of the 'research' that has gone on in the past on this important issue, which he labels, 'unethical, invalid, racist and inhumane'. Unfortunately current practice, in his opinion, is in danger of not learning from the mistakes of the past. He details a series of recommendations which can help to make ethnicity a sound epidemiological variable and positively assist in the planning of health services.

11

Healthy Public Policy

Fran Baum

Healthy public policy is characterised by an explicit concern for health and equity in all areas of policy and by accountability for health impact. The main aim of healthy public policy is to create a supportive environment to enable people to lead healthy lives (World Health Organization, 1988)

Healthy public policy covers a broad range of activities in most sectors of society, and aims to alter the socioeconomic and physical environments in which we live, and ultimately to affect individual behaviours so that quality of life, well-being and health are enhanced. It is distinct from health policy, which is concerned with those policies that determine the financing and operation of sickness care services (Brown, 1992).

Pederson and Edwards (1988) note that healthy public policy seems to have been plagued by both conceptual ambiguity and terminology. They suggest the following definition: 'public policy for health using health in the broadest, ecological sense'. It is difficult to imagine policy areas that do not have implications for health. Their view of healthy public policy recognizes the complex factors that affect health and illness, and the complex relationships between different sectors in society. Draper (1991) defined six features of healthy public policy:

- Public health issues are invariably multisectoral and involve a range of interest groups. For instance, attempts to control drink-driving involve the police, hospital emergency departments, alcohol producers and retailers, schools and workplaces.
- Healthy public policy should involve commerce and industry, voluntary organizations, the community and all three tiers of government.
- Increasingly, risks to public health are international and not confined within regional or national boundaries. This is particularly true of environmental problems.
- The aim should be 'educational and persuasive rather than dictatorial or puritanical' (Draper, 1991: 18) and should aim to 'make the healthy choices the easy choices'. However, health legislation may be necessary in some circumstances.

First published in *The New Public Health: an Australian Perspective*. Oxford: Oxford University Press, 1998, pp. 364–85.

- Action for healthy public policy takes many forms, through formally organized lobby groups or the actions of local community health initiatives.
- Healthy public policy is an intrinsically political activity.

Some commentators have suggested that the broad aims of healthy public policy smack of health imperialism and may end up irritating other sectors who do not see health as a legitimate player in their policy environment. In response to this concern, Pederson and Edwards (1988: 6) suggest that 'the objective of healthy public policy is not to make health the only goal of public policy but to put health higher on the political agenda'.

POLICY FORMULATION

'Policy' is a nebulous term, used in many different contexts from general references to the foreign policy of a country to the particular policies of an organization. It has been defined as 'a set of principles guiding action towards predetermined ends' (Titmus, 1974). The simplicity of this definition is appealing, and it makes clear that policy should lead to action. Inevitably, creating policy is complex, and can take years or decades. Legge and Butler (1995) suggest that policy should be viewed as a narrative that provides guidelines for co-ordinated action across sectors and institutions. They state:

> The policy narrative tells of a set of problems and contextual issues; it tells of a world in which these problems could be resolved or ameliorated and it tells of actions that people will take that will lead to changes (or avoid changes) and that in doing so will help to create the better situation envisaged. (Legge et al., 1995: 7)

This fits well with Walt's (1994) assessment of policy as involving the decision to act on a particular problem, but as also including subsequent decisions on implementation and enforcement. She points out that a government's decision not to do something may represent policy, so policy 'must include what governments say they will do, what they actually do, and what they decide not to do' (Walt, 1994: 41).

Phases in policy-making

Policy-making usually involves a series of phases, such as this framework offered by Walt (1994: 45):

- **problem identification and issue recognition**: analysis asking which issues do and do not get on the policy agenda, and why;
- **policy formulation**: determining who formulates policy and how, and where the initiatives come from;

- **policy implementation**: asking how policies are implemented, what resources are available, and how implementation is enforced;
- **policy evaluation**: asking how the policy is monitored, whether it achieves its objectives, and if it has unintended outcomes.

It would be very rare for policy stages to follow such a rational or ordered linear process in reality. Policy-making and implementation are usually more iterative, subjective, and are affected by the social environment. Walt (1994) quotes Leichter's (1979) ordering of the factors that influence policy into four areas:

- **situational factors** that are transient, changing and possibly idiosyncratic, and which depend on local conditions or circumstances;
- **structural factors** that are the relatively stable elements of society and its political system;
- **cultural factors** that are the various value systems evident in a community;
- **environmental factors** that are events, structures and values lying outside the boundaries of a policy decision-making environment, but which influence decisions within it.

Approaches to policy formulation

Most literature on policy formulation identifies three main approaches:

Rational-deductive start with a problem and work through to its solution in a rational and linear way. The approach has its origins in the early part of the twentieth century when modernism held that scientific approaches and technology would lead to rational policy-making. The approach has been described as involving policy-makers in:

> identifying the goals or objectives that should govern the choice of solutions to the problems, and in undertaking a comprehensive analysis of all possible alternatives and their consequences. On this basis, a solution is chosen as a master plan for maximising the objectives chosen. (Wiseman, quoted in Ziglio, 1987)

The main features of this approach are its rationality, following a logical sequence to arrive at decisions and making use of as much information as possible. Policy-making tries as far as possible to follow a deductive approach to decision-making, which is akin to the traditional scientific method.

Incremental an opportunistic approach which recognizes that all implications are never known at the outset and so there is a constant need to reflect and amend. Lindblom (1959) characterized the approach as 'muddling through'. Policy decisions are never the definitive option but the ones that make sense at a particular point in time. Policies need to be adapted to suit new or changed circumstances. The approach relies heavily on the judgements of key players and reflects a pluralistic society in which there are multiple influences. Interest groups play a key role in shaping and reshaping the policy environment. Ziglio (1987) points out that incremental policy-making will tend to be reactive and likely to reinforce the status quo, rather than lead to innovation and change.

Mixed-scanning This aims to combine the best features of the previous two. It is based on the understanding that the rational-deductive approach does not pay sufficient attention to the politics and values of any policy environment and that the incremental approach tends to be overly reactive. The main proponent of mixed-scanning is Etzioni (1967), who suggested that an overall scan of the policy environment is useful to identify those decisions that can be taken incrementally and those which are strategic. For the latter, information should be gathered and analysed in a way that takes into account the value and political issues. By doing this, policy-makers are able to retain a long-term vision and respond to immediate issues that require policy amendment. Hancock (1992) suggested that in the new public health, planning requires 'goal directed muddling through'. This sits well with the mixed-scanning approach. After reviewing the three models, Ziglio (1987) recommends a mixed-scanning approach for healthy public policy.

Policies and power

Milio (1983) defined the public policy environment in which policies for health come about. Key players are politicians, bureaucrats, media representatives and interest groups, and the process involves struggles between groups to ensure their desired policy ends are achieved in preference to those put forward by other groups. Inevitably, policy formulation is entangled with issues of power and influence. Different groups have different amounts of power and influence with which they can influence policy decisions.

   Analysis of power is complex. Political science has presented an increasingly sophisticated understanding of how it operates in pluralist societies. Lukes (1974) pointed out that power does not just involve one person or group persuading another to act in a particular way, but also influencing the actual wants and desires of another person or group. People's views may be manipulated by those possessing power in such a way that their judgement about their real interests may become clouded. Foucault (1984) has also pointed out how power in modern societies is exercised through numerous interactions in everyday life. Medical knowledge, in particular, was seen as being very powerful in affecting people's behaviour. Bachrach and Baratz (1970) argue that 'non-decision' making can also influence policy processes. People with power may manipulate the decision-making process so that certain issues are not even raised. In Australia, it could, for instance, be argued that the power of parts of the medical profession and the private health insurance industry operate to ensure that the concept of an exclusively public health insurance scheme is not canvassed.

These perspectives on power make it imperative for policy analysts to go beyond obvious conflicts (or agreements) in any situation to determine how it is being manipulated. In analysing policy it is crucial to ask whose interests will be served or threatened by a policy change and their power to affect the policy formulation process. An equally important question is to consider involved groups that have no power or influence to affect policy. The move towards more consultative processes in bureaucracies was partly motivated by a desire to introduce less powerful voices.

PUBLIC HEALTH ADVOCACY

One of the most important ways of influencing policy is advocacy. Chapman (1994: 6) notes that public health advocacy is used 'most often to refer to the process of overcoming major structural (as opposed to individual or behavioural) barriers to public health goals'. Broad public acceptance of public health policy can result from lobbying through the media and other avenues at the local, state, national or international level (see Box 11.1). Advocacy has seen an alliance between public health practitioners and activists in the growing consumer movement.

Box 11.1: Examples of public health advocacy

- A group of brain surgeons who lobby for safer road design with the aim of preventing brain injury.
- Local residents who work together to persuade their local council to reduce the speed limit and implement traffic calming measures to make their suburb safer for pedestrians.
- The international movement against buying products from the Nestlé company in protest against their marketing of breast milk substitutes in developing countries.
- A group of local residents lobbying against the diversion of a polluted river to their coastal suburb because of the marine pollution and environmental degradation.
- International Physicians Against Nuclear War.

Advocacy strategies

Successful strategies should set an agenda, frame the issue for public consumption and advocate specific solutions. Wallack et al. (1993) suggest that public health advocates can catalyse public opinion, bolster the public's willingness to support the proposed solution and gain access to key opinion leaders and community decision-makers. The campaign against Nestle's promotion of their product as preferable to breast milk is an example of successful advocacy (Wallack et al., 1993). The problem of declining breastfeeding in Third World countries was initially seen as the failure of the mothers, until Infant Formula Coalition Action (INFACT) used strategies such as a boycott of Nestle's products, a CBS documentary and lobbying of the WHO to adopt the International Code of Marketing Breast Milk Substitutes.

Strategies used by advocates are as varied as the imagination of activists. The BUGAUP (Billboard Utilizing Graffitists Against Unhealthy Promotions) campaign in the 1980s organized its members to change the message of advertising billboards in a humorous way (for instance, changing 'Welcome to Marlborough Country' to 'Welcome to Cancer Country'). The organization's members were often arrested during their activities, which led to free publicity, especially when medical practitioners were in the group (Egger et al., 1993).

Media advocacy

Media advocacy has become an increasingly important public health activity because of the influence of mass print and electronic media. According to Walt (1994: 66) mass media serve a number of functions in contemporary society:

- as agents of socialization by transmitting society's culture, values and norms;
- as sources of information;
- as propaganda mechanisms in that they seek to persuade people to support particular policies or buy consumer goods;
- as agents of legitimacy for the dominant political and economic institutions.

Maibach and Holtgrave (1995: 226) define media advocacy as the strategic use of the mass media to advance a social or public policy initiative. Wallack et al. (1993) suggest that media advocacy addresses power gaps between powerful and less powerful groups in society. They see advocacy as a public health strategy quite different in focus to the use of mass media to persuade individuals to change their behaviours. Instead, it can reshape public agendas so that, instead of public health issues being continually individualized (Tesh, 1988), the underlying structural and environmental issues can be highlighted. Advocacy becomes a powerful tool of the new public health:

> Advocacy is necessary to steer public attention away from disease as a personal problem to health as a social issue, and the mass media are an invaluable tool in this process. Advocacy is a strategy for blending science and

politics with a social justice value orientation to make the system work better, particularly for those with least resources. (Wallack et al., 1993: 5)

Public health advocates often work against lobbyists from business interests with far more resources and access to powerful media and influential decision-makers. Tobacco companies have long employed lobbyists to persuade politicians and the public that the dangers of tobacco have not been proven beyond doubt.

The communications and information revolution

There was a revolution in communication and information technologies and capabilities in the 1990s. New technologies such as the world wide web, internet, computer bulletin boards, on-line information databases and distance learning technologies have speeded up access to information and communication around the globe. Computer-based information technologies may play an important role in increasing the information available to advocacy groups in the future. The implications for public health advocacy are considerable.

The potential of the internet as an advocacy mechanism was demonstrated recently by a concerted campaign by non-government organizations around the world against the Multilateral Agreement on Investment (MAI). These groups used web sites to publicize the details of the proposed MAI and analyses of its likely impact. The internet was used to maintain communication between NGOs around the world and to spread the latest details of the negotiations. These techniques enabled protest groups to pool their information so that 'they have broken through the wall of secrecy that traditionally surrounds international negotiations, forcing governments to deal with their complaints' (Drohan, 1998). The immediacy of internet communication offers considerable benefits to advocacy and protest groups.

Information is crucial to public health, and gathering it can now be done far quicker than before, as the electronic networks enable public health practitioners to communicate more easily. They also encourage community participation in public health, as groups have easier access to information about any public health topic, but this obviously depends on their access to the new technology. The equity with which it is available determines the equity with which it can be used.

Food and nutrition policies as an example of healthy public policy

Food and nutrition are basic elements of human survival, and policies to influence them are crucial aspects of public health. Globally, food and nutrition present a paradox in that the rich countries suffer from problems of excess food consumption and poor countries often from insufficient food. We examine food and nutrition policy issues in developed countries, and then look at malnutrition.

Food and nutrition policies in rich countries Australia, like other rich countries, has dietary patterns that contribute to a high prevalence of chronic disease. Diet has been implicated in the aetiology of cardio-vascular disease, obesity, a number of cancers and diabetes. In recent years, food safety has re-emerged as a significant policy issue. Mad cow disease in the UK and outbreaks of salmonella in a number of Australian states have increased interest in policies relating to food and nutrition that are relevant for local, state and Commonwealth governments.

Local government is required by legislation to perform regulatory functions relating to food production and retailing. The existence of legislation to regulate food production, consumption and retail prices reflects developments from the nineteenth century onwards. Most local food and nutrition policies relate to ensuring the maintenance of food safety standards, but some local policies go further to promote health and strive for equity. One of the most comprehensive initiatives reported is the Knoxville (Tennessee, USA) Food Policy Council (See Box 11.2).

Box 11.2: Knoxville (Tennessee, USA) Food Policy Council

The Food Policy Council was established by the local city council and was jointly responsible to the mayor, city council and people. It represented people with existing public roles, those working in the food business and people active in neighbourhood and consumer issues. The aim of the Food Council was to:

- ensure that an adequate and nutritious food supply is equally available to all citizens
- strengthen the economic viability of the private food industry
- improve the quality of food available to all citizens
- encourage citizens to accept and consume nutritious food (Petrey, 1990: 76).

The Food Policy Council had no formal powers but sought to influence policies in a wide range of areas. It provided a forum for discussion and problem-solving of food-related issues and acted as an advocate. It was able to work with officials from a broad range of sectors. The changes the Council was reported to have brought about included the introduction of a breakfast programme, changing bus routes to provide better access to food purchasing for low-income residents, ensuring the Metropolitan Planning Commission identified food distribution facilities and considered the location of food stores in its planning, lobbying for policy changes to improve food access for low-income people (such as the removal of sales tax from food), the local transport company developing a grocery bus with racks to hold bags of groceries that would carry groups of people between their neighbourhood and a quality food store.

(*Source:* Petry, 1990)

Milio (1989) has contrasted two approaches to policies in this area: the Norwegian interventionist, comprehensive public policy and the USA *laissez-faire*, market-oriented strategy. Norway has had a Food and Nutrition Policy since 1975 and so provides one of the few opportunities to evaluate the effectiveness of such policies. The three goals of the policy were to (Milio, 1989: 417):

- promote a healthy national diet, reducing fat consumption to 35 per cent (from 42 per cent) of food energy, by reducing pork, vegetable and other fats – except butter and milk; changing the P/S ration to 0.5 (from 0.3), increasing fibre, fresh produce, fish and low fat foods and decreasing sugar and sodium;
- promote domestic food production and consumption, especially in outlying, disadvantaged regions and reduce dependence on food imports to 48 per cent (from 61 per cent) of total national food energy supplies, giving priority to grains;
- contribute to world food security through international grain reserves and Third World farm and food production aid and trade.

Overall, Milio determines that the Food and Nutrition Policy made significant progress towards its goals. The food self-sufficiency goals were met and exceeded in some cases. Norway, through the 1970s and 1980s, made a significant contribution to world food security, particularly given the size of the country. Evaluation of the dietary objectives showed a more complex picture with some improvements but a continued high intake of saturated fats. There were declines in cardiovascular deaths, but these could also be linked to stringent smoking control. Nevertheless, Norwegian death rates from cardiovascular disease were more favourable than those from other Nordic countries that had not had comparable nutrition policies. Milio's analysis of the USA's market-driven approach to food and nutrition was not as favourable. She found the food and nutrition policies to 'be piecemeal, influenced by political and commercial interests, and consequently inconsistent, tending to neutralise or confound support for healthy nutritional patterns' (1989: 420). Market interests took precedence over those of health. The effects of the absence of national policies were particularly clear in terms of equity. In the 1980s disparities grew between rich and poor in diet-related low-birthweight babies and infant mortality, dietary risk factors and diet-related disease and deaths (Milio, 1989: 420). Overall, Milio concludes that the 'invisible hand' of the market is less effective than public policy in promoting healthy food choices for a population.

Food and nutrition policy formulation and implementation in all settings demonstrate the importance of competing interests and agendas on policy. The food and agriculture industry is extremely powerful and dominated by multinational companies who have at their disposal powerful advertising mechanisms and access to governments, because of

their ability to affect national economic issues. Inevitably there are conflicts between the interests of these companies in maximizing their profits
and in contributing to national goals for healthy diets. Policy formulation
and implementation are generally done in an environment in which the
voices of these industries are clearly heard. Governments, including
successive Australian ones, seek to make partnerships with industry
when dealing with policy. Grossman and Webb (1991: 276) recognize the
necessity of this in a pluralistic society, but also offer this warning:

> It is true that the industry is a power to be tapped, especially as health
> promotion grows out of its past concentration on education of the population
> into a more politically aware, structural phase. Nevertheless, what must be
> remembered in working with the food industry is that on many topics there is
> a straightforward conflict of interest between those of us who are (broadly
> speaking) working for the population as a whole and those who are paid to
> represent corporate interests. The syllogism which says that the public health
> lobby, once committed to intersectoral action, must court the food industry at
> all costs is foolish: it encourages the worst sort of appeasement.

Public health interests must be continually alert to the dangers of co-
option by interests whose primary concerns are other than health. Such
considerations ensure that healthy public policy will remain complex,
challenging and far more of an art than a science.

WHAT MAKES FOR HEALTHY PUBLIC POLICY?

The processes needed for the successful adoption of healthy public
policies are:

- an issue over which there is clear evidence about adverse effects on
  health;
- effective lobby groups in favour of policy and legislation to control
  the source of the adverse effects on health;
- winning of support for policy and legislation change from key
  opinion leaders, including the media and politicians, in spite of
  opposition from groups which favour the status quo;
- supportive bureaucratic players in key positions;
- a policy environment that supports government intervention to
  change social and economic structures in order to promote health.

An effective new public health relies on policies that do restrict the
freedom of individuals, but which can be justified in terms of the gains in
health status in the population as a whole. The extent to which the power
of policy and legislation can continue to be harnessed to improve health
depends on the acceptance of restrictions on the freedoms of individuals.
The likelihood of such restrictions being acceptable is increased when
community values are seen as a crucial component of a healthy society.

REFERENCES

Bachrach, P. and Baratz, M.S. (1970) *Power and Poverty: Theory and Practice.* Oxford: Oxford University Press.

Brown, L.R. (1992) 'Launching the environmental revolution', in L. Starke (ed.), *State of the World.* New York: W.W. Norton. pp. 174–246.

Chapman, S. (1994) 'What is public health advocacy?' in S. Chapman and D. Lupton (eds), *The Fight for Public Health.* London: BMJ Publishing Group.

Draper, P. (ed.) (1991) *Health Through Public Policy.* London: Green Print.

Drohan, M. (1998) 'How the net killed the MAI. Grassroots used their own globalization to derail deal', *The Globe and Mail,* 29 April.

Egger, G., Spark, R. and Donovan, R. (1993) *Health and the Media.* Sydney: McGraw-Hill.

Etzioni, A. (1967) 'Mixed-scanning: a third approach to decision-making', *Public Administrative Review,* 27: 385–92.

Foucault, M. (1984) 'Space knowledge and power', in P. Rabinow (ed.), *The Foucault Reader: an Introduction to Foucault's Thought.* New York: Pantheon Books.

Grossman, J. and Webb, K. (1991) 'Local food and nutrition policy', *Australian Journal of Public Health,* 15 (4): 271–6.

Hancock, T. (1992) 'The healthy city: utopias and realities', in J. Ashton, *Healthy Cities.* Buckingham: Open University Press. pp. 22–9.

Legge, D. and Butler, P. (1995) *Policies for a Healthy Australia.* Canberra: Commonwealth Department of Human Services and Health.

Leichter, H.M. (1979) *A Comparative Approach to Policy Analysis: Health Care Policy in Four Nations.* Cambridge: Cambridge University Press.

Lindblom, C.E. (1959) 'The science of muddling through', *Public Administration Review,* 19: 79–88.

Lukes, S. (1974) *Power: A Radical View.* London: Macmillan.

Maibach, E. and Holtgrave, D.R. (1995) 'Advances in public health communication', *Annual Review of Public Health,* 16: 219–38.

Milio, N. (1983) *Promoting Health Through Public Policy.* Philadelphia: F.A. Davis.

Milio, N. (1989) 'Nutrition and health: patterns and policy perspectives in food-rich countries', *Social Science and Medicine,* 29 (3): 413–23.

Pederson, A.P. and Edwards, R.K. (1988) *Co-ordinating Healthy Public Policy: An Analytic Literature Review and Bibliography.* Toronto: Department of Behavioural Science, University of Toronto.

Petrey, D.L. (1990) 'The Knoxville Food Policy Council: a case study', in A. Evers and W. Farrant (eds), *Healthy Public Policy at the Local Level.* Frankfurt am Main: Campus Verlag. pp. 67–82.

Tesh, S. (1988). *Hidden Arguments: Political Ideology and Disease Prevention Policy.* New Brunswick: Rutgers University Press.

Titmus, R. (1974) *Social Policy: an Introduction.* London: Allen and Unwin.

Wallack, L., Dorfman, L., Jernigan, D. and Themba, M. (1993) *Media Advocacy and Public Health: Power for Prevention.* Newbury Park, CA: Sage.

Walt, G. (1994) *Health Policy: An Introduction to Process and Power.* London and New Jersey: Zed Books.

World Health Organization (1988) *Healthy Public Policy Adelaide Recommendations.* Geneva: WHO.

Ziglio, E. (1987) *Policy Making and Planning in Conditions of Uncertainty: Theoretical Considerations for Health Promotion Policy.* Research Unit in Health and Behavioural Change, University of Edinburgh.

12

Rethinking Environment and Health

Anthony J. McMichael

The scale and complexity of ongoing changes in the world's environment are obliging epidemiologists to rethink the scope and priorities in environmental health. The inherently elastic word 'environment' applies particularly to ambient external exposures that are predominantly involuntary and shared. The two important dimensions to the external environment are: (1) the local physico-chemical and microbiological environment; and (2) the ecological and geophysical infrastructure that sustains life-supporting environmental conditions.

Environmental exposures can be differentiated on another axis, occurring as either natural or human-made phenomena. Natural environmental influences include: seasonal and latitudinal variations in solar ultraviolet irradiation, extremes of weather, locally resident infectious agents, physical disasters, and local micronutrient deficiencies that reflect soil composition. For example, almost one-fifth of the world population lives on ancient, leached, and often mountainous soils where they are at consequent risk of dietary iodine deficiency (Hetzel, 1994). Likewise, there are pockets of high-risk exposure to selenium deficiency in China (causing Keshan disease of the heart muscle in young adults and Kashin-Beck disease of bones and joints in older persons); and of soil-and-water arsenic exposure (causing skin lesions, cardiovascular disorders and cancers) in southwest Taiwan, the Obuasi region of Ghana, and West Bengal (Appleton et al., 1996; Mazumder et al., 1998).

The distinction between natural and human-made can be fuzzy. Gopalan, for example, describes several situations in India where natural environmental, nutritional health hazards have, in recent decades, been made unexpectedly better or worse by human intervention in the wider environment (Gopalan, 1999). Those interventions have disturbed geochemical processes in soil and water, causing altered human ingestion of certain metals and trace elements. Both pellagra (tryptophan deficiency) and lathyrism (exposure to neurotoxin in lathyrus seeds) were alleviated in the 1980s by basic, social/economic-driven changes in India's production and market price of alternative cereal grains. Wheat and, to a lesser

First published as 'From hazard to habitat: rethinking environment and health', in *Epidemiology and Society*, 10 (4), July 1999: pp. 460–464 extent, rice substantially displaced pulses and jowar. Meanwhile, goitre and intellectual stunting due to iodine deficiency and skeletal fluorosis both increased their geographic range – the former because both the spread of irrigation and expanded sugar-cane production depleted soil iodine levels; the latter because the use of dams and tubewells resulted in mineral disturbances within surface and subterranean drinking water composition, leading to increased fluoride content or increased bio-activity of water fluoride.

Our pre-eminent 'environmental' concern as epidemiologists, how-ever, has been with overt human-made hazards in the ambient environ-ment. In industrialized countries the focus has been on chemical contaminants entering the air, water, soil and food and various physical hazards such as ionizing and non-ionizing radiation, urban noise and road trauma. In less developed countries, the persisting environmental concerns are with the microbiological quality of drinking water and food, the physical safety of housing and work, indoor air pollution, and hazardous local roadways. Environmental epidemiologists have thus mostly concentrated on estimating risks attributable to locally generated exposures that cause direct toxicity, injury or infection, such as the relations between ionizing radiation and leukaemia, blood lead concentration and child IQ, and tropospheric ozone levels and attacks of asthma.

Today we are beginning to embrace a broader view of 'environment'. This emerging shift in our conceptualization of the population–environment–health relation reflects a new awareness of the working of the 'earth system' and its component ecosystems, and of how long-term population health depends upon the integrity of those systems (Last, 1998; McMichael, 1993). The important recent insights include:

1   Recognition of the pervasive and cumulative consequences of many human-made toxic environmental contaminants that accumulate in the world's environment. Various persistent semi-volatile organic chemicals (such as PCBs, DDT and toxaphene) undergo a type of global distillation that redistributes them from low latitudes to high latitudes, where they finally condense out from the atmosphere at heightened concentrations and enter the human food chain (World Resource Institute, 1998). Certain organic chemical pollutants appear to have endocrine-disrupting effects in wildlife and perhaps in humans (Sharpe and Skakkebaek, 1993). Others impair immune system functioning or impede intellectual development in children (World Resource Institute, 1998).

2   Awareness of how worldwide mass urbanization is affecting environ-mental quality, social relations, consumer culture, microbial 'traffic' and, therefore, human well-being and health. In particular, we under-stand better the complex ecological influences upon infectious disease patterns (Wilson, 1995).

3   Awareness of the potential health impacts of global environmental changes. The best known are climate change and stratospheric ozone depletion. Other signs of planetary overload include a widespread loss of biodiversity (Pimm et al., 1995), an apparent recent plateauing in the productivity of our main terrestrial and marine food-producing ecosystems (Doos, 1994; FAO, 1995), and regional depletion of fresh water (Watson et al., 1998).

HISTORICAL CHANGES IN OUR PERCEPTION OF ENVIRONMENT AND HEALTH

Historians discern several distinct stages in Western society's relationships to nature. During much of the seventeenth and eighteenth centuries, disease was deemed to arise from nature as God's judgement on the human condition. The wages of sin were disease. Then, in the wake of the Enlightenment and the rise of more humane and egalitarian social ideologies in the early nineteenth century, the view emerged that populations were affected by their social and physical environment. There was much talk of miasmas (foul emanations arising from decay and putrefaction), especially within urban environments. After the crisis of urban-industrial blight and increased mortality in the 1830s in Britain, the sanitary idea emerged and became, temporarily, linked with ideas of urban sustainability including ideas of recycling sewage, maintaining fertile adjoining soils, attaining local self-sufficiency in food production, and achieving full employment. This new belief in the possibilities for enlightened collective action and for the general technocratic management of nature challenged the inherent selfishness of the *laissez-faire* ideology of the age.

From around mid-nineteenth century, however, 'environmental health' increasingly became an analytic form of knowledge pursued by biomedical scientists. Statistics were collected on exposures, disease and deaths, and public authorities were urged to engineer particular offending places to reduce the risks to health. The rise of bacteriology in the 1880s caused further divergence from the earlier ecological perspective. Microbes were deemed a ubiquitous cause of disease. This germ theory, along with the new theories of cell biology and of heredity, new concern over micronutrient deficiencies, and the medicalization of childbearing and child rearing, all refocused the health sciences on the individual. Ideas of shared environmental exposures and their risks to health receded.

In the latter third of the twentieth century, we became aware of pervasive forms of biologically damaging environmental contamination. Rachel Carson radically changed our perceptions, contemplating a *Silent Spring* induced by ecologically damaging pesticides. Then we became aware of acid rain, and, later, of how cumulative exposures to various families of environmental contaminants could disrupt the workings of the immune system, the reproductive system and the neurological system. These were harbingers of today's systems-oriented concerns about environmental change and population health.

We now see that humankind is causing various new and unprecedentedly large-scale environmental changes to the stratosphere, the troposphere, the forests, the soils, the oceans, and the world's biotic repertoire (McMichael, 1993). These changes reflect the impact of population increase and escalating levels of material consumption. In the twentieth century global economic activity increased twentyfold and the human population has, in absolute terms, been growing faster than ever, achieving a remarkable fourfold increase from around 1.5 to 6 billion in the last century. Consideration of how global environmental change does, or in the future may, affect human health expands how we think about environmental influences on human population health. The world around us is much more than a repository of potential environmental hazards; it is also our habitat.

POTENTIAL HEALTH CONSEQUENCES OF GLOBAL ENVIRONMENTAL CHANGE

Climate change provides an instructive example of how a global environmental change can influence health risks in populations around the world. The anticipated health effects of climate change encompass direct and indirect, immediate and delayed effects (McMichael and Haines, 1997). While some health outcomes in some populations would be beneficial (for example, some tropical regions may become too hot for mosquitoes or other disease vector organisms, or winter cold-snaps may become milder in temperate zones), the available evidence and reason indicate that most health effects would be adverse. Long-term changes in background climatic conditions would alter the functioning of various biophysical and ecological systems that naturally stabilize and underpin human population health.

The anticipated direct effects include altered mortality and morbidity from a change in exposure to thermal extremes (for example heat waves), the physical hazards of an altered pattern of storms, floods and droughts, and, perhaps, the respiratory health consequences of increased exposure to photochemical pollutants and aeroallergens (spores, moulds, etc.).

Indirect health effects would include alterations in the range and intensity of vector-borne infectious diseases (for example malaria, dengue fever, leishmaniasis, tick-borne encephalitis, and Lyme disease). Predictive mathematical modelling has shown that the geographic zone and seasonality of potential transmission of malaria, and of dengue fever, might increase in many parts of the world (Intergovernmental Panel, 1996; McMichael and Haines, 1997). The increase of about 0.4°C in average world temperature since the 1970s, thought likely to be an early manifestation of anthropogenic climate change (Intergovernmental Panel, 1996), may have contributed to the ascent of malaria, dengue fever, or their mosquito vectors to higher altitudes on all continents (Epstein et al., 1998).

Other indirect effects would include altered transmission of person-to-person infections (especially summer-season food poisoning and water-borne pathogens); the nutritional health consequences of regional declines in agricultural productivity in poorly resourced populations, especially in South Asia, northern Africa and Central America; and the various physical, microbiological and psychological health consequences of rising sea levels and population displacement.

In the 1950s, René Dubos indicated that technological innovation, whether industrial, agricultural or medical, disrupted natural ecological balances and unleashed infectious diseases (Dubos, 1959). Subsequently, forest clearance has exposed rural populations in countries around the world to new infective organisms, such as the several haemorrhagic fever viruses now widely encountered in rural Latin America (Morse, 1993). Continued over-fishing of oceans will reduce per capita supplies of seafood, unless the formidable ecological problems with aquaculture are overcome. Further production pressure on vulnerable agroecosystems will increase undernutrition in food-insecure regions, and will exacerbate rural-to-urban migration and the attendant health risks faced by slum dwellers. These sorts of problems have afflicted human societies before, but in localized and occasional fashion. Today they are becoming global and concurrent (Watson et al., 1998).

THE GLOBAL PHENOMENON OF 'NEW AND RESURGING' INFECTIOUS DISEASES

Infectious diseases receded in Western countries throughout the latter nineteenth and most of the twentieth centuries. The receding tide may have turned within the last quarter of the twentieth century, however. An unusually large number of new or newly discovered infectious diseases have been recorded in the past 25 years, including rotavirus, cryptosporidiosis, legionellosis, the Ebola virus, Lyme disease, hepatitis C, HIV/AIDS, Hantavirus pulmonary syndrome, *Escherichia coli* 0157, cholera 0139, toxic shock syndrome (staphylococcal), and others (Heymann and Rodier, 1997; Morse, 1995).

This apparent increase in the spectrum and incidence of infectious diseases most probably reflects the rapid changes in human ecology and environmental impact in today's globalizing world (McMichael et al., 1999; Wilson, 1995). Populations everywhere are becoming interconnected economically, culturally and physically, enhancing the mixing of people, animals and microbes from all geographical areas. Human mobility has escalated dramatically, in volume and speed, between and

within countries. Long-distance trade facilitates the geographical redis-
tribution of pests and pathogens, well illustrated in recent years by the
HIV pandemic, the worldwide dispersal of rat-borne hantaviruses,
the rapid dissemination of a new epidemic strain of bacterial meningitis
along routes of travel and trade, and the cargo ship-borne introduction of
the Asian tiger mosquito, *Aedes albopictus*, a vector for yellow fever
and dengue, into South America, North America, Africa and Europe
(Morse, 1995).

Climate change may foster the spread of cholera via the warming-
induced proliferation of coastal and estuarine aquatic planktonic organisms within which the cholera vibrio naturally shelters and multiplies
(Colwell, 1996). Environmental changes, in some settings, reduce the
risks of infectious disease. For example, forest clearance for extension
of agriculture in South-east Asia has been associated with reductions
in malaria transmission because of the destruction of the mosquito
(*Anopheles dirus*) habitat, as also happened with *Anopheles darlingi* in
South America (Gomes et al., 1998; WHO, 1996).

Rapid urbanization is expanding the traditional role of cities as
gateways for infections; new vistas of possibility are thus opened to
otherwise marginal and obscure microbes. This facilitation may have
been critical in the launching of the poorly transmissible HIV/AIDS virus
in the 1980s (Morse, 1995). Meanwhile, infectious disease patterns are
increasingly being affected by the intensification of food production and
processing methods, well illustrated by the meat-borne spread of *E. coli*
0157 and by the ongoing BSE/CJD episode in Britain (McMichael, 1996).

In the late twentieth century the globalization of economic activities
and culture, the escalation of travel and trade, and our increasing use of
intensified food production and processing, other technologies, antibiotics, and various medical procedures are all reshaping the world of
microbial relations. Pathogens live today in a world of changing, mostly
increasing, opportunity.

HEALTH AS A 'SUSTAINABLE STATE'

The prospect of global environmental change affecting human health
into the future raises a radical question about the *sustainability* of
population health. Conventionally, we measure population health cross-
sectionally, in tally-card fashion, as an *achieved* entity. Those tally-card
measures resemble our conventional assessment of society's economic
performance: we measure the accrued wealth and achieved output, not
the sustainability of economic activity.

To conclude that things must actually be getting better since life
expectancies are increasing may be to misunderstand this sustainability
dimension. In nature, gains in population size and life expectancy
tend to happen when the immediate carrying capacity (supply) of the

environment exceeds the number of dependent individuals (demand). Correspondingly, recent gains in human life expectancy indicate that, in an immediate sense, the life-supporting capacity of the human-modulated environment has been increasing. But at what cost, and at what future risk?

These gains in health and longevity in the twentieth century have depended primarily on reductions in early-life deaths from infectious disease. Basic gains in food security and in sanitation, supplemented by advances in vaccination, antibiotic treatment and oral rehydration therapy, have changed the profile of infectious disease mortality. These and other more recent life-lengthening technical and social improvements have been closely bound up with the processes of urbanization, industrialization and increasing material wealth. They, and the resultant gains in life expectancy, have therefore proceeded in parallel with the increasing levels of depletion and contamination of our ambient environment. For how long can we maintain these parallel increasing trends in consumption, life expectancy and environmental damage?

In the past, questions about 'sustainable health' have only been asked when the limits of local environmental carrying capacity are reached. Such limits tend to be reached first in poor overcrowded populations where environmental infrastructure is consumed or degraded, where food supplies become inadequate, and where external support (via trade or aid) is lacking (King, 1990). Now, the sustainability question is becoming more general. How can we assess the long-term sustainability of good health in large urban populations, particularly those with increasingly pervasive and damaging impacts upon local, regional and global systems?

Indices of the sustainability of population health would focus, in particular, upon the integrity and productivity of the biosphere's life-supporting systems. Such indices would assess the extent to which current human health needs are being met by the sustainable consumption of natural resources. They would need to address dynamic processes, not static conditions. They would monitor selected bioindicators known to be predictive of human disease risk, such as indices of vegetation and ground water in relation to infectious disease vectors (mosquitoes, tsetse flies, etc.), and indices of soil fertility and crop growth. Perhaps the experience of assessing the 'health' of aquatic systems is instructive. Over recent decades, water quality has been conventionally assessed in terms of measured levels of each of a list of itemized toxic chemical and microbiological hazards. More recently, there has been a turning back to more integrative measures such as the 'index of biological integrity' (Karr, 1998).

The pursuit of good population health makes little sense unless it is sustainable over future generations. This century's gains in life expectancy have derived, to some (as yet unquantified) extent, from increasingly intensive, often ecologically damaging modes of food production, from reliance on energy-intensive urban infrastructure and medical technology, and from overuse of antibiotics and chemical pesticides. Manifestations of this erosion of natural capital include the increasingly large proportion of the world's net primary (photosynthetic) product being co-opted by humans and the various global environmental changes that are now becoming manifest (Vitousek et al., 1997).

SEEKING SOLUTIONS

The apparent erosion of life-support systems at a global level is a serious public health issue. We are living in an important transitional period, in which we must reconceptualize the natural environment and humankind's relationship with it. In simpler times, not long past, we could generally rely on the continuation of nature's goods and services, and therefore could focus our concerns on the health hazards arising from man-made contamination of that external environment. Today, we also see that the provision of those goods and services is under threat (Daily, 1997), and that the natural environment, as habitat, is becoming less able to support life.

Thus, at the end of the twentieth century, we extended our environmental health concerns from hazard to habitat, from the idea of humans as targets of toxicants to one of humans fundamentally dependent on the sustained function of now-threatened nature. This view extends the scale of environmental health concern from risks to certain local groups or communities to risks to whole populations and their future generations. This thinking becomes particularly relevant today as we approach the post-genome age and must decide how best to apply our new, technologically dazzling, molecular genetic knowledge. Should we, as some agribusiness transnationals are urging, engage in a reductionist transgenic re-engineering of selected single species, manipulated without regard for their normal ecological context and for the possible knock-on consequences? Or should we find ways of using this new knowledge to work *with* nature to modulate, sustainably, the function of ecosystems? It is only the latter approach that is compatible with the idea of biosphere as 'habitat'.

The environmental health risk assessment task before us is formidable. The special incentive is this: if global environmental changes do, indeed, pose a substantive prospective risk to human health, knowledge of this will be an extremely important contribution to the policy-making process. Over the next few decades, humankind may well need to achieve more rapid social, economic and political change than ever before. As Rudolf Virchow, the famous nineteenth-century pathologist and public health advocate, might have said, this type of environmental health will be politics writ very large indeed.

REFERENCES

Appleton, J.D., Fuge, R. and McCall, G.J.H. (1996) *Environmental Geochemistry and Health*. Special Publication no. 113. London: The Geological Society.

Colwell, R. (1996) 'Global climate and infectious disease: the cholera paradigm', *Science*, 274: 2025–31.

Daily, G.C. (ed.) (1997) *Nature's Services*. Washington, DC: Island Press.

Doos, B.R. (1994) 'Environmental degradation, global food production and risk of large-scale migrations', *Ambio*, 23: 124–30.

Dubos, R. (1959) *Mirage of Health: Utopias, Progress, and Biological Change*. New York: Harper & Row.

Epstein, P.R., Diaz, H.F., Elias, S., Grabherr, G., Graham, N.E., Martens, W.J.M., Mosley-Thomson, E. and Susskind, J. (1998) 'Biological and physical signs of climate change: focus on mosquito-borne diseases', *Bulletin of the American Meteorological Society*, 78: 409–17.

FAO: Food and Agriculture Organization (1995) *State of the World's Fisheries*. Rome: FAO.

Gomes, M., Linthicum, K. and Haile, M. (1998) 'Malaria: the role of agriculture in changing the epidemiology of malaria', in K. De Cock and B. Greenwood (eds), *New and Resurgent Infections. Prediction, Detection and Management of Tomorrow's Epidemics*. Chichester: Wiley. pp. 87–100.

Gopalan, C. (1999) 'The changing epidemiology of malnutrition in a developing society. The effect of unforeseen factors', *Bulletin of the Nutritional Foundation of India*, 20: 1–5.

Hetzel, B.S. and Pandav, C.S. (1994) *SOS for a Billion. The Conquest of Iodine Deficiency Disorders*. Bombay: Oxford University Press.

Heymann, D.L. and Rodier, G. (1997) 'Reemerging pathogens and diseases out of control', *The Lancet*, 349 (suppl. III): 8–9.

Intergovernmental Panel on Climate Change (1996) *Second Assessment Report. Climate Change 1995*, Vols I, II, III. New York: Cambridge University Press.

Karr, J.R. Chu (1998) *Restoring Life in Running Waters: Better Biological Monitoring*. Washington, DC: Island Press.

King, M. (1990) 'Health is a sustainable state', *The Lancet*, 336: 664–7.

Last, J.M. (1998) *Public Health and Human Ecology*. Stamford, CT: Appleton & Lange.

McMichael, A.J. (1993) *Planetary Overload: Global Environmental Change and the Health of the Human Species*. Cambridge: Cambridge University Press.

McMichael, A.J. (1996) 'Bovine spongiform encephalopathy: wider implications for population health' (Editorial), *British Medical Journal*, 312: 313–14.

McMichael, A.J. and Haines, A. (1997) 'Global climate change: the potential effects on health', *British Medical Journal*, 315: 805–9.

McMichael, A.J., Bolin, B., Costanza, R., Daily, G.C., Folke, C., Lindahl-Kiessling, K., Lindgren, E. and Niklasson, B. (1999) 'Globalization and the sustainability of health: an ecological perspective', *BioScience*, 49: 205–10.

Mazumder D.N.G., Haque, R., Ghosh, N., De, B.K., Santra, A., Chakraborty, D. and Smith, A.H. (1998) 'Arsenic levels in drinking water and the prevalence of skin lesions in West Bengal, India', *International Journal of Epidemiology*, 27: 871–7.

Morse, S.S. (1993) 'Examining the origins of emerging viruses', in S.S. Morse (ed.), *Emerging Viruses*. New York: Oxford University Press.

Morse, S.S. (1995) 'Factors in the emergence of infectious diseases', *Emerging Infectious Diseases*, 1: 7–15.

Pimm, S.L., Russell, G.J., Gittleman, J.L. and Brooks, T.M. (1995) 'The future of biodiversity', *Science*, 269: 347–54.

Sharpe, R.M. and Skakkebaek, N. (1993) 'Are oestrogens involved in falling sperm counts and disorders of the male reproductive tract?' *The Lancet*, 341: 1392–5.

Vitousek, P.M., Mooney, H.A., Lubchenco, J. and Melillo, J.M. (1997) 'Human domination of Earth's ecosystems', *Science*, 277: 494–9.

Watson, R.T., Dixon, J.A., Hamburg, S.P., Janetos, A.C. and Moss, R.H. (1998) *Protecting Our Planet. Securing Our Future. Linkages among Global Environmental Issues and Human Needs.* UNEP, USNASA, World Bank.

WHO (1996) *World Health Report 1996. Fighting Disease, Fostering Development.* Geneva: WHO.

Wilson, M.E. (1995) 'Infectious diseases: an ecological perspective', *British Medical Journal*, 311: 1681–4.

World Resource Institute (1998) *1998–99 World Resources. A Guide to the Global Environment. Environmental Change and Human Health.* Oxford: Oxford University Press.

13

Globalization of International Health

Gill Walt

Co-operation between countries on health issues has a long history. The first international meeting was held in Paris, France, in 1851, and collaboration this century was formalized through the United Nations (UN) and its various agencies, such as WHO. Resources for health development have been channelled by the multilateral organizations of the UN, by bilateral organizations such as the UK Department for International Development, and by non-governmental organizations through grants, loans and technical assistance. These resources have benefited both rich and poor countries (Institute of Medicine, 1997).

But circumstances have changed since these institutions were founded. There will have been many direct and indirect challenges to health care and health in the year 2000 compared with 1950, when the UN was established. Although the processes of change are complex, increasing interdependence and globalization are clearly challenging national control of health policy. The issue of how well the bodies established to promote international health are meeting those challenges must therefore be raised. This chapter first sets out the context of change, then questions the potential impact of these challenges on international organizations concerned with health. Although some of these challenges are recognized, how they are best met is more elusive. This chapter does not provide solutions, but opens a debate that needs airing.

BACKGROUND

WHO, once the main player in 'directing and coordinating international health work' is now one of many. Other UN organizations are concerned with health; the World Bank now plays an increased financial and technical role in the sector, and bilateral agencies make significant contributions to health both at global and at national level. The private sector – consisting of a wide range of non-profit organizations, such as non-governmental bodies (e.g. Oxfam) or foundations (e.g. Rockefeller), and profit-making organizations (such as pharmaceutical firms or insurance companies) –

First published in *The Lancet*, 351, 7 February 1998: 434–7.

has a firm niche in international health. In so far as financial resources confer power and influence, overall bilateral aid (government to government) is more influential than multilateral aid (through the UN system); the former provided about US$55 billion net disbursements in 1996, the latter roughly $5 billion (Overseas Development Institute, 1997).

Global comparisons of official development assistance specifically for health are difficult, but about 10 per cent of total development assistance is spent on health activities (Raymond, 1997). Although most activities assist countries of low and middle income, it must be recognized that – with a few important exceptions – less than 20 per cent of funds spent on health and health care in those countries comes from international sources (World Bank, 1997); most resources are generated nationally. The concern nevertheless remains that, despite rapid growth in the global economy, overall aid is falling – official development assistance decreased by 17 per cent between 1992 and 1997 (Organisation for Economic Cooperation and Development, 1997), a fall which puts greater pressure on international organizations to ensure that multilateral resources focus on international collective action, and avoid tasks that can be financed by national resources.

The UN and many of its organizations, such as WHO, have faced a barrage of criticism over the past decade (Lee et al., 1996; Nordic UN Reform Report, 1996). However, an increasingly, interdependent world working within a global economy, and the entry of new players such as the World Trade Organization, suggest a greater role rather than a diminished one for the multilateral organizations of the UN system (Department for International Development, 1997; Overseas Development Institute, 1997). Specialized agencies, such as WHO, are perceived as neutral (Lucas et al., 1997), and cannot be replaced by bilateral organizations that are directly bound by domestic and foreign policy. Non-governmental organizations are increasingly involved and active within the UN, since they see the UN as a vehicle for broader representation and pressure for change (Krut, 1997). Although a shift in approach towards global co-operation might have taken place – from high expectations in 1950 to a more critical and detached view in industrialized countries in the late 1990s – this shift has not been reflected in the withdrawal of financial resources (except perhaps in the case of US non-payment of contributions to the UN). Financial support from countries belonging to the Organization for Economic Cooperation and Development (OECD) to UN organizations dispensing multilateral aid has not significantly changed since 1975, fluctuating between 9 per cent and 11 per cent of overall aid (Overseas Development Institute, 1997) – although more control is being exercised by means of the balance of contributions made through extrabudgetary or non-core funding, by which countries can specify where and on what they want their money spent.

Despite criticisms, therefore, many still see a role for international organizations, in terms of both self-interest and international development. The

Table 13.1 Perceived challenges to health in 1950 and 2000

Issues	1950	2000	Challenges
Health care			
Predominant disease pattern	Communicable	Non-communicable; Resurgence of old diseases; New and emerging infections	Some countries face significant levels of both; Known treatments not always effective; costs of drugs high; No current cures
Interventions			
Drugs	Promising and inexpensive drugs	Drugs resistance	Poor prescription practices; pharmaceutical innovation slower
Technology	Limited	Increasingly sophisticated	New ethical, financial and medical-legal resource issues (e.g. gene therapy, fertility treatment, transplantation, euthanasia)
Indirect			
Trade and markets	Regional, national (colonial networks)	Liberalized, privatized, global, multinational	New winners and losers within and between countries; financial instability; increasing unemployment possible; pressure on natural resources; increasing pollution, global warming
Transport, mobility of people	Ship, rail, fairly limited	Air, car, increasing travel	Spread of disease through greater contact; food exchange; road accidents; pollution
Illegal and legal drugs, arms sales	Largely limited to regions	Increasingly multinational, global	Increasing availability of legal (e.g. tobacco) and illegal substances, rise in related illness, conflict and violence
Population	Population growth	Ageing, refugees, and displaced people	Pressure on resource allocation, conflict between groups
Communications	Radio	Film, television, electronic networks	Widespread cultural diffusion leading to increased expectations and demand
Approach to international co-operation	High expectations for international co-operation through UN; end of period of global conflict	UN heavily criticized, growth of civil society groups (non-governmental organizations); growth in conflict, emergencies	Rich countries more detached from world issues; self-interest defined in domestic terms; attention on relieving conflicts

question is, what kinds of changes are needed for these institutions? They no longer have a dominant position in international co-operation, but are players in a complex and rapidly changing arena. The elimination of polio, for example, has been spearheaded by several governments, the WHO, and Rotary International working together for an agreed end; the Intergovernmental Panel on Climate Change, on the other hand, is a multidisciplinary body of scientists established by the UN in 1988, which has a continuing concern with the effects of climate change, including its implications for human health. Several global networks exist on health research, working independently or with international organizations. Is there a danger that the growth in different methods of organization at international level – made possible by the telecommunications revolution – will lead to marginalization of some countries (and individuals), duplication of activities, and wastage of resources? What role do international organizations have in the monitoring and promotion of international co-operation in this changed world?

Direct challenges to health care in the year 2000

Although many of the direct challenges to health noted in Table 13.1 will be met by domestic health policies, some will depend heavily on international collaboration. Health care will be affected directly by predominant disease patterns, such as emerging infections, and by interventions to address them; health care will be affected indirectly by issues such as increased pollution. The understanding, monitoring and treatment of emerging infections and resistance to existing drug therapy will demand global co-operation and exchange of information. Monitoring and surveillance systems (especially for infectious diseases) need updating and modernizing. Surveillance into the next century, once the task of WHO, will require co-operation between different organizations – co-operation that the telecommunications revolution should facilitate, and which WHO is already exploring. Yach and Bettcher (1998) suggest the establishment of a transnational organization: a Global Health Watch to advance global awareness and vigilence in this area. The difficulty will be to overcome institutional interests.

Old scourges remain in many countries and are imported into others. Malaria and tuberculosis are the main diseases of global concern, and treatment is complicated by resistance, lack of resources, and poverty. As technical interventions improve and populations age, new issues about ethical, financial and human resources must be addressed, not just nationally, but globally. New challenges will arise, ranging from the management of 'healthy ageing' to intensified debates over euthanasia, the right to control end of life (Warnock, 1994), and gene patenting and manipulation.

All these challenges demand broad public health discussion and political courage. Although some international organizations have helped raise awareness about the magnitude of these challenges, they have been less active in advocating specific policies to meet them. Such challenges highlight issues of national and global concern, and call for international leadership and vision (thereby supporting and legitimizing national policies). Tobacco-related morbidity, disability and mortality, for example, should be at the top of WHO's agenda (WHO, 1997). In future, the WHO may need to lobby the World Trade Organization to exempt tobacco sales from free-trade principles on the grounds of tobacco's serious consequences for health. The UK government justified its policy reversal to allow tobacco sponsorship for Formula One motor racing by arguing that a global ban is needed to prevent the sport moving to another country in which advertising is permitted. Stimulation of debate, the building of consensus on controversial policy issues, and acceleration of exchange of information and experience can be brought about by international (or regional) organizations through training, research, conferences, and other methods (McKee et al., 1997).

Indirect challenges to health

Globalization is increasingly acknowledged as a force that is changing many aspects of life far beyond financial markets and trade. Although some indirect challenges to health in the next century will not necessarily result from globalization, changes in trade and markets, the movement of people, goods and services (including trade in legal and illegal substances and in military arms), and communications over the past half-century will have consequences on health in the next 50 years.

The greatest indirect challenges to health probably occur through global liberalization of trade, and the resulting movement of goods and services within a world economy. Although increased exchanges bring benefits, they also carry risks, such as the international trade in illegal products and contaminated foodstuffs, inconsistent safety standards, and the indiscriminate spread of medical technologies (Institute of Medicine, 1997). Electronic media and the internet may provide opportunities for rapid communication, but they also allow, for example, the sale of prescription drugs that have not been approved by national drug-monitoring bodies (Siegel-Itzkovich, 1997). International regulations to control some of the risks associated with a global economy are limited (Yach, 1998).

As capital, trade and markets open up, the policies of different countries and sectors affect one another. 'Poison fog blanket threatens world climate' was typical of newspaper headlines in 1997 (Vidal, 1997); such headlines referred to Indonesia's forest fires, which, coupled with unfavourable winds and drought, polluted the atmosphere of several South-East Asian countries, and led to an increase in respiratory disorders. Deregulation, privatization and weak governmental regulations have led to the loss of more than 1 million hectares of Indonesian forest per year through logging for provision of paper and palm oil. The health disorders caused by the smog may have been short-lived compared with the long-term disturbances to the ecosystem from carbon dioxide released by slow-burning peatlands, species loss, and food chains broken by non-pollination (Economist, 1997).

Trends to liberalize trade and increase privatization are also cause for concern, since they could accelerate the destruction of the regenerative capacities of ecosystems on which future generations will depend. Excess carbon dioxide, methane and other gas emissions are widely acknowledged to contribute to global warming. Climatic change will have both direct effects (ranging from respiratory disorders and infections caused by contaminated drinking water and food, to changed transmission of vector organisms) and indirect effects (through alteration of the range, proliferation and behaviour of a large number of vectors, intermediate hosts, and the viability of infectious agents) (McMichael and Haines, 1997). Such changes affect groups differently, depending on levels of poverty, age, nutritional status and geographical location.

Changes in modes of transport and greater access to them have increased the mobility of people, goods and services; how far these developments have affected health and health care, however, is unclear. On the one hand, health systems tend to be distinctive (Moran and Wood, 1995), health policy the domain of national governments, and the mobility of patients across borders limited. Although the migration of providers from lower-income to higher-income countries has been significant, this migration may be slowing with increasing immigration restrictions and unemployment of indigenous health professionals. Even in the European Union, health professionals have made limited use of their rights to practise in other European countries (McKee et al., 1996). 'Medical tourism', on the other hand, may increase as patients seek effective or less expensive care, especially if the internet provides information on available facilities. The Australian government has introduced a 'medical visa' for those from abroad seeking health care in Australia, and an excess of hospital beds in the USA has prompted major marketing campaigns to reach potential foreign patients. As trade restrictions are lifted, more foreign investment in health services is being allowed, although often with national partners (United Nations Conference on Trade & Development, 1997). The implications of greater freedom and deregulation of trade on the practices of health professionals are only just being explored.

Winners and losers in the global economy – emerging health inequalities

Although the extent to which globalization is affecting health is unclear, winners and losers in the world economy will undoubtedly emerge – both between and within countries. During the past two decades, for example, the least developed countries – which make up 10 per cent of the world's population – have halved their share of world trade, and today account for only 0.3 per cent of it (United Nations Development Programme, 1997). Whether or not such inequalities result primarily from globalization, they have potentially severe repercussions for relations between countries, including economic migration, political instability, violent conflict and social unrest.

Inequalities within countries continue to take their toll on health, and may be widening (*Soc Sci Med*, 1997). Wilkinson (1996a) has argued that egalitarian societies are healthier (and socially more cohesive) than those with large income differences between groups. Although quantification of such social relations is difficult, few would disagree that levels of health and well-being depend on the quality of these relations. The fall in life expectancy of Russian men (from 64 years in 1989 to 59 in 1993) resulted partly from a reduction in real income, increased stress, stress-related behaviour (e.g. alcohol consumption), and a breakdown in health services (Goldstein, 1997; Leon, 1997); but it may also have been exacerbated by a loss in the longer term of egalitarian ethics, public spirit and comradeship (Wilkinson, 1996b).

Inequalities within countries have increased partly because employment opportunities have diminished. Although the relation between globalization and unemployment is not precise, little doubt exists that the labour market is rapidly changing. In the UK, Hutton (1995) has drawn attention to what he calls the '40:30:30 society', in which 40 per cent of the working population are in full-time, long-term employment; 30 per cent are in part-time, insecure jobs; and another 30 per cent are unemployed or working for poverty wages. Though unemployment may be a short-term difficulty, as individuals adjust to demands for greater flexibility and technological competence in the global workplace, it may also signal 'the end of work' as we know it (Rifkin, 1995), the repercussions of which could deepen inequalities between social groups. The term 'social exclusion' is increasingly used to highlight the implications of long-term unemployment and the move from universal to targeted welfare provision (Macintosh, 1997). Low-income countries are affected similarly by changes in the global division of labour, which are altering the nature of work worldwide.

Evidently, challenges to health in the next century are many. What can international organizations do to meet these challenges?

Rethinking the role of international organizations

In view of the challenges that affect health care directly and indirectly, priorities need reordering and hard choices must be made. More attention needs to be paid to which functions international organizations are best able to undertake, and what national governments should be doing. Some functions may be better organized through intergovernmental networks than through multilateral organizations (issues of public health regulation, for example).

International organizations may have to increase their advocacy roles – on medical-legal issues, for example. The results of trade liberalization and World Trade Organization decisions in relation to tobacco or pharmaceutical production and trade may need to be monitored and challenged when their health effects are clearly deleterious, or when grave inequalities between countries are exacerbated. Just as the United Nations Children's Fund (UNICEF) challenged the World Bank over structural adjustment policies with its 1987 publication *Adjustment with a Human Face* (Cornia, 1987), so WHO or the World Bank may need to question decisions made by the World Trade Organization. Clearly, international organizations must make broader links and partnerships with groups in civil society, from academic and research institutions to interest groups at the community level. Many have begun to do so. International organizations will need to keep up with the burgeoning network of new groupings in international co-operation, to avoid duplication and waste.

Finally, international organizations need to regain lost moral ground. There are still significant and influential groups in all nations that recognize the need for global co-operation, leadership from international organizations, venues for debate and advocacy, and the exchange and monitoring of information. International organizations must respond to the demands of such groups by avoiding domination by a handful of countries, or by being blinded by conventional wisdom. But before the role of international organizations can be rethought, every nation – rich or poor – must recognize that it is not in its interest to retreat into a domestic sphere, or to detach itself from global responsibility.

REFERENCES

Cornia, A., Jolly, R. and Stewart, F. (1987) *Adjustment with a Human Face*. Oxford: Clarendon.

Department for International Development (1997) *Eliminating World Poverty: A Challenge for the 21st Century: White Paper on International Development*. London: Department for International Development.

Goldstein, E., Preker, A., Adeyi, O. and Chellaraj, G. (1997) *Trends in Health Status, Services and Finance: The Transition in Central and Eastern Europe*. World Bank technical paper 341, vol 1. Washington: World Bank.

Economist (1997) 'An Asian pea-souper', September 27: 82.

'Health inequalities in modern societies and beyond' (1997) *Soc Sci Med*, 44 (special issue): 6.

Hutton, W. (1995) *The State We're In*. London: Jonathan Cape.

Institute of Medicine (1997) *America's Vital Interests in Global Health*. Washington: National Academy Press.

Krut, R. (1997) *Globalization and Civil Society: NGO Influence in International Decision-making*. Geneva: UN Research Institute for Social Development.

Lee, K., Collinson, S., Walt, G. and Gilson, L. (1996) 'Who should be doing what in international health: a confusion of mandates in the United Nations?', *British Medical Journal*, 312: 302–27.

Leon, D., Chenet, L., Shkolnikov, V. et al. (1997) 'Huge variation in Russian mortality rates 1984–94: artefact, alcohol, or what?', *The Lancet*, 350: 383–88.

Lucas, A., Mogedal, S., Walt, G. et al. (1997) *Cooperation for Health Development: The World Health Organisation's Support to Programmes at Country Level: Synthesis Report*. London: London School of Hygiene and Tropical Medicine.

McKee, M., Mossialos, E. and Belcher, P. (1996) 'The influence of European law on national health policy', *Journal of European Social Policy*, 6: 263–86.

Mackintosh, M. (1997) 'Public management for social inclusion: keynote paper for conference on public management for the next century,' Manchester, June 29–3 July.

McMichael, J. and Haines, A. (1997) 'Global climate change: the potential effects on health', *British Medical Journal*, 315: 805–9.

Moran, M. and Wood, B. (1995) 'The globalization of health care policy?', in P. Gummett (ed.), *Globalization and Public Policy*. Vermont: Edward Elgar.

Nordic UN Reform Report 1996.

Organisation for Economic Cooperation and Development (1997) Development assistance committee: report in *Aidwatch*, 14, May and June. Somerset: Development Initiatives.

Overseas Development Institute (1997) *The UN's Role in Grant-financed Development*, briefing paper 2, May. London: Overseas Development Institute.

Raymond, S. (ed.) (1997) *Global Public Health Collaboration: Organizing for a Time of Renewal*. New York: New York Academy of Sciences.

Rifkin, J. (1995) *The end of work*. New York: Tarcher/Putnam.

Siegel-Itzkovich, J. (1997) 'WHO calls for tighter controls on Internet', *British Medical Journal*, 314: 1504.

United Nations Conference on Trade & Development (1997) 'International trade in health services: difficulties and opportunities for developing countries.' UN conference on trade and development, background note by secretariat, TD/B/COM.1/EM.1/2.

United Nations Development Programme (1997) *Human Development Report*. Oxford: Oxford University Press.

Vidal, J. (1997) 'Poison fog blanket threatens world climate', *Guardian*, Sep 27: 3.

Warnock, M. (1994) 'Some moral problems in medicine', *Health Economics*, 3: 297–300.

WHO (1997) *Think and Act Globally and Intersectorally to Protect National Health*. Geneva: WHO.

Wilkinson, R. (1996a) *Unhealthy Societies*. London and New York: Routledge.

Wilkinson, R. (1996b) 'Health and civic society in Eastern Europe before 1989', in C. Hertzman, S. Kelly and M. Bobak (eds), *East-west Life Expectancy Gap in Europe: Environmental and Non-environmental Determinants*. Dordrecht: Kluwer Academic Publishers.

World Bank (1997) *Human Development Network and Sector Strategy*, Health Nutrition and Population Division, Washington: World Bank.

Yach, D. and Bettcher, D. (1998) 'The globalization of public health: the convergence of self-interest and altruism', *American Journal of Public Health*, 5: 735-7.

14

Health Impact Assessment

Alex Scott-Samuel

Health impact assessment (HIA) builds on the now generally accepted understanding that a nation's or community's health is determined by a wide range of economic, psychosocial and environmental influences, as well as by heredity and health care. Once this is accepted, it is clearly important to evaluate the health effects of these influences. This is the aim of health impact assessment, which has been defined as *the estimation of the effects of a specified action on the health of a defined population* (Scott-Samuel, 1998).

The actions concerned may represent big or small public policies ranging from major governmental policies such as Welfare to Work, to locally determined programmes such as the decisions regarding water metering or urban regeneration projects. Ideally, HIAs should be prospective – in other words, they should precede the introduction of the policy concerned, in order that any potential negative health effects can be avoided or reduced, and any positive ones enhanced.

The elements of this approach have much in common with those underlying the established field of environmental impact assessment (EIA). In essence, they involve the following elements:

- screening to select policies or projects for assessment;
- profiling the areas, communities and interest groups likely to be affected by the policy or project;
- obtaining data from key informants and stakeholders to identify potential health impacts;
- evaluating the importance, scale and likelihood of potential impacts;
- option appraisal and recommendations for action.

Key principles of HIA include an explicit focus on social and environmental justice (it is usually the already disadvantaged who suffer most from negative health impacts); a multidisciplinary, participatory approach; both qualitative and quantitative assessment methods; explicit values and politics; and openness to public scrutiny.

BACKGROUND

During the last two decades a series of publications have documented the evidence showing that public policy is the most important determinant of the public's health, and the concept of healthy public policy has become central to health promotion discourse. (Doyal, 1996; Milio, 1981; Townsend et al., 1992). The WHO European health for all strategy (WHO, 1985) also made a key contribution. But while such reports have created a climate where it is now universally acceptable to talk of the health impact of housing, unemployment or poverty, few if any of them attempt to assess the scale of that impact.

Meanwhile, in the 'less developed' countries of the South, where the health effects of public policy are often painfully evident, the prospective assessment of unintended health impacts of development projects – such as road building, agricultural or sanitation schemes – has gone on for well over a decade (Birley, 1995).

In the 'developed' world, environmental impact assessment first took off in the USA following the National Environmental Policy Act of 1969, which made it a mandatory component of the planning process. EIA was soon complemented by social impact assessments (and later by health impact assessments) of the effects of environmental projects – such as a potentially hazardous factory, a motorway or a nuclear plant. This 'environmental HIA' concept was also developed in Canada, Australia (Ewan et al., 1994) and New Zealand.

The first formal example of prospective HIA in the UK was the assessment of the health impact of the proposed second runway at Manchester Airport undertaken by Manchester and Stockport Health Commissions and submitted to the Manchester Airport public inquiry in 1994 (Will et al., 1994). This pioneering HIA used methods specially developed by the authors for assessing and estimating potential impacts.

The UK Department of Health issued its *Policy Appraisal and Health* report in December 1995. The concept of HIA which this report describes is based on the Treasury's economic appraisal model. It relies heavily on the quantification and valuation of predicted impacts. However, qualitative impacts may be every bit as important as quantitative ones – and valuations of actual impacts or their opportunity costs may be very hard to come by. Despite this, the report represented a major advance in terms of the then government not only recognizing the crucial importance of public policy as a determinant of public health, but also acknowledging the need to routinely assess its potential health impact.

Following the election in May 1997, the Labour government's commitment to addressing the health impacts of its public policies has become clear. All four national consultative documents on public health strategy have referred to the necessity for health impact assessment of both national and local policies and projects (Secretary of State for Health, 1998;

Secretary of State for Northern Ireland, 1997; Secretary of State for Scotland, 1998; Secretary of State for Wales, 1998). In addition to the present exercise, the English health department is supporting a special interest group, funding research and development into health impact assessment, and it co-sponsored a national conference in November 1998. The Scottish Office Department of Health has circulated a discussion paper on the development of health impact assessment in Scotland (Douglas, 1998) to directors of public health, and is funding a research programme.

METHODS

This section applies the Liverpool Observatory's general approach to HIA to the assessment of public sector policy. Box 14.1 shows the key elements of the proposed method.

Box 14.1: Liverpool Public Health Observatory EQUAL (Equity in Health Research and Development Unit)

Prospective health impact assessment of public policy – key principles

1 Application of screening criteria for policy selection
2 Policy analysis
3 Profiling of affected areas/communities
4 Identification of stakeholders and key informants
5 Identification of potential positive and negative health impacts

- with stakeholders and key informants
- using qualitative methods
- by phase of policy implementation
- by key health determinants, using socio-environmental model of health

6 Assessment of extent of mediation of impacts

- by community vulnerability ('at risk' groups from environmental/social equity perspectives)
- by environmental factors
- by capacity and capabilities of health-relevant public agencies

7 Assessment of health risks posed by health impacts

- estimation of probability of occurrence
- categorisation of measurability

8 Quantification and valuation of health/health care impacts (where possible)
9 Ranking of most important impacts
10 Assessing and actioning information/research needs for highest priority impacts
11 Option appraisal
12 Health risk management recommendations
13 Implementation, monitoring and evaluation

Box 14.2: Health impact assessment screening procedure

Economic issues
- size of the policy and of the population(s) affected
- costs of the policy, and their distribution

Outcome issues
- nature of potential health impacts of the policy (crudely estimated)
- likely nature and extent of disruption caused to communities by the policy
- existence of potentially cumulative impacts

Epidemiological issues
- degree of certainty (risk) of health impacts
- likely frequency (incidence/prevalence rates) of potential health impacts
- likely severity of potential health impacts
- size of any probable health service impacts
- likely consistency of 'expert' and 'community' perceptions of probability (i.e. risk), frequency and severity of important impacts. The greater the likely consistency – i.e. the greater the likely agreement between expert and lay perceptions of important impacts – the greater the need for a HIA.

Strategic issues
- the need to give greater priority to policies than to programmes, and to programmes than to projects, all other things being equal. (This results from the broader scope – and hence potential impact – of policies as compared to programmes and to projects)
- Timeliness:
  - ensuring that HIA is prospective wherever possible
  - Planning Regulations and other statutory frameworks
- Relevance to local decision-making

Screening

Since resources for HIA will always be scarce, it is necessary to be selective about what work is undertaken. Screening is the process whereby policies are selected for health impact assessment. The procedures used are shown in Box 14.2 (they are not in priority order). While the process is necessarily crude, it can give a useful indication of how resources for HIA can be most effectively deployed.

Policy analysis

Once a policy has been selected for HIA, an initial policy analysis should be carried out; this may build on or use material already available from earlier policy development work. Elements of this stage may include, for example, policy content and dimensions; sociopolitical and policy context; policy objectives, priorities and outputs; trade-offs and critical sociocultural impacts.

Profiling of affected areas/communities

A profile of the areas and communities likely to be affected by the policy should be compiled using available sociodemographic and health data and other relevant information. The profile should include an assessment of the nature and characteristics of groups whose health could be enhanced or placed at risk by the policy's effects. Vulnerable and disadvantaged groups require special consideration. It will often be possible to use specially collected survey or other information in the profile in addition to routine data.

Depending on the nature of the policy being assessed, affected communities may be defined by geography, age, sex, income, or other social, economic or environmental characteristics; they may also be communities of interest, e.g. arts or sport enthusiasts, vegetarians, cyclists.

Identification of stakeholders and key informants

The process of HIA must be participatory if a comprehensive picture is to be established. A steering group will be required to give advice and support to the project, agree its terms of reference (including all inputs and outputs) and ensure their fulfilment. Its membership should include representatives of the commissioners of the HIA, the researchers carrying it out, the policy's proponents (i.e. those developing and/or working on it), affected communities, and other interested parties as appropriate. In addition to these stakeholders, the identification of potential health impacts will also require the co-operation and expertise of key informants such as staff involved in implementing the policy, primary care and other community staff familiar with the groups likely to be affected by the policy, and possibly technical experts on relevant specialist issues. Community participation throughout the HIA is essential to ensure that local concerns are fully addressed.

Identification of potential positive and negative health impacts

Clearly the range of health impacts identified in HIA is dependent on the definition of health which is employed. We use a socio-environmental model of health derived from the work of Labonté (1998) and Lalonde (1974). This model is similar to that currently being applied by the UK government (DoH, 1995; Secretary of State for Northern Ireland, 1997; Secretary of State for Scotland, 1998; Secretary of State for Wales, 1998) and other bodies such as the World Health Organization. The elements of this model can be used to generate detailed lists of health determinants which have been demonstrated to influence health status.

The collection of data on potential health impacts involves qualitative research with the stakeholders and key informants identified above. The nature and number of subjects involved will obviously depend on the nature and scope of the policy under study, as well as on sampling considerations and practical constraints. The range of potential methods includes semi-structured interviews, focus groups, Delphi exercises and with- and without-policy scenarios.

The first step involves the provision to informants of a summary of the proposed policy which is sufficiently detailed to elicit an adequate response. Timeliness is crucial; assessment should ideally take place early enough in policy development to permit constructive modifications to be carried out prior to implementation, but late enough for a clear idea to have been formed – and documented – as to the nature and content of the policy.

While in some contexts open-ended questions will be sufficient to facilitate the identification of potential health impacts, in others it may help to ask closed questions. Issues which have been highlighted in initial interviews can also be explored in greater depth in focus groups or brainstorming sessions. Interviews are more appropriate where sensitive or confidential issues are involved.

Data are recorded on a form which is designed to record the following information separately:

- potential health impacts during policy development and implementation phases;
- positive and negative health impacts (for example, a potential negative impact: increased levels of asthma);
- health categories and determinants resulting in the impacts identified (e.g. physical environment and air pollution);
- policy activities altering determinants (e.g. increased traffic flow)
- nature and size of potential impacts;
- measurability of potential impact – qualitative, estimable or calculable;
- certainty (risk) of potential impact – definite, probable or speculative.

In addition to considering the views of stakeholders and key informants (and judging these against the available evidence base), it will often be necessary to assess the extent to which predicted impacts are modified by factors specific to the policy being studied. There may be particular groups affected by the policy whose resistance or vulnerability differs from that of the population at large. Environmental conditions (such as wind direction, water courses, or pre-existing local conditions) may modify health impacts – sometimes in the long term and/or over long distances. Similarly, long latent periods prior to the development of certain diseases may mean that some impacts are distant in time from the intervention under study. The quality and quantity of health care and other health-relevant services (e.g. environmental health, social services) may also mediate impacts.

Assessment of health risks posed by health impacts

As outlined above, perceptions of risk are, when possible, recorded at the time of identification of potential impacts. While in some instances existing evidence (which may require to be researched) will permit precise assessment of risk, it will frequently be necessary to record subjective perceptions – especially in the case of non-expert informants such as community members. Assuming adequate sampling, such sub-jective risk data are no less valid than are more 'objective' technical data, and merit equal consideration – particularly where sensory perceptions (such as increased noise or smell, or deterioration of outlook) are concerned.

Risk perceptions are recorded using simple three-point scales of meas-urability (potential impacts are characterized as qualitative, estimable or calculable) and of probability of occurrence (definite, probable or spec-ulative). The temptation to quantify such scales (as has been suggested by some practitioners of EIA) should be resisted – such numbers could not be commensurable and would carry a wholly spurious authority.

It should also be pointed out that definite, calculable risk data are in no sense superior to speculative, qualitative data. For instance, a definite increase of, say, 0.5 per cent in levels of the common cold is arguably less important than a speculative risk of a less attractive outlook from the windows of a block of houses.

Ranking and researching the most important impacts

In almost all health impact assessments it will prove impossible to consider all potential impacts in detail; informants should be encouraged to prioritize or rank those they identify. Once all the initial evidence has been collected, a priority-setting exercise should be carried out – the HIA steering group will usually be best placed to undertake this. Because of differential perceptions of risk there will rarely be complete consensus; criteria may need to be agreed so that the views of all informants are adequately reflected. The number of priorities to be pursued will vary with the size of the HIA, the importance of the policy and the nature of the impacts identified. Once this has been done, available information and relevant evidence concerning priority impacts will need to be collated.

Option appraisal and health risk management recommendations

Although it will occasionally prove possible to define a single clear solution which will optimize the health impact of the policy being assessed, in most cases a series of options will have to be defined and presented. Formal option appraisal according to Treasury guidelines will health implications) will require the application of these methods in their entirety.

Prospective and retrospective HIA

While ideally, HIA should take place early enough in the development of a policy to permit constructive modifications to be carried out prior to its implementation, but late enough for a clear idea to have been formed as to its nature and content, circumstances will often make this unrealistic. In many cases it will be desirable to retrospectively assess the past or continuing health impact of an existing policy; in others, there will be some smaller departure from the ideal situation outlined. Methods need to be sufficiently flexible to accommodate the range of possibilities.

It is also important to recognize that the knowledge base for prospective studies essentially derives from existing retrospective assessments of the health impacts of public policies. While some attempts have been made to collate this literature (CPHA, 1997; Koivusalo et al., 1997), more systematic work will be required.

Values, equity and participation

Much research claims to be value-neutral – which usually means that its values are implicit rather than stated. The aims of public policy dictate that HIA should openly declare its values – and that social, material and environmental equity should feature strongly among them. This is because public policy impacts disproportionately on the already disadvantaged. Consistent with the adoption of an equity-focused approach are the use of participatory methods which fully involve those affected by public policy at every stage of assessment, and openness of all stages of the HIA process to public scrutiny.

ACKNOWLEDGEMENTS

I acknowledge the intellectual contributions to the material in this paper of Kate Ardern, Martin Birley, Mike Eastwood, Nigel Fleeman and Lyn Winters.

REFERENCES

Birley M.H. (1995) *The Health Impact Assessment of Development Projects*. London: HMSO.

CPHA: Canadian Public Health Association (1997) *Health Impacts of Social and Economic Conditions: Implications for Public Policy*. Ottawa: CPHA.

Department of Health (1995) *Policy Appraisal and Health*. London: Department of Health. (Issued under cover of EL(95)129 / CI(95)47.)

Douglas, M. (1998) *Health Impact Assessment: a Way Forward for Scotland*. Edinburgh: Scottish Office Department of Health.

Doyal, L. (1979) *The Political Economy of Health*. London: Pluto Press.

Ewan, C., Young, A., Bryant, E. and Calvert, D. (1994) *National Framework for Environmental and Health Impact Assessment. National Health and Medical Research Council*. Canberra: Australian Government Publishing Service.

Koivusalo, M., Ollila, E. and Santalahti, P. (1997) *Intersectoral Action for Health in Finland*. Themes 7/1997. Helsinki: Health Services Research Unit, National Research and Development Centre for Welfare and Health.

Labonté, R. (1998) *A Community Development Approach to Health Promotion*. Health Education Board for Scotland/Research Unit on Health and Behavioural Change, University of Edinburgh.

Lalonde, M. (1974) *A New Perspective on the Health of Canadians*. Ottawa: Ministry of Supply and Services.

Milio, N. (1981) *Promoting Health through Public Policy*. Philadelphia: F.A. Davis.

Milner, S. and Marples, G. (1997) *Policy Appraisal and Health Project. Phase 1 – a Literature Review*. Newcastle: University of Northumbria.

Population Health Resource Branch (1994a) *Health Impact Assessment Toolkit. A Resource for Government Analysts*. Victoria, British Columbia: Ministry of Health.

Scott-Samuel, A. (1998) 'Health impact assessment – theory into practice', *Journal of Epidemiology and Community Health*, 52: 704–5.

Secretary of State for Health (1998) *Our Healthier Nation: a Contract for Health*. Cm 3852. London.: HMSO.

Secretary of State for Northern Ireland (1997) *Well into 2000*. Belfast: Department of Health and Social Services.

Secretary of State for Scotland (1998) *Working Together for a Healthier Scotland*. Cm 3584. Edinburgh: The Stationery Office.

Secretary of State for Wales (1998) *Better health – Better Wales*. Cm 3922. London: HMSO.

Townsend, P., Davidson, N. and Whitehead, M. (eds) (1992) *Inequalities in Health*. Harmondsworth: Perguin.

Will, S., Ardern, K., Spencely, M. and Watkins, S. (1994) *A prospective health impact assessment of the proposed development of a second runway at Manchester International Airport*. Written submission to the public inquiry. Manchester and Stockport Health Commissions.

World Health Organization Regional Office for Europe (1985) *Targets for Health for All*. Copenhagen: WHO.

> Some streets are OK. We don't use the parks. There are a lot of them but nobody uses them because the muggers hang out there. (Boy, inner city Birmingham)

> I feel pretty safe round here. I usually walk up on my own to the park or cycle. But it's pretty friendly and I feel safe. (Boy, Northampton suburb)

> I'm allowed to go everywhere round here because everywhere is quite normal. (Girl, Kettering district)

Even within areas that were perceived as generally low risk clear distinctions were made between different areas and times of day. Compared with familiar home areas, town centres in both medium- and low-density locations were seen by some young people as threatening and unsafe after dark. A distinction was often made between the 'other' – scary and exciting places to which access was limited – and the 'familiar' – safe and essentially boring local areas.

> The local area is not threatening. In busy areas with gangs such as the town centre it may be. (Boy, Northampton suburb)

> You have to go into Kettering to do anything. Not everyone wants to go to places like that. I mean some of the mums won't let them go out on their own. So if they're only let out in their area there's nothing to do. (Boy, Kettering district)

SCARY PEOPLE

Scary people differed between locations. In high-density areas they were often known and lived locally: the older boy who threatened a younger one into giving up his bike; the local gang hanging out in the local park. There were also unknown muggers and gangs of older teenagers on the fringes of the local area who presented a danger to the unwary. For Asian girls in mid-suburban Birmingham, racial and sexual harassment was an added threat.

> It happened to me one Sunday. I was walking down to the Mosque, and it was the first time I'd been on my own. Because I usually walk down there with my mum. And there was this man. And I was walking down across the bridge. And then, as soon as he saw me, he just took off his trousers. And they were a bit like. . . . And I just closed my eyes. I didn't even want to go to the Mosque. And when it was time to pray, I couldn't pray. I just ended up crying as well. (Girl, middle suburb, Birmingham)

In medium- and low-density areas there were few known local sources of danger. As a boy from a village in Kettering district noted, 'everyone knows everyone else, even know the milkman'. The risks were from those perceived as outsiders. 'Gypsies' were usually blamed for vandalism, but they overlapped as a group to accuse with the 'others' who existed on the fringes of the safe local areas. Sometimes, the accounts made clear that vandals actually were known; they were older teenagers, especially boys trying to impress their peers.

Part of the scary quality of town centres in the medium- and low-density locations derived from the people who frequented them. Older teenagers, often with cars, were a source of constant worry to the young people's parents.

> My mum she doesn't trust anybody around us like. I mean she came over here to pick me up from a disco and she looks around and there's tons of like older boys in cars and stuff and she thinks, they're going to grab you and push you into a car, that they're going to be really like mad. (Girl, Northampton)

ASSESSING AND MANAGING RISK

In all locations, young people actively engaged in the work of assessing and managing risk. Risk arose partly from their own worries about scary places, spaces and people but another potent source was parental concern. Asian girls in Birmingham reported that their parents saw them as needing much more protection than their brothers. Mothers' views about lack of safety and accounts about needing to satisfy maternal concerns were most common. In some cases young people reported that 'my mum trusts me and everything but she doesn't trust other people' (Girl, inner Birmingham).

Perceptions of environmental danger influenced risk management. For example, 48 per cent of Asian girls at the middle ring comprehensive were driven to school by car, as against 12 per cent of non-Asian girls. While walking was the most favoured mode of travel almost every-where, only about a third of this was unaccompanied. In all areas, both on school journeys and for out-of-school activities, walking with peers was the dominant mode for both boys and girls. Boys were more likely to travel alone than girls, but the difference was much less marked in the low-density area, where 29 per cent of boys and 20 per cent of girls regularly travelled alone. Girls in all areas were less likely to travel alone after dark. Cycling to school was rare, although cycle ownership was high in both the medium- and low-density areas and boys everywhere nominated cycling as their preferred transport mode.

CONSTRUCTING SAFETY

Young people moved beyond managing risk to a more elaborate process of 'constructing safety'. Whereas managing risk focused on minimizing risky activities, constructing safety was concerned with creating situ-ations in which safety was maximized without loss of independence. Its cornerstone was the use of 'groups'. According to young people, adults were unable to distinguish between 'gangs' and 'groups' and saw them all as potentially dangerous whereas for young people groups afforded necessary protection and formed part of constructing safety.

> I think like parents have got this stereotype attitude, if you're with a group they think like, oh there's a gang over there. But you might not be in a gang, you might just be with a group of friends and they think oh we'll stay away from there and all this sort of thing, and they put their cars in garages and everything, but you're not doing anything wrong, you're just standing there with your friends or having a game of football. (Girl, Northampton)

These were not the small, functional groups used for school travel but larger and less homogeneous. In most cases they were mixed, based on the peer group but with some older and younger participants. Groups offered young people freedom from fear of verbal and physical assault. They were an essential resource for young people themselves rather than part of a parentally approved system for keeping safe.

> We go [into town] at the weekend. Nobody is really worried because you go around in big groups, twenty to thirty people, and you . . . just hang around shops and stuff. (Boy, Northampton)

> Also you don't get picked on by other people if you are in a group. If you are in a big group no one will like come along and push you and stuff but if you are on your own and you go past big groups that's tricky (Boy, Kettering district)

NEGOTIATING ACCESS

Many young people acknowledged the legitimacy of parental fears and rules. Forty per cent of Asian-origin girls in mid-suburban Birmingham said they obeyed rules even if they disagreed with them. One commented: 'I sometimes disagree with my parents, but I don't want to break their heart so I just agree with them'. Other teenagers, especially girls, worked to maximize freedom of movement. They developed a discourse to cope with parents, using elaborate types of evasion and collusion. As one boy in Kettering district commented, parents 'don't need to know'. Here is a typical account from Northampton:

> *Girl 1:* There was a weirdo last night. We were up the park. I seen him, he was lying down, he was a drunk or something, he had a bottle of cider with him, and he started flashing, and I thought, ugh, go away. You've got nothing to show, go away.
> *Interviewer:* Did you tell your parents that?
> *Girl 1:* No, they'd never let you out.
> *Girl 2:* If they knew about like some of the things you've seen like, they'd never let you out.

Collusion between young people in the cause of allaying parental fears was widely reported, especially by girls. This involved building trust by releasing some plausible details about planned activities, while screening out elements that would be likely to alarm parents.

> I think what she doesn't know won't hurt her, so I just tell her I'm going up the park and I go somewhere else and she won't know about it. And then, I come back and she'll say 'oh, where have you been?' and I'll say 'I've been over the park' and she'll say 'oh, all right'. But if I tell her where I've been she'll go mad. (Girl, Northampton)

> They think they know but we just don't tell them. If I go down [town] I don't say. I walk around up town by McDonald's and that but she doesn't know what else I get up to. (Girl, Kettering district)

HANDLING THE TENSIONS

Young people reported various types of tensions, mainly relating to boredom, hassle from adults and lack of respect. A strong sense of the early teenage years as the 'in-between years', plagued by boredom, permeates their accounts. The risks of inactivity were noted as young people recorded their views about staying healthy. Most described health in terms of a healthy appearance and physical fitness. Health was a visible dimension, evidenced for boys by muscle tone and physical stamina, and for girls by a slim body, white teeth and shining hair. Having 'bought into' the dominant discourse about physical health they were well aware that it was difficult to deliver.

> How can we be healthy if there's nothing to do? (Girl, Birmingham)

> They say you've got to be healthy and they give you lectures but then there's nothing to do that is healthy. (Girl, Northampton)

Their ideas for change almost all focused on enabling them to be more active while staying safe. Young people in Birmingham called for cycle paths, safer parks, pedestrian areas and traffic restraint. In other areas the demand was for more leisure facilities (such as improved skateboarding equipment) and better, cheaper public transport. In all areas they called for greater security in parks. Vandalism was seen as bound up with boredom and adult inaction. While acknowledging that some young people did 'cause trouble', they rejected adult accounts which stereotyped them as vandals rather than as teenagers with time on their hands.

> If there were more things to do people wouldn't hang around on the streets and everything, so much.
> When they get bored, they want to do things like smash windows, just to entertain themselves. (Two boys, Northampton)

In medium- and low-density areas adults were held responsible for causing the tensions, partly by demonizing teenagers. Threatening to 'call the police' was a widely reported adult tactic. In all areas, teenagers described being watched in local shops and 'only being allowed in two at a time'. They felt that adult complaints were attended to whereas theirs were ignored. One teenager produced the following analysis of the generation gap:

> I hate the way people think, well they treat you like a kid, because maybe all right 30 or 40 years ago when you were 13 or 14 you wouldn't know so many things about drugs and you wouldn't act the way like we do now, like in the 90s and everything. I hate the way that people treat you like 10-year-olds. But we're not, we're young adults, we should be treated with a bit more respect. (Girl, Northampton)

CONCLUSIONS

Young people and their parents routinely engaged in managing risk (Adams, 1995; Backett-Milburn et al., 1999; Beck, 1992; Lupton, 1995). While parents were generally reported as trying to avoid risk by creating barriers to their children's independent mobility, teenagers sought to compensate for risk by 'constructing safety'. Scary places, spaces and people could not be entirely avoided, even in the safest areas; fears about racist attacks and sexual assault were grounded in real experience. Thus, in all locations young people had developed strategies to deal with risk: in particular membership of large mixed groups.

Although activities that involve negotiating the external environment have been seen as essential to children's development (Hillman et al., 1990), many teenagers were unable to cycle freely, use local parks or even travel safely by themselves in their local areas. A strong sense of being 'the in-between years' – neither 'kids' any more nor grown up enough to gain acceptance in the adult world – pervades the findings. They felt themselves excluded from adult activities so that hanging around in the street became the main option, provoking the distrust of adults and helping to confirm the view that teenagers weren't to be trusted. When they proposed practical ideas for change such as building leisure facilities or bike paths, which they argued could help to transform their local areas into safer, more accessible environments, they felt their voices were not heard.

The findings should be of concern to health educators and promoters, indeed to anyone involved at national or local level in developing new public health agenda policies for young people. Teenagers in this study asked for safe places to go outside the home rather than to be corralled within it. Their perception was of managing environmental risk while policy-makers ignored their voices and adults criticized from the side-lines. Yet the ideas and insights they provide suggest that young people should be seen not as a nuisance but as a rich resource to enable health educators and policy-makers to make more constructive and appropriate policy decisions about healthy living in communities.

NOTE

1. For details of the four locations see Birmingham City Council, *Small Area Statistics*. Birmingham: Birmingham City Council, 1996; Northamptonshire County Council, *Census Atlas of Northamptonshire*. Northampton: NCC, 1995; OPCS, *Ward and Civil Parish Monitor* (Census 1991). London: OPCS, 1994. Information was also obtained from relevant Education Departments.

REFERENCES

Adams, J. (1995) *Risk*. London: UCL Press.

Backett-Milburn, K., Harden, J., Scott, S. and Jackson, S. (1999) 'Risk anxiety, safety and health: everyday accounts of children and their parents'. Paper presented at the Researching for Health Conference, Edinburgh, Heriot-Watt University, September.

Beck, U. (1992) *Risk Society: Towards a New Modernity*. London: Sage.

Davis, A. and Jones, L. (1996a) 'Children in the urban environment: an issue for the new public health agenda', *Health and Place*, 2 (2): 107–13.

Davis, A. and Jones, L. (1996b) 'Environmental constraints on health: listening to children's views', *Health Education Journal*, 55: 363–74.

Davis, A. and Jones, L. (1997) 'Whose neighbourhood? Whose quality of life? Developing a new agenda for health in urban settings', *Health Education Journal*, 56: 363–74.

Department of Health (1999) *Saving Lives: Our Healthier Nation*. London: HMSO.

Hillman, M., Adams, J. and Whitelegg, J. (1990) *One False Move: A Study of Children's Independent Mobility*. London: Policy Studies Institute.

Jones, L. (1998) 'Inequality in access to local environments: the experiences of Asian and non-Asian girls', *Health Education Journal*, 57: 313–28.

Jones, L. (1999) 'Young people at risk? Researching the impact of transport policy on health and wellbeing'. Paper presented at the Researching for Health Conference, Edinburgh, Heriot-Watt University, September.

Jones, L., Davis, A. and Eyers, T. (in progress) 'Young people, risk and health: comparing access and independent mobility in high, medium and low density environments'.

Joshi, M.S. and Maclean, M. (1995) 'Parental attitudes to children's journeys to school', *World Transport Policy and Practice*, 1 (4): 29–36.

Lupton, D. (1995) *The Imperative of Health: Public Health and the Regulated Body*. London: Sage.

Roberts, I. and Coggan, C. (1994) 'Blaming children for child pedestrian injuries', *Social Science and Medicine*, 38 (5): 749–53.

communities, and recommends a framework for developing the role of participatory arts initiatives in public policy.

BACKGROUND

Over the last 10 years it has increasingly become accepted that the arts play an important role in the economic life of the country. These arguments have informed public policy, especially in urban renewal, and underpin much recent political thinking on the arts. But they have two flaws:

- They tend to focus on financial issues rather than on economics in its deeper sense as the management of society's resources.
- They miss the real purpose of the arts, which is not to create wealth but to contribute to a stable, confident and creative society.

Those who work in the arts, especially in the participatory sector, have long argued that they produce positive social impacts. But they have had very little independent evidence with which to support that contention. Indeed, some argue that such qualitative benefits cannot be evaluated at all.

This research was designed to add a dimension to existing economic and aesthetic rationales for the arts by looking at their role in social development and cohesion. Given the complexity involved, the study was undertaken as a first step into this area, with two aims:

- to identify evidence of the social impact of participation in the arts at amateur or community level;
- to identify ways of assessing social impact which are helpful and workable for policy-makers and those working in the arts or social fields.

To this end, case study research was undertaken in Batley, Bolton, Hounslow, London, Nottingham, Sandwell, Portsmouth, Northern Scotland, Derry, Helsinki and New York. Additional research included the use of a questionnaire for participants. A series of working papers on various aspects of social impact of the arts, including research in Australia and the USA, was published. The methodology included questionnaires, interviews, formal and informal discussion groups, participant observation, agreed indicators, observer groups and other survey techniques, as well as desk research. None was satisfactory in itself, but each contributed to a multidimensional understanding of project outcomes.

PRINCIPAL RESEARCH FINDINGS

The research divided the social impact of participation in the arts into six different themes, relating to people as individuals or community change; there is obviously a degree of overlap between them.

Personal development

Participation in the arts can have a significant impact on people's self-confidence, and as a result on their social lives. Many participants go on to become involved in other community activities or personal development through training. In some cases, like the V & A Mughal Tent project, people feel they have gained more control over how they are seen by friends and family. In others, the arts work has provided groups with an opportunity to think about their rights and social responsibilities. Most participants have gained practical and social skills which they feel will help them in their working and home lives. Teachers identified educational benefits to schoolchildren in several areas including language development, creativity and social skills. A significant proportion of adult participants have been encouraged to take up training or education opportunities. Some people, especially those working with digital technology, have found work as a result of being involved, while many more believe that their new skills and confidence will make it easier for them to get jobs. The research found that among adult participants:

- 84 per cent feel more confident about what they can do
- 37 per cent have decided to take up training or a course
- 80 per cent have learnt new skills by being involved

Social cohesion

Participatory arts projects can contribute to social cohesion in several ways. At a basic level, they bring people together, and provide neutral spaces in which friendships can develop. They encourage partnership and co-operation. Some projects, like Portsmouth's home festival, promote intercultural understanding and help recognize the contribution of all sections of the community. The arts are also important means of bringing young and old together, and projects in Batley showed the value of these intergenerational contacts, especially in reducing anxiety about young people. There was also evidence that the community development aspects of participatory arts projects could help reduce fear of crime and promote neighbourhood security. Projects involving offenders in the UK, the United States and Australia also show important rehabilitation benefits. The research found that among adult participants:

- 91 per cent have made new friends
- 54 per cent have learnt about other people's cultures
- 84 per cent have become interested in something new

Community empowerment and self-determination

Taking part in local arts projects is a popular way of becoming involved in community activities; (it is one of the top six reasons for volunteering in the UK). As a result it helps build organizational skills and capacity, as seen, for example, in almost 30 *feisean* (Gaelic festivals) which have grown up recently across the Scottish Highlands and Islands. Skills learnt in the arts can be applied to other local projects: in South Uist, the *feis* organizer has gone on to establish a major women's training organization with EU funding. Participatory arts projects can also be empowering, and help people gain control over their lives – sometimes, as with Acting Up's work with severely disabled people, in a very practical sense. They can also play a vital role in the regeneration process, facilitating consultation and partnership between residents and public agencies. Arts projects can nurture local democracy. They encourage people to become more active citizens, and strengthen support for local and self-help projects. The research found that among adult participants:

- 86 per cent want to be involved in further projects
- 21 per cent have a new sense of their rights

Local image and identity

Participatory arts projects have an important role in celebrating local cultures and traditions such as the York Mystery Plays. In new areas they can help develop local identity and belonging, as the living Archive project in Milton Keynes has sought to do. The arts can affirm the pride of marginalized groups, and help improve their local image. Participatory projects can encourage people to become involved in environmental improvements and make them feel better about where they live. They can also help transform perceptions of public agencies and local authorities, renewing the public image of cities for their own citizens, as well as outsiders. The study found among adult participants:

- 40 per cent feel more positive about where they live
- 63 per cent have become keen to help in local projects

Imagination and vision

Participating in the arts made a big difference in developing people's creativity and confidence about the arts. For many, this was simply enjoyable and liberating, but professionals in teaching, social services, health, housing, countryside services and other areas said it had changed how they saw their work. Workers in Batley, Nottingham, Portsmouth and elsewhere intended to change their practice to use the arts in future. Projects had also helped public bodies to be more responsive to the views and interests of their users. Their creativity and openness encouraged people to take positive risks, both personally and organizationally, with far-reaching benefits. Arts projects could embody people's values and raise their expectations. The study found that:

- 86 per cent of adult participants have tried things they haven't done before
- 49 per cent think taking part has changed their ideas
- 81 per cent say being creative was important to them

Health and well-being

The research did not look at arts in health care, but there was considerable evidence that participating in arts projects could make people feel better. Projects in Nottingham, Durham and Portsmouth were making very positive contributions to supporting mental health service users and other vulnerable people. In Batley, Sandwell and London, arts work with young people produced important health education resources. Finally, it was very clear that people derived great pleasure from being involved in arts activities, and that it added greatly to their quality of life. The study found that among adult participants:

- 52 per cent feel better or healthier
- 73 per cent have been happier since being involved

Counterweight

The study found some costs and problems to set against these positive impacts. Participatory arts projects can fail or underachieve for a variety of reasons, including inexperience and under-resourcing. Since they are part of a continuum of experience, positive outcomes can turn sour if the work is not built on. It must also be recognized that people can experience personal costs (e.g. in relationships) especially where their lives do change and growth puts existing situations under pressure.

Economic impacts

Although the study did not address economic impacts, some issues arose, including the contribution to local economies made by the invisible voluntary labour of all the people who make participation in the arts possible. At a time when education and training are at the top of the political agenda, this represents a boost to the country's education resources worth hundreds of millions of pounds. It is also a significant contributor to other public services, including child care, social services, health promotion and crime prevention, sometimes directly and sometimes through expenditure savings. The work is often paid for (where there is a financial transaction) out of communities' existing resources, with marginal support from the state.

Social policy and the arts

The study concludes that participatory arts projects are essential components of successful social policy, helping to turn houses into homes. They can open critical dialogue between service users and providers, and avert costly mistakes. They involve people missed by other initiatives and introduce creativity, meaning and communication into the equation. They offer flexible, responsive and cost-effective solutions: a creative, not a soft option. Social policy would benefit from a marginal repositioning of priorities to make use of them.

The arts and social policy

The arts also have a responsibility, at least so long as they are in receipt of public funds, to consider their existing or potential contribution to society's wider goals. They should recognize their dependence on the audiences, new talent and creative ideas which the participatory sector develops. They have nothing to fear from such projects, especially not falling standards: a culture which needs protecting from people's participation is not worth the name.

Building a creative environment

The study reached a number of conclusions about the social impact of participation in the arts, the most important of which being that:

- participation in arts activities brings social benefits;
- the benefits are integral to the act of participation;
- the social impacts are complex but understandable;
- social impacts can be assessed and planned for.

In short, it concludes that the arts have a serious contribution to make in addressing contemporary social challenges. Rather than the cherry on the policy cake to which they are so often compared, they should be seen as the yeast without which it fails to rise to expectations.

The study sees the creativity, openness and elasticity of the arts as the roots of their social impacts. Since these may appear hard to integrate into public policy the study recommends focusing on planning an environment in which participatory arts projects can succeed. It suggests that this could be based on seven core principles:

1   clear objectives
2   equitable partnership
3   good planning
4   shared ethical principles

5   excellence
6   proportional expectations
7   joint evaluation

Participatory arts projects built on these principles lay sound foundations of internal success and are most likely to produce positive social
outcomes. Indicators of social impact are not difficult to establish or use
in this framework, and arts projects can be evaluated consistently and
integrated with mainstream public policy.

FIFTY SOCIAL IMPACTS OF PARTICIPATION IN THE ARTS

This list has been drawn up to give a sense of the range of social
outcomes which the study has shown can be produced by participatory
arts projects. Naturally, it is not complete, and there are many others
which might emerge from a different analysis. Equally, no single project
should be expected to deliver all of them, or to produce outcomes in the
same way or to the same degree.

The study shows that participation in the arts can

1   Increase people's confidence and sense of self-worth
2   Extend involvement in social activity
3   Give people influence over how they are seen by others
4   Stimulate interest and confidence in the arts
5   Provide a forum to explore personal rights and responsibilities
6   Contribute to the educational development of children
7   Encourage adults to take up education and training opportunities
8   Help build new skills and work experience
9   Contribute to people's employability
10 Help people take up or develop careers in the arts
11 Reduce isolation by helping people to make friends
12 Develop community networks and sociability
13 Promote tolerance and contribute to conflict resolution
14 Provide a forum for intercultural understanding and friendship
15 Help validate the contribution of a whole community
16 Promote intercultural contact and co-operation
17 Develop contact between the generations
18 Help offenders and victims address issues of crime
19 Provide a route to rehabilitation and integration for offenders
20 Build community organizational capacity
21 Encourage local self-reliance and project management
22 Help people extend control over their own lives
23 Be a means of gaining insight into political and social ideas
24 Facilitate effective public consultation and participation
25 Help involve local people in the regeneration process

PRIMARY PREVENTION: POPULATION OR INDIVIDUALS

Examples from primary prevention can be used to show how prevention may benefit the whole population or merely individuals. Most people remain healthy, so preventative measures applied to the whole population can prove very expensive when, compared to treating only those who develop the disease, only a few benefit. However, primary prevention includes public health schemes aimed to benefit every individual in the community. An example of this is the addition of fluoride to water supplies to try to reduce the incidence of dental decay. Even though such a scheme may be expensive, it benefits very large numbers of people so is more likely to be most cost-effective. This type of environmental manipulation contrasts with personal preventative measures like vaccination. Tuberculosis is now relatively rare in Britain but the policy of mass vaccination of children with BCG vaccine assumes that all people are equally susceptible to the illness. In the past, more children would have been expected to benefit from this prevention. Now, since the disease is less common, fewer are likely to derive benefit in terms of preventing an infection that would otherwise have occurred. However, all are exposed to the risks such as side effects of the vaccine. It has been estimated that in 1968, 750 children needed a BCG vaccination to prevent one notified case of tuberculosis but by 1978 this number had risen to 3000 children (Barker and Rose, 1990). Nowadays it may be more cost-effective merely to vaccinate high-risk children, such as Asians, and to treat the few cases that occur outside such groups. This illustrates the fact that health promotion schemes need to be constantly evaluated, as well as initially validated, to ensure that they are still more cost-effective than treatment.

SCREENING: POPULATIONS OR INDIVIDUALS

Screening the whole population can be less expensive than treating cases of disease even if not everyone would have developed the disease without the measures taken after a positive result on a screening test. Examples of this occur in the field of pre-natal diagnosis and neonatal testing. However, before this is considered, it is useful to be aware of the requirements of a screening test. These are:

- ability to detect disease at a stage when early treatment will provide a superior prognosis to treatment at a later stage;
- sufficient sensitivity to detect the disease at an early stage;
- sufficient specificity to distinguish the disease from non-specific changes;

- cost-effectiveness;
- simpleness of administration;
- acceptability to those undergoing screening.

Two diseases, congenital dislocation of the hip and phenylketonuria, demonstrate how prevention by screening the whole population can be less expensive than curing or treating the condition. Phenylketonuria is a rare inborn error of metabolism leading to learning disability. Since it is so rare, with an incidence of only one in 20,000, it may be thought that screening the whole population of babies with the Guthrie test may not be cost-effective. Indeed, Carter (1976) has estimated the cost of detecting a single case of the disease as being £6,000 and the follow-up treatment to result in a cost of £37,000. But phenylketonuria imposes a significant need for lifelong care due to the resultant learning disability. An affected individual, in an institution for 30 years, was estimated to need £46,800 worth of institutional care. When this whole idea of treatment of the disease is considered, it is clearly seen that prevention of phenylketonuria is less expensive than dealing with the condition once it is established. Congenital dislocation of the hip is more common, with an incidence of around one in 600, and treatment of the condition in childhood is relatively successful. However, it is still better to employ secondary prevention by screening for dislocation during routine neonatal clinical examinations. At this time treatment is fairly simple; the legs merely requiring splinting. If the condition is not detected until the child walks, then surgery is needed and poorer results tend to be obtained. The preventative measure in neonates is cheap and easy to employ. It avoids substantial extra costs and emotional pain involved in trying to cure an established dislocation of the hip.

However, not all population screening is less expensive than cure of the disease. This varies for each condition and each test. It can be illustrated with an example from pre-natal screening. Pre-natal diagnosis does not fit the criteria for a screening test in that it does not allow treatment as such for the condition. However, it is preventative in that a positive result enables the chance to abort the foetus. It is for this reason that pre-natal diagnosis is regarded as a screening procedure. Amniocentesis is often used to detect cases of Trisomy 21, Down's syndrome, in high-risk pregnancies, especially those of mothers over the age of 40 years. Since numerically more Down's syndrome babies are born to so-called low-risk mothers under the age of 35, it may be argued that it would be cost-effective to offer amniocentesis to all pregnant women. However such a scheme would be extremely expensive. The cost of investigation would be less than the potential cost of caring for affected individuals due to the low incidence and greater number of pregnancies occurring in younger women (Hagard and Carter, 1976).

also illustrates the fact that it is not always possible to directly extrapolate the results of clinical trials to the whole population.

Further factors relating to prevention and treatment can be discussed by comparing ovarian and endometrial cancer with cancer of the cervix. In the former two conditions mass screening programmes have not yet been found to be cost-effective compared to treating the disease. In the case of endometrial cancer this is more related to the success of treatment since the disease tends to present early, at a stage when many patients can be cured. However, for ovarian cancer the disease tends to present late when permanent cure is unlikely. In this case the lack of a preventative approach relies more on the lack of technique to detect the cancer much earlier. As yet, there is no known pre-malignant form of ovarian cancer and screening tests are not very successful at picking up small, non-metastatic deposits. Various studies have used ultrasound or tumour markers to screen for ovarian lesions. Due to the relatively low incidence of the disease, it was uneconomical to screen the entire female population. It was more cost-effective to screen high-risk women, those with a positive family history of ovarian cancer in close relatives, but this still does not yet appear to be better than treatment on a national scale. However, clinical trials on secondary preventative schemes are currently continuing so the situation may change in the future.

PREVENTATIVE IDEAS APPLIED TO TREATMENT

So far prevention and cure have been considered basically as separate issues. However, it is often less expensive to employ preventative measures than treatments. This is the basis of prophylaxis as compared to managing acute exacerbations of conditions as they occur. An illustration of this point can be found in the case of asthma. Blainey et al. (1990–91) looked at the costs of treating asthmatics and the treatment of their condition. It was estimated that there was unnecessary morbidity and mortality from asthma, largely due to the underuse of preventative therapy. This was found to lead to an increased admission rate. The problem was not just due to patients – apparently in only five of 35 patients presenting to their GP in the week prior to emergency hospital admission, had appropriate prophylactic changes to the medication been made. Using 1988 costs Blainey and his colleagues estimated the daily cost of an acute medical bed to be £88.30. Extrapolated nationally this led to a potentially preventable £3 million. Although the study did not indicate whether the extra cost of prophylactic drugs was deducted from the cost of hospital stay, the increased cost (let alone increased anxiety and social disruption) is likely to have been substantial. Such a study demonstrates the need to consider prevention even if a specific preventative scheme, in terms of screening for a disease, is not in operation.

CONCLUSIONS

There is a widespread belief that, because it reduces the need for high-cost treatment, prevention is cheaper than cure but this is not necessarily true. It cannot be assumed that even if a disease is detected before symptoms occur, the prognosis following treatment is necessarily improved. The optional strategy for prevention or treatment needs to be decided. Costs and benefits of prevention can vary markedly according to the size of the programme, selection of individuals, frequency of intervention and technological innovation or changing health trends.

REFERENCES

Barker, D.J.P. and Rose, G. (1990) *Epidemiology in Medical Practice*. London: Churchill Livingstone.

Blainey, D., Lomas, D., Beale, A. and Partridge, M. (1990–91) 'The cost of acute asthma – how much is preventable?', *Health Trends*, 22 (4): 151–3.

Carter, R.A. (1976) 'The value of screening in paediatrics', *Journal of the Royal College of Physicians*, 10 (2): 153–60.

Fowler, G. and Mant, D. (1990) 'Health checks for adults', *British Medical Journal*, 300: 1318–20.

Hagard, S. and Carter, F.A. (1976) 'Preventing the birth of infants with Down's Syndrome: a cost-benefit analysis', *British Medical Journal*, 1: 753–6.

Hypertension Detection and Follow-up Program Co-operative Group (1979) 'Five-year findings of the hypertension detection and follow-up program', *Journal of the American Medical Association*, 242 (2): 2562–71.

McCormick, J.S. (1989) 'Cervical smears: a questionable practice?' *The Lancet*, 2: 207–9.

MRC Working Party (1985) 'MRC trial of treatment of mild hypertension', *British Medical Journal*, 291: 97–104.

Royal College of Physicians of London (1991) *Preventative Medicine*. London: Royal College of Physicians.

18

Is Research into Ethnicity and Health Racist, Unsound, or Important Science?

Raj Bhopal

Epidemiology aids health policy and planning and helps discover the laws governing health and disease. As with other sciences (Osborne et al., 1978), epidemiology has been beguiled by ethnicity and race (Polednak, 1989) and has become racialized. Racialization consists of the idea that race is a primary, natural and neutral means of grouping humans and that racial groups are distinct in other ways, such as their behaviour (Ahmad, 1993). Racialism is the belief in the superiority of some races. In this chapter I draw lessons from the racialized research of the nineteenth century, discuss the terms *race* and *ethnicity*, and analyse the value of and problems with research into ethnicity and health.

RESEARCH ON RACE: A HISTORICAL LOOK

Racialized research has an inglorious history: scientists have been besotted by race and ethnicity, while politicians and social commentators have encouraged them. In the nineteenth century scientists ranked races on their biological and social worth, particularly using measurements of the size and shape of the head and the contents of the brain to measure intelligence (northern European groups always ranked top) (Barkan, 1992; Gould, 1984; Stepan, 1982). Such research was used to justify slavery, imperialism, anti-immigration policy, and the social status quo (Ahmad, 1993; Barkan, 1992; Stepan, 1982). One underlying value of this research was that biology determined social position – that is, biological determinism. The power behind scientific racism is shown by the prowess of some of the researchers, who included Louis Agassiz, Francis Galton, Paul Broca and John Down (see Gould for details of their contributions).

Medical practitioners contributed to racialized science. 'Diseases' such as drapetomania (irrational and pathological desire of slaves to run away) and dysaethesia Aethiopica (rascality) were invented. To quote a textbook, 'the pelves becomes increasingly lower and broader the more

First published in *British Medical Journal*, 314, 14 June 1997: 1751–6.

civilised the race from which it is obtained', and, 'coloured children weigh considerably less than white, a fact which, in large cities at least, is indicative of the physical degeneration which characterises the race' (Whitridge Williams, 1926). The importance of race research and the innate inequality of races was considered self-evident, and few scientists questioned whether their work was ethical (Barkan, 1992).

CURRENT VIEWS ON RACE AND ETHNICITY

Humans are one species: races are not biologically distinct, there is little variation in genetic composition between geographically separated groups, and the physical characteristics distinguishing races result from a small number of genes that do not relate closely to either behaviours or disease (Kuper, 1975). Massive effort over 150 years to classify races has largely failed, though we use crude classifications which trace their heritage to Linnaeus, based on the division of populations as *Homo Afer* (synonyms: black, Negro, Negroid), *Homo Europaeus* (synonyms: white, Caucasian, Caucasoid), *Homo Asiaticus* (Mongoloid), and *Homo Americanus* (American Indian). Variants of these classifications also have a grouping for Australian Aborigines (Kuper, 1975; Osborne et al., 1978). Most complex classification has been forgotten.

Haddon and Huxley recommended that the race be replaced by ethnic type (Stepan, 1982), an idea enjoying much support and some criticism. None the less, race remains important in modern thinking, though increasingly it reflects geographical, social and class divisions rather than biological ones (Smaje, 1995). The term 'race' is often used alongside ethnicity (Ahmad, 1993; Polednak, 1989). While arguing for abandoning race, Huth did not see problems with ethnic identification (Huth, 1995).

Ethnicity

The taboo surrounding research into race (Barkan, 1992), greater under-standing of social and cultural factors in health and disease (Ahmad, 1993; Senior and Bhopal, 1994; Smaje, 1995), and the need to describe the health and health care of people from ethnic minorities created the spur for new terminology (Senior and Bhopal, 1994), and ethnicity is at the fore. In the context of health it means a group that people belong to because of shared characteristics, including ancestral and geographical origins, cultural tradition and languages (Senior and Bhopal, 1994; Smaje, 1995). Ethnicity is a complex idea that has become a euphemism for race, and writers have not separated the concepts clearly. For example, a paper by Hopkinson constructed around race uses the ethnic groups as classified by the census (Hopkinson et al., 1994). Inability to use a clear definition of ethnicity echoes the past, when a consensus on the definition of race could not be achieved but was too important an idea to discard.

Ethnicity is a fluid concept and depends on context. For practical and theoretical reasons, the current preference is for self-assessment of ethnicity (Senior and Bhopal, 1994; Smaje, 1995). People change their self-assessment over time, as is their prerogative. The alternatives include skin colour, birthplace, ancestry, names, geographical origins, or a mixture of these. Ethnicity is not measurable with accuracy or validity (Senior and Bhopal, 1994). The question on ethnicity in the 1991 census worked only to the extent that people were willing to answer it, and the classification was arbitrary.

RESEARCH INTO ETHNICITY AND HEALTH

Expectations of researchers

Scientists want to discover the causes and processes of disease, while health policy-makers and planners want to meet the needs of ethnic minority groups. Historical analysis reveals motives such as a wish to reverse the health and social disadvantages of ethnic minority groups, curiosity about racial and ethnic variation, and an interest in ranking races and ethnic groups.

Studies of migrant groups help to separate the effects of environmental and genetic factors (Polednak, 1989). Leaving aside problems of bias and the difficulties of making comparable measurements across long distances, studies of migration could be a powerful means of generating and testing hypotheses. When both migrants and their offspring are compared with other ethnic groups the design is enriched. Changing circumstances within and between generations in different migrant and ethnic groups can be linked to changing health.

The message from most publications on ethnicity and health is that this opportunity must not be missed (Polednak, 1989). In *Biocultural Aspects of Disease* Henry Rothschild offered ethnicity as a paradigm for understanding diseases of complex aetiology (Rothschild, 1981). Marmot and colleagues' report *Immigrant Mortality in England and Wales* opens with the statement: 'Studies of mortality of immigrants are useful for pointing to particular disease problems of immigrants, investigating aetiology and validating international differences in disease.' (Marmot et al., 1984)

Black box epidemiology

Does such research discover aetiology? Thousands of associations between racial and ethnic groups and disease have been published with the promise that they will help in elucidating aetiology. The data are usually published in the style of aetiological epidemiology to show relative frequency of disease by means of standardized mortality ratios or similar measures (see Senior and Bhopal (1994) for a fuller discussion). Few variations have been explained in a way that gives new insight into aetiology (Smaje, 1995).

Most ethnicity and health research is 'black box' epidemiology – what Skrabanek described as epidemiology where the causal mechanism behind an association remains unknown and hidden ('black') but the inference is that the causal mechanism is within the association ('box') (Skrabanek, 1994). Skrabanek argued that science must open and understand the black box. He cited a review of 35 case-control studies of coffee drinking and bladder cancer which failed to provide important information and likened such epidemiology to repeatedly punching a soft pillow. David Savitz defended black box epidemiology, particularly for exploring new subjects, arguing that epidemiology may not be needed when other sciences have elucidated causal paths (Savitz, 1994).

Many studies have investigated patterns of cancer in immigrant, racial and ethnic minority populations (Barker and Barker, 1990; Bhopal and Rankin, 1996; Polednak, 1989). Marmot and colleagues' analysis of cancers in immigrants in England and Wales found many differences, but, overall, immigrants had lower cancer rates (Marmot et al., 1984). The researchers' aetiological focus is illustrated by their emphasis on causal hypotheses, of which many of interest were developed. They noted that international data for cancers of the large intestine and female breast showed high correlations with heart disease and fat consumption. Their observation of low rates of these two cancers in Indian immigrants but high rates of heart disease led them to question the assumption that dietary fat was the common factor in cancer of the large bowel and breast, and they queried whether the high fibre content of the Indian diet modified the effect of fat on large bowel cancer.

Balarajan and colleagues' study of immigrant populations by region of origin also found many differences from which they developed aetiological hypotheses, and they urged that data on ethnicity and health be used to develop more (Balarajan et al., 1984). Donaldson and Clayton found numerous ethnic differences in patterns of cancer registration in Leicestershire health district (Donaldson and Clayton, 1984). The authors rightly concluded: 'The results indicate the need for formal epidemiological study to test specific aetiological hypotheses which may account for these apparent differences.' This type of work has been repeated – for example, by Barker and Baker (1990) in Bradford, by Matheson et al. (1985) in Scotland, and by Balarajan and Bulusu (Osbourne et al., 1978). Similar work has been done on children. The conclusion is almost invariate – differences exist and need detailed study (Bhopal and Rankin, 1996).

However, there has been little progression beyond this black box epidemiology, since few studies have explored the ideas generated. One exception is the study of diabetes and insulin resistance in south Asian communities as the possible basis of their surprisingly high rates of coronary heart disease. Marmot et al. observed that 'The high rate of diabetes could contribute to the high rate of ischaemic heart disease in Indians. This explanation would then pose the problem of why immigrants from the Caribbean, with their high rate of diabetes, do not also have a high rate of ischaemic heart disease' (Marmot et al., 1984). This question is being pursued tenaciously.

We need to move from the repetitious demonstration of disease variations that have already been shown in research into ethnicity and health or in work on international variations or in social and sex variations – that is, stop punching the pillow – and move to new territory. Studies of ethnicity and health should be able to provide models and contexts for advancing aetiological knowledge if questions for research are clearly articulated and pursued with sound methods.

Is such research unsound epidemiology?

Much research into ethnicity and health is unsound (Stepan, 1982). The key variables of ethnicity and race are vaguely defined, and the underlying concepts are poorly understood and hard to measure (Senior and Bhopal, 1994). There is inconsistent use of terminology: for example, Asian, white, Caucasian, and Hispanic are common terms in research but have inconsistent and non-specific meanings (Bhopal et al., 1991). There are difficulties in collecting comparable data across cultural groups: for example, do questions on stress or alcohol consumption have equivalence across cultures? There are problems in recruiting representative and comparable population samples.

Data need to be adjusted for known confounding variables and interpreted with the recognition that adjustment is probably incomplete. These issues have been detailed elsewhere (Bhopal, 1990; Senior and Bhopal, 1994) Rigour is needed for sound epidemiology in ethnicity and health, but the literature is littered with elementary errors (Box 18.1).

There is little evidence that criticism of the methods and concepts of research into ethnicity and health (Bhopal, 1990; Senior and Bhopal, 1994; Smaje, 1995) has paid dividends. For example, while Marmot and colleagues' analysis of mortality in immigrants attempted to analyse ethnicity because country of birth was too crude (Marmot et al., 1984), an update using mortality data for 1980–82 did not even though there were then far more British-born people in ethnic minority groups (Balarajan et al., 1984).

While methodological errors may be apparent, it is more difficult to judge whether the research questions are valuable and whether the conceptual basis of the research (largely comparative) is sound.

Harm from such research

Osborne (1992) answered yes to the disturbing question of whether race-based research in medicine is racist. His review cites projects that focused on differences between blacks and whites in diseases associated with

---

Box 18.1: Basic errors in epidemiological studies of ethnicity

- *Inventing ethnic groups* – A study labelled a group as Urdus on the basis of the language spoken, thus inventing an ethnic group (Melia et al., 1998).
- *Not comparing like with like* – Inner city populations are different from whole population samples, but studies of ethnicity and health continue to focus on them for convenience – as in the recent Health Education Authority survey, in which the comparison population was not an inner city sample (Health Education Authority, 1994)
- *Lumping groups together* – A paper on smoking and drinking habits in British residents born in the Indian subcontinent did not describe sex and regional variations, creating the impression that smoking and drinking were unimportant in the 'Asian' population. As has been shown (Health Education Authority, 1994), and long known by people knowledgeable about populations of Indian origin, smoking and drinking are important problems in some subgroups. Heterogeneity in the prevalence of disease and risk factors has even been shown among different Hindu castes in one city in Tanzania. Yet journals still publish comparisons as crude as white and non-white (Smaje, 1995). The British attitude before 1940 was to blur the racial specificity of colonial populations (Barkan, 1992).
- *Not adjusting for confounding factors* – Inferences can change radically once interacting and confounding factors are accounted for: Lillie-Blanton et al. (1993) challenged the observation that crack smoking was commoner in African-Americans and Hispanic Americans and showed that once social and cultural factors were accounted for there were no differences.

---

promiscuity, underachievement and antisocial behaviour and which implied that the underlying explanation lay in race rather than class, lifestyle or socioeconomic status.

Perceiving ethnic minorities as unhealthy – The perception that the health of ethnic minority groups is poor can augment the belief that immigrants and ethnic minorities are a burden. The perception is at least partially false for some migrant groups, especially men, as shown in Table 18.1 (Balarajan et al., 1984; Marmot et al., 1984). There are variations by cause of disease, but overall standardized mortality ratios hover around the average for England and Wales. Bearing in mind inaccuracy in the denominator, the fact that those born in Britain have not usually been included, and that some deaths and illnesses are among visitors rather than residents, it is not clear whether the true rates are higher in most ethnic minority groups. The perception of poorer health arises from a focus on differences where the excess of disease is in the ethnic minority population (Senior and Bhopal, 1994). For many causes, morbidity and mortality are lower.

The focus on a few 'ethnic' problems (such as high birth rates, 'Asian' rickets', the haemoglobinopathies, and congenital defects said to be

Table 18.1 *Standardized mortality ratio (standardized to population of England and Wales) for all causes of death in England and Wales among people aged 20–69 by country of birth*

Country of birth	Men	Women
Indian subcontinent		
During 1970–72*	99	111
During 1979–83[†]	106	105
Caribbean Commonwealth countries		
During 1970–72*	95	131
During 1979–83[†]	79	105
African Commonwealth countries		
During 1970–72*	133	133
During 1979–83[†]	109	114

* Data from Marmot et al. (1984)
[†] Data from Balarajan and Bulusu (1984)

linked to consanguinity) has been at the expense of major problems (Bhopal and Donaldson, 1998; Senior and Bhopal, 1994). Health education material for ethnic minority groups in the 1980s tackled birth control, lice, child care and spitting, but there was nothing on heart disease and little on smoking and alcohol (Bhopal and Donaldson, 1998). The idea of a package of specific 'ethnic' diseases has echoes in history: Negro susceptibility to particular diseases such as leprosy, tetanus, pneumonia, scurvy and sore eyes was instrumental in 'branding blacks as an exotic breed', and the differences were explained by nonsensical hypotheses on causation (Kiple and King, 1981).

The comparative approach – Most research into ethnicity and health (including mine) is based on the comparative paradigm and presents data using the 'white' population as the standard (Senior and Bhopal, 1994). Inevitably, attention is focused on diseases that are commoner in ethnic minority groups than in the white population, thereby displacing problems like cancer and respiratory disease that are very common but less so than in the white population from their rightful place as high priorities for ethnic minority groups. A bibliography by Karmi and McKeigue stated: 'Although cancer is one of the key areas specified in the Health of the Nation white paper, it is not especially relevant to ethnic groups in Britain' (Karmi and McKeigue, 1993). This shows the danger of the comparative approach. Cancers are a major cause of death and disability in ethnic minority groups, and there is an opportunity to prevent some cancers reaching the high levels seen in the general population (Bhopal and Rankin, 1996).

Ignoring quality of services – The implications of comparative research, including the risk of ethnocentrism, is discussed in more detail elsewhere (Senior and Bhopal, 1994), and a strategy for setting priorities for ethnic minority groups is forthcoming (Bhopal, in press). The misperception that the needs of ethnic minorities are so different from those of the majority that separate strategies are necessary (but which may not materialize) provides a rationale for national strategy to exclude consideration of ethnic minority groups. The promise of aetiological understanding has meant a focus on variation in diseases, as opposed to the quality of services. There is a huge gap in the research record on the quality of care received by ethnic minority groups (Smaje, 1995).

Fuelling racial prejudice – Finally, racial prejudice is fuelled by research portraying ethnic minorities as inferior to the majority. Infectious diseases, population growth and culture are common foci for publicity. Following the release of statistics on the ethnicity of single mothers, the *Sunday Express* of 13 August 1996 had the headline 'The ethnic time bomb.' Toni Morrison wrote that 'A whip of fear broke through the heart chambers as soon as you saw a Negro's face in a paper', for this signalled exceptionally bad news (Bhopal et al., 1991). Researchers cannot be responsible for media reporting but must be aware of the potential impact of their work on race relations.

CONCLUSION

With hindsight, we can see that much race-oriented science in the past was unethical, invalid, racist and inhumane though it was perceived to be of great importance. *The Bell Curve* is a reminder that research which purports to demonstrate the innate inferiority of some racial groups continues and that race science is alive (Bhopal, 1990). Researchers need to understand how research into race and health was misused in the past. Epidemiologists should remember that warnings from disciplines incorporating anthropology and psychology may be based on harsh experience, for these disciplines played a leading part in racializing science (Barkan, 1992). Epidemiologists who remain unpersuaded that racial prejudice could influence science should read about the Tuskegee syphilis study, which examined the natural course of syphilis in 600 poor 'negroes' in Alabama, denying them effective treatments and hastening many deaths (Brandt, 1978).

Knowledge of the interplay of cultural, genetic and environmental factors is valuable, and research into race and ethnicity is one way to achieve it. Contemporary researchers also justify such research as necessary to help meet the needs of ethnic minority groups and point out that lack of data can hinder health policy. Inequalities in the health status of ethnic minority groups demand attention (Balarajan et al., 1984; Huth, 1995; Marmot et al., 1984). For these reasons, scientists' interest in the relation between race, ethnicity and health will increase.

Participation by ethnic minorities in research, policy-making and the development of services might be one safeguard against repeating the mistakes of the past. The American College of Epidemiology has called

Barkan, E. (1992) *The Retreat of Scientific Racism*. Cambridge: Cambridge University Press.

Barker, R.M. and Barker, M.R. (1990) 'Incidence of cancer in Bradford Asians', *J. Epidemiol Community Health*, 44: 127–9.

Bhopal, R.S. (1990) 'Future research on the health of ethnic minorities: back to basics. A personal view', *Ethnic Minorities Health*, 1 (3): 1–3.

Bhopal, R.S. (in press) 'Health needs assessment: setting priorities for health care for minority ethnic groups', in S. Rawaf and B. Vahl (eds) *Health Needs Assessment for Ethnic Minority Groups*. London: Department of Health.

Bhopal, R.S. and Donaldson, L.J. (1998) 'Health education for ethnic minorities: current provision and future directions', *Health Educ. J.*, 47: 137–40.

Bhopal, R.S. and Rankin, J. (1996) 'Cancer in ethnic minorities: setting priorities based on epidemiological data', *Br. J. Cancer*, 74: 522–32.

Bhopal, R.S. Kohli, H. and Rankin, J. (in press) 'Editor's practice and views on terminology in ethnicity and health research', *Ethm. Health*.

Bhopal, R.S., Phillimore, P. and Kohli, H.S. (1991) 'Inappropriate use of the term "Asian": an obstacle to ethnicity and health research', *J. Public Health Med*, 1: (13) 224–6.

Brandt, A.M. (1978) 'Racism and research: the case of the Tuskegee syphillis study', *Hastings Cent Rep.*, 8 (6): 21–9.

Donaldson, L.J. and Clayton, D.G. (1984) 'Occurrence of cancer in Asians and non-Asians', *J. Epidemiol Community Health*, 38: 203–7.

Gould, S.J. (1984) *The Mismeasure of Man*. London: Pelican.

Health Education Authority (1994) *Health and Lifestyles: Black and minority ethnic groups in England*. London: HEA.

Hernstein, R.J. and Murray, C. (1994) *The Bell Curve*. New York: Free Press.

Hopkinson, N.D., Doherty, M., Powell, R.J. (1994) 'Clinical features and race-specific incidence/prevalence rates of systemic lupus erythematosis in a geographically complete cohort of patients', *Ann. Rheum. Dis.*, 53: 675–80.

Huth, E.J. (1995) 'Identifying ethnicity in medical papers', *Ann. Intern. Med.*, 122: (6) 19–21.

Karmi, G. and McKeigue, P. (eds) (1993) *The Ethnic Health Biography*. London: North East and North West Thames Regional Health Authority.

Kiple, K.F. and King, V.H. (1981) *Another Dimension to the Black Diaspora*. Cambridge: Cambridge University Press.

Kuper, L. (ed.) (1975) *Race, Science and Society*. London: Allen and Unwin.

Lille-Blanton, M., Anthony, J.C. and Schuster, C.R. (1993) 'Probing the meaning of racial/ethnic group comparisons in crack cocaine smoking', *JAMA*, 269: 993–7.

Marmot, M.G., Adelstein, A.M. and Bulusu, L. (1984) *Immigrant Mortality in England and Wales 1970–78*. London: HMSO.

Matheson, L.M., Dunnigan, M.G., Hole, D. and Gillis, C.R. (1985) 'Incidence of colo-rectal, breast and lung cancer in a Scottish Asian population', *Health Bull. (Edinb.)*, 43: 245–9.

Melia, R.J.W., Chinn, S. and Rona, R.J. (1998) 'Respiratory illness and home environment of ethnic groups', *BMJ*, 296: 1430–40.

Morrison, T. (1993) *Beloved*. London: Chatto and Windus.

Osborne, N.G. and Feit, M.D. (1992) 'The use of race in medical research', *JAMA*, 267: 275–9.

Osbourne, R.T., Noble, C.E. and Wyel, N. (1978) *Human Variation: the Bio-Psychology of Age, Race and Sex.* New York: Academic Press.

Polednak, A.P. (1989) *Racial and Ethnic Differences in Disease.* Oxford: Oxford University Press.

Rothschild, H. (1981) (ed.) *Biocultural Aspects of Disease.* London: Academic Press.

Savitz, D.A. (1994) 'In defence of black box epidemiology', *Epidemiology*, 5: 550–2.

Senior, P. and Bhopal, R.S. (1994) 'Ethnicity as a variable in epidemiological research', *BMJ*, 309: 37–9.

Skrabanek, P. (1994) 'The emptiness of the black box', *Epidemiology*, 5: 553–5.

Smaje, C. (1995) *Race, Ethnicity and Health.* London: King's Fund Institute.

Stepan, N. (1982) *The Idea of Race in Science.* London: Macmillan Press.

Whitridge Williams, J.A. (1926) *A Text-Book for the Use of Students and Practitioners.* New York: D. Appleton.

PART IV

THE HUMAN SIDE OF HEALTH

This part of the book attempts to explore some of the interfaces between individualized views of health and health systems, and the more public or official accounts that cover the same subject areas. The papers selected have been chosen to represent a variety of *methodologies* or approaches that might throw light on these issues. Statistics, reflective practice, sociopolitical analysis, even physiological study and critical self-examination, all have their part to play in the study of human health, and these various modalities are sampled in this part of the reader. Some chapters here take individual experience of health concerns and explore their wider significance for health services and health policy. Others look more widely at global trends and pictures and use these to focus on possible meanings and implications for individual people. It is apparent, once again, that no single methodology or academic discipline can adequately cope with the complexity of 'human health', but together all these approaches have their part to play.

Kathy Davis (Chapter 19: 'My Body Is My Art') presents a challenging picture using descriptions of potentially disturbing 'performance art' to explore current conceptions of the 'perfect body' and its relation to health. This chapter describes the work of Orlan, a French performance artist who has had a series of plastic surgery operations 'performed' on her. The possibly cosy relationship between health and beauty is almost literally dissected and challenged as part of the feminist project to expose the fact that women are usually the subjects of manipulation and experimentation in the field of health. Orlan (and Davis) set out to 'shock, disrupt convention and provoke people into discussing taboo subjects'. It is probable that no change in attitudes or health care systems will indeed be possible without an element of confrontation and the stripping away of preconceptions.

Stephen Pattison (Chapter 20: 'User Involvement and Participation in the NHS') sets about the task of disrupting any conventional notions that public participation and involvement in decision-making within the NHS is straightforward, or even attainable. As a 'lifelong NHS user' at various levels, he uses his personal experience, as well as evidence from a considerable volume of published research, to outline the barriers, pitfalls and 'practicalities' of the use and abuse of 'ordinary' people within the health care decision-making system.

Donald M. Berwick (Chapter 21: 'Quality Comes Home') uses a similar methodology to explore the changes that would need to be made to a health care system to make it more likely to meet the needs of individual patients. In this instance he uses the experience of observing the 'care' that his father received while in various health institutions to draw widespread conclusions and make important strategic, policy and quality recommendations for those organizations. Although this chapter is based on experiences in the health care system within the USA, its observations, insights and conclusions are universally applicable.

The entirety of the experience of human health cannot be adequately explained by the use of statistics, but the detailed study of officially collected statistics is an important area from which significant insights can be gleaned.

Sarah Payne (Chapter 22: 'Masculinity and the Redundant Male') uses statistical material to focus on a major human problem. The individual experience of men, particularly young men, growing up in contemporary society is changing and this is reflected in various statistical data sets. 'By the end of the 1990s, figures show a continuing excess of young men in figures for both institutional psychiatric treatment and legal control in the criminal justice system.' Statistics can also act as pointers or indicate possible explanations for these social phenomena, which Payne does using the concept of 'redundancy'. Being considered redundant both at the workplace and increasingly in the home, the conjecture is that young men take solace in increasing numbers in 'more public expression of masculinity . . . one result may be an increased risk of being drawn in by the penal system. The other may be an increased risk of being hospitalized in the psychiatric system'.

Julie Taylor et al. (Chapter 23: 'Social, Economic and Political Context of Parenting') use a less statistical, but similarly broad social science perspective to explore intimate human interactions within their fullest context. For these authors the human experience of parenting, as a child and as a parent, must be 'understood in its social and economic context'. Those who would seek to judge parents and attribute various features of social disorder to 'poor parenting', should consider that, 'These families have experienced both acute and chronic material deprivation and it is reasonable to suppose that parenting styles have been directly affected by these factors'.

Aamra R. Darr (Chapter 24: 'Communicating the Implications of Genetic Disease') explores several issues concerned with increasing knowledge about the genetic basis of health and disease. For every human being, their genetic make-up is a central component of their individual, and possibly their entire family's, experience of health and illness. But how is information about this fundamental, but newly recognized, factor communicated? Darr uses quotations from a series of intimate interviews to draw out many of the relevant themes and discussions. This technique, largely taking the 'patient's' perspective, allows us to share some of the human experience involved in the discovery of genetic problems. The diverse cultural and ethnic complexities only serve to highlight the need for improved communication between people who might be affected and the professionals charged with looking after them.

Professionals may be more comfortable dealing with the component parts of human beings than with the complexities of the whole person in front of them. But when studying the human side of health, detailed physical and physiological pathways are also important to understand.

Gonneke Willemsen and Cathy Lloyd (Chapter 25: 'The Physiology of Stressful Life Experiences') looks at the way that stress and other features of living may actually create human illness, or indeed serve to protect people from disease. A review of the evidence of the 'psycho-biological' links between stress and disease leads these authors to conclude that, in humans at least, 'whilst the relationship between stress and disease has become more accepted by those working in health care provision, the exact nature of the links remains to be clarified.'

surgery viewable as an understandable and even unavoidable course of action in light of their particular biographical circumstances. I learned of their despair, not because their bodies were not beautiful, but because they were not ordinary – 'just like everyone else'. I listened to their accounts of how they struggled with the decision to have cosmetic surgery, weighing their anxieties about risks against the anticipated benefits of the surgery. I discovered that they were often highly ambivalent about cosmetic surgery and wrestled with the same dilemmas which have made cosmetic surgery problematic for many feminists. My research gave a central role to women's agency, underlining their active and lived relationship with their bodies and showing how they could knowledgeably choose to have cosmetic surgery. While I remained critical of the practice of cosmetic surgery and the discourse of feminine inferiority which it sustains, I did not reject it as an absolute evil, to be avoided at any cost. Instead I argued for viewing cosmetic surgery as a complex dilemma: problem and solution, symptom of oppression and act of empowerment, all in one.

Given my research on cosmetic surgery, I was obviously intrigued by Orlan's surgical experiments. While I was fascinated by her willingness to put her body under the knife, however, I did not immediately see what her project had to offer for understanding why 'ordinary' women have cosmetic surgery. It came as a surprise, therefore, when my research was continually being linked to Orlan's project.

In particular, two questions have begun to occupy my attention. The first is to what extent Orlan's aims coincide with my own; that is, to provide a feminist critique of the technologies and practices of the feminine beauty system while taking women who have cosmetic surgery seriously. The second is whether Orlan's project can provide insight into the motives of the run-of-the-mill cosmetic surgery recipient.

In this chapter I am going to begin with this second question.

ORLAN'S BODY ART

Orlan came of age in the 1960s – the era of the student uprisings in Paris, the 'sexual revolution' and the emergence of populist street theatre. As a visual artist, she has always used her own body in unconventional ways to challenge gender stereotypes, defy religion and, more generally, to shock her audience (Lovelace, 1995). For example, in the 1960s, she displayed the sheets of her bridal trousseau stained with semen to document her various sexual encounters, thereby poking fun at the demands for virgin brides in France.

Her present project in which she uses surgery as a performance is, by far, her most radical and outrageous. She devised a computer-synthesized ideal self-portrait based on features taken from women in famous works of art: the forehead of Da Vinci's *Mona Lisa*, the chin of

Botticelli's *Venus*, the nose of Fontainebleau's *Diana*, the eyes of Gérard's *Psyche* and the mouth of Boucher's *Europa*. She did not choose her models for their beauty, but rather for the stories which are associated with them. Mona Lisa represents transsexuality for beneath the woman is – as we now know – the hidden self-portrait of the artist Leonardo da Vinci; Diana is the aggressive adventuress; Europa gazes with anticipation at an uncertain future on another continent; Psyche incorporates love and spiritual hunger; and Venus represents fertility and creativity.

Orlan's 'self-portraits' are not created at the easel, but on the operating table. Each operation is a 'happening'. The operating theatre is decorated with colourful props and larger-than-life representations of the artist and her muses. Male striptease dancers perform to music. The surgeons and nurses wear costumes by top designers and Orlan herself appears in net stockings and party hat with one breast exposed. She kisses the surgeon ostentatiously on the mouth before lying down on the operating table. Each performance has a theme (like 'Carnal Art', 'This is My Body, This is My Software', 'I Have Given My Body to Art', 'Identity Alterity'). Orlan reads philosophical, literary or psychoanalytic texts while being operated on under local anaesthesia. Her mood is playful and she talks animatedly even while her face is being jabbed with needles or cut ('producing', as she puts it, 'the image of a cadaver under autopsy which just keeps speaking').

All of the operations have been filmed. The seventh operation-performance in 1993 was transmitted live by satellite to galleries around the world (the theme was omnipresence) where specialists were able to watch the operation and ask questions which Orlan then answered 'live' during the performance. Under the motto 'my body is my art', she has collected souvenirs from her operations and stored them in circular, plexi-glass receptacles which are on display in her studio in Ivry, France. These 'reliquaries' include pieces of her flesh preserved in liquid, sections of her scalp with hair still attached, fat cells which have been suctioned out of her face, or crumpled bits of surgical gauze drenched in her blood. She sells them for as much as 10,000 francs, intending to continue until she has 'no more flesh to sell'.

Orlan's performances require a strong stomach and her audiences have been known to walk out midway through the video. Reactions range from irritation to – in Vienna – a viewer fainting. While Orlan begins her performances by apologizing to her audience for causing them pain, this is precisely her intention. As she puts it, art has to be transgressive, disruptive and unpleasant in order to have a social function. ('Art is not for decorating apartments, for we already have plenty of that with aquariums, plants, carpets, curtains, furniture'). Both artist and audience need to feel uncomfortable so that 'we will be forced to ask questions'.

For Orlan, the most important question concerns 'the status of the body in our society and its future . . . in terms of the new technologies' In

Thirdly, a utopian response ignores women's suffering with their appearance. The visions presented by both Orlan and Morgan involve women who are not dissatisfied with their appearance as most women are; nor, indeed, do they seem to care what happens to their bodies at all. For women who have spent years hating their excess flesh or disciplining their bodies with drastic diets, killing fitness programmes or cosmetic surgery, the image of 'injecting fat cells' or having the breasts 'pulled down' is insulting. The choice of 'darkened skin' for a feminist spectacle which aims to 'valorize the ugly' is unlikely to go down well with women of colour. At best, such models negate their pain. At worst, they treat women who care about their appearance as the unenlightened prisoners of the beauty system who are more 'culturally scripted' than their artistic sisters.

Fourthly, a utopian response discounts the everyday acts of compliance and resistance which are part of ordinary women's involvement in cosmetic surgery. The surgical experiments put forth by Orlan and Morgan have the pretension of being revolutionary. In engaging in acts which are extraordinary and shocking, they not only entertain and disturb, but also distance us from the more mundane forms of protest. It is difficult to imagine that cosmetic surgery might entail *both* compliance *and* resistance. The act of having cosmetic surgery involves going along with the dictates of the beauty system, but also refusal – refusal to suffer beyond a certain point.

In conclusion, I would like to return to the young woman I mentioned at the beginning of this chapter. At first glance, her reaction might be attributed to her failure to appreciate the radicality of Orlan's project. She is apparently unable to go beyond her initial, 'gut level' response of horror at the pictures and consider what Orlan's performances have to say in general about the status of the female body in a technological age. She is just not sophisticated enough to benefit from this particular form of feminist 'shock therapy'.

However, having explored the 'ins' and 'outs' of surgical utopias, I am not convinced that this is how we should interpret her reaction. Her refusal to take up Orlan's invitation may also be attributed to concern. She may feel concern for the pale woman before her whose face still bears the painful marks of her previous operations. Or she may be concerned that anyone can talk so abstractly and without emotion about something which is so visibly personal and painful. Or she may simply be concerned that in order to appreciate art, she is being required to dismiss her own feelings.

Her concern reminds us of what Orlan and, indeed, any utopian approach to cosmetic surgery leaves out: the sentient and embodied female subject, the one who feels concern about herself and about others. As feminists in search of a radical response to women's involvement in cosmetic surgery, we would do well to be concerned about this omission as well.

REFERENCES

Davis, K. (1995) *Reshaping the Female Body. The Dilemma of Cosmetic Surgery.* New York: Routledge.

Lovelace, C. (1995) 'Orlan: offensive acts', *Performing Arts Journal*, 49: 13–25.

Morgan, K.P. (1991) 'Women and the knife: cosmetic surgery and the colonization of women's bodies', *Hypatia*, 6 (3): 25–53.

20

User Involvement and Participation in the NHS: A Personal Perspective

Stephen Pattison

How is it that despite statements by Health and Local Authorities that they consult users, users of mental health services still feel that they have little or no control over most of service planning or provision? (Garcia Maza, 1996)

The NHS was five years old when I was born in one of its maternity hospitals to one of its staff, 46 years ago. This makes me a lifelong NHS user. Occasionally, I have been a direct consumer, paying intermittent visits to my dentist or general practitioner. However, I have had more prolonged types of engagement with the service in other ways. During the 1970s and 1980s I worked as a part-time chaplain in the acute sector and mental health institutions. From 1988 to 1990 I was the paid chief officer of a Community Health Council (CHC), a much-criticized body established to represent patients' views and interests locally within the NHS (Coote and Hunter, 1996; Seale, 1993). Between 1990 and 1998, I worked at the Open University writing learning materials for health and social care professionals. Under the aegis of the consumerism that became fashionable around that time (Seale, 1993; Winkler, 1995), these materials on cancer prevention, disability, health and mental health attempted to model and provide a user-centred approach. Most recently, I have been appointed by my local health authority, after application and interview, to be the sole 'lay member' of the new Primary Care Group covering the area I live in. Together with seven GPs, two nurses, a social services representative, a Health Authority representative, and a senior manager, I am required to shape and take responsibility for health planning and services to meet the needs of the local population.

I guess all this experience should make me an expert about, and an enthusiast for, concepts like user participation, user involvement and public accountability in the NHS. I am pleased that the service has moved from seeing itself as medically run, ostensibly for the benefit of a faceless national population of 'patients', to regarding itself as having some responsibility for directly taking into account the views and preferences of its users, actual or potential. It seems correct in principle that the public should not be regarded as 'objects' of pro-fessionally determined health care. As users, citizens and taxpayers, the population of the country has a right and a responsibility to be involved in the shaping of health and health care in one of our largest public institutions.

That said, I find myself curiously unconvinced and uneasy about this whole area. The ideological transition from passive, invisible patients through consumerism to shared partnership with health care institutions and workers is mostly to be welcomed (Coulter, 1999; Johnson, 1977; NHS Management Executive, 1992). Nor do I doubt the value of the increasing number of effective techniques such as user panels, citizens' juries and focus groups that are now on offer for increasing user involvement, participation and consultation (Adams and Barnes, 1998; Audit Commission, 1999; Cooper et al., 1995; Coote, 1993). My unease stems from the suspicion that wishful thinking and idealistic myth rather than widespread, useful performance continue to characterize this area. As in religion (Pattison, 1997), one is required to have faith in user involvement and participation despite there being little hard evidence for its prevalence or effectiveness.

In this chapter I want to point up some of the continuing barriers to user participation and involvement from a personal perspective. Ideally, of course, it would be good to draw on extensive empirical evaluations. Unfortunately, these are relatively few and far between. Although there are isolated examples of 'good practice' and of projects where much was achieved, it is not clear that such projects are easily replicable (Audit Commission, 1999). Good practice in this area seems to require huge amounts of energy, determination and goodwill. The process is always vulnerable to misunderstanding, mistrust and misuse. This perhaps helps to account for the sense that while user participation is indeed possible and desirable, it is fragile and, like healing miracles, it often seems to happen 'somewhere else' rather than in one's own locality. Even when one has been urged to look at a 'beacon' of good practice somewhere, what one often sees is something different from what was claimed to be happening, or just the smouldering embers of a project that was once doing something useful.

OBSTACLES TO USER PARTICIPATION AND INVOLVEMENT

Who is the 'user'?

> (T)here is no single monolithic or uniform public but rather several publics each with its own particular values and preferences. (Hunter, 1997: 82)

Within a universally provided service, potentially every member of the population is, has been, or will be a NHS user. Those who are not active users now may well be in the future. Realistically, then, who is to be taken as the 'user' whose involvement and participation is to be sought and encouraged?

This immediately poses problems of selection, representation and legitimacy. If everyone is qualified by birth and citizenship to participate in the NHS, how is it possible to ensure that that participation is real and effective?

This problem is partly addressed in other public services by direct democratic control. Users of council services can be deemed to have a voice and some control because they directly elect representatives who supervise and monitor provision. In the NHS, there is a measure of direct democratic accountability through the Secretary of State for Health, himself accountable to Parliament. However, local Trust, Health Authority and Primary Care Group board members have no direct accountability to the local public. Nor do CHC members who are nominated through various means, none of which involve the ballot box. The net result is a 'democratic deficit' (Cooper et al., 1995). Accountability is upwards, ultimately to the Secretary of State, while the responsibility for shaping and delivering local services is to the local population.

Even if there were more effective *representative* local and national democracy within the NHS, this does not get over the problem of the lack of *participative* democracy whereby citizens really get involved with helping to shape health and health care services (Cooper et al., 1995). Particularly in the case of more informal, active participative democracy, the question arises, Who should be involved and in what ways? This is a surprisingly difficult issue to tackle once one moves away from direct election and accountability through the ballot box.

Although many citizens feel that public views should be taken into account in NHS policy-making and priority-setting, there is a significant proportion who feels that their active responsibility ends with electing democratic representatives to do this (New, 1999: 37). Understandably, most citizens do not wish to be users, yet alone shapers, of the NHS. They are often largely ignorant of or indifferent to a complex, professionally led service and may have little wish to be involved in it more than they absolutely need to be to get the care they need when they need it. They may want to avoid thinking about services associated with illness, death and unhappiness. It cannot be assumed, then, that people want actively to participate in debates about policy, particularly if they lack the information and knowledge they need to understand those debates (Hunter, 1997: 131).

If a cross-section of the general public is asked to opine about health and health services, their opinions may be of limited value. For example, they may tend to overvalue the importance of life-saving high technology as against other elements of service provision (Hunter, 1997: 82). They do not necessarily have the understanding required to make informed comments or decisions about complex services and issues. Furthermore, they may fail to have regard to the needs of minority groups such as people with mental health problems or learning difficulties (Hunter, 1997: 129). A 'dictatorship of the uninformed' majority can never be a substitute for the effective accountability of elected agencies (cf. Hunter, 1997: 86, 91).

If ordinary people do want to participate in the shaping of services, they may be overwhelmed by the complexity of a professionally oriented, large organization replete with jargon and esoteric vocabulary. Some people transcend these problems to become knowledgeable, articulate experts on services. They may then have much to contribute. However, by becoming experts, they are then no longer representative of the population at large. Furthermore, some of the 'wisest' consumers are people who have come to knowledge because they have had occasion to use the NHS in specific ways, e.g. for children, for mental health problems. This means that their knowledge may be very specialized – they may know little of cardiac or elderly care services. Furthermore, they may actually have a bias in favour of the services they use and implicitly against others. This makes them not only unrepresentative of the citizenry in general but also *parti pris* so that they may potentially damage the legitimate interests of other citizens with different needs.

Similar points could be made about groups of users. It can be argued that it is only when users get together that they are likely to have any chance of influencing service provision and decisions at all, because individuals can easily be picked off, dismissed or demoralized (Gabriel and Lang, 1995: 152ff.). However, powerful and effective user groups can easily be regarded by professionals, managers and policy-making groups as ignorant, unrepresentative, self-interested and partisan. This diminishes their perceived legitimacy.

Ordinary, averagely informed citizens and 'wise' consumers, whether singly or in groups, are unlikely to feel that the needs of minority groups, whether categories of user or cultural groups, are their most pressing concern. Thus people from numerically small ethnic groups such as Vietnamese people, or people who suffer from relatively rare diseases such as sickle cell anaemia, might find that their needs were neglected if the majority interest entirely determined priorities. Clearly this would be morally unacceptable to minorities and health workers alike. However, it would be equally unacceptable to run a health service whose shape and priorities were solely determined by vociferous minorities. The 'silent' majority, together with 'silent' or invisible minorities, must have their interests balanced and protected within the NHS.

It can be very difficult, practically and philosophically, to identify both individuals and types of user who should have a voice in the NHS. This problem precedes thinking about how participation might be enabled more effectively. Everyone is entitled to have their voices and interests taken acount of. But how should these be balanced out? Despite the proliferation of involvement and consultation methods, no one has been able to produce a formula that can guarantee the 'right' kind of balanced participatory democracy in the NHS or demonstrate the extent to which different kinds of users or citizens should be consulted or taken into account.

Levels of participation

Beyond trying to identify users to participate in various ways in the NHS there are important decisions about how and at what level they might be involved. Most users would expect to have some say in their own individual treatment as 'customers'. This is embodied in the need for informed consent. Minimally, there is some obligation upon health bodies to consult in some way with the public about plans and major service changes. However, such consultation can range from the cursory to the exhaustive. Some bodies set up patient panels to advise them on an ongoing basis about health issues and problems. Others tell people after plans have been made what their intentions are, and only then ask for feedback. Focus groups, citizens' juries, public meetings, information distribution, polls, referendums, questionnaires and electronic conferencing are just some possible ways of gathering public opinions about policies and services (Adams and Barnes, 1998; Audit Commission, 1999; Coote, 1993). However, in many instances even cursory methods of consultation are not well prosecuted and the results of consultation may have limited influence on final decisions and outcomes.

Beyond the consultative role lies that of greater accountability to users, and even user power. In this scenario, users might expect to be able to exercise some kind of direct choice and/or veto over plans and services provided. Although there are instances of users controlling their own services (usually by means of taking over the management of them), this is not a widespread option. It is difficult, for example, to envisage any advantage from users directly managing, say, casualty services. Yet it seems sensible, given their long experience and expertise, for people with long-term medical conditions to have a primary day-to-day role in shaping and running their own services (Garcia Maza, 1996; Wilson, 1999).

Over recent years, the impetus to user involvement and participation has mostly been directed at involving them in thinking about particular services or the needs of specific localities. However, local planning and provision is carried out within the framework of nationwide policies in a national service (Secretary of State for Health, 1992). This imposes strain and tension between localities and central government, and between the values of democracy and equity (New, 1999: 47f.). Local populations may have different ideas about what is desirable from national policy-makers and politicians. Within a sensitive, politically controlled service headed by a Secretary of State, it is unrealistic to think that decision-making, planning and service provision will ever be devolved entirely to users in particular localities. There are very good reasons why it should not be; some kind of equity and comparability across the country needs to be maintained. This poses limits to user participation and involvement that remain rather hazy, perhaps for reasons of political expediency.

Using and abusing user involvement and participation

Once appropriate users have been identified and the right levels and kinds of participation have been determined, there is still the issue of how users are used and abused within the system.

A potent inhibitor to increased user involvement and participation consists of the various kinds of low-key exploitation and abuse that users may be exposed to. At a basic level, users who do become involved in shaping policies and services may be unpaid while professionals are well rewarded for their input. They may have to attend meetings at times and places which are inconvenient to them and find they are outnumbered or patronized as 'token' users by professionals articulately representing vested interests. Their representativeness or integrity may be questioned (Crepaz-Keay, 1996) and their voices may be unheard or, worse, ignored. Subsequently, they may find that their engagement produces no tangible result that benefits them. At the same time, professionals and managers may legitimize their plans and service provision by reference to extensive user participation and consultation. All of which leads to disillusion, cynicism, and a sense of being exploited to no good purpose. Some users withdraw from consultation and participation exercises, worn down by the process and discontented with the outcome. A 'user-centred' high-level mental health policy steering group in one English city was unable to recruit a user to participate in its deliberations because user activists felt they would be better able to make an effective contribution to it by retaining total independence and lobbying from outside.

Another kind of user abuse is to be unclear as to the nature, extent, purpose and planned outcomes of user involvement. It is not uncommon for public authorities to consult or involve users on policy or operational issues without being clear about what users may expect as a result of their participation. Thus users may be consulted as to the closure of health facilities only to find that their views, however strongly stated or well reasoned, have already been discounted. At other times, users may feel that they have been promised influence or services only to have their wishes subverted by the authorities concerned.

In this context, there is only one thing worse than not being asked one's opinion, and that is to be asked – and then ignored. This, unfortunately, is a common experience for individuals and groups of users in the NHS. Sometimes, well-articulated user views are simply ignored outright; this does nothing to enhance the prospects of future involvement. At other times, users can find that their collaboration in creating plans and giving information brings about exactly the opposite result from the one that they had hoped for, leaving them with a feeling of having been duped or traduced. One group of people with learning difficulties who co-operated fully in plans for their resettlement found that once the plans were available they were then accelerated and modified, to their discomfiture and dismay (Malby and Pattison, 1999: 22).

Frequently, users are asked to opine on trivial things that do not matter or to which the solution is obvious, while they are allowed no say in larger matters such as planning and priorities. This may be appropriate because, in practice, health purchasing and providing bodies may have very little choice in what they are able to do (Hunter, 1997: 67). Much of their budget is irrevocably committed to basic services already. There is little point in involving users in decision-making and -shaping if there is little or no scope for real change.

A final, more subtle form of user abuse is to consult or involve users with a view to passing on to them difficult or unpopular decisions, for example about rationing. This kind of abuse can be a manipulative process which is neither rational nor moral, and it risks creating a 'dictatorship of the uninformed' while absolving duly appointed authorities from taking proper responsibility for decisions that should be theirs (cf. Hunter, 1997: 86f.). At least one English city has an unelected and uninformed panel of voters who 'vote' on all the policies passed by elected councillors. The outcomes of this second 'vote' either legitimize the councillors' actions or cause policy revision. Either way, this seems an unsubtle, wasteful and irresponsible way of gaining public participation. Politicians and policy-makers are supposed to lead public opinion, not just to reflect it.

Creating trusting, non-exploitative relationships between users and health care planners and providers is not easy. Trust can easily be violated or destroyed. This leaves an unfortunate and lasting legacy for the future.

Professional obstacles

There are probably few health care managers and professionals who would dare dismiss the idea of the importance of user participation and involvement in the NHS. Superficial assent to the concept is, however, a very different thing from active commitment and possessing the necessary skills to enable participation to happen. Thus Lamont notes of participation between patients and professionals that 'Regardless of the genuine intention to help and empower people, the reality of the participatory processes is often contradictory to the empowering principle' (Lamont, 1999: 783).

Few general practices or health care institutions have established user involvement or consultative groups, or do much to foster participation in consultation, planning or decision-making. None of the 23 general practices in my own Primary Care Group, for example, have such institutions.

Behind this reality lies a set of factors that are inimical to user involvement. Clearly, there are organizational and professional imperatives and changes that may make it difficult to find the time and energy to take on the views and interests of users more directly. Additionally, there is still vast ignorance, indifference, and even fear of users as active participants or partners in health care. One GP of my acquaintance recently volunteered that he saw CHCs as 'public enemy number one' because he perceived them to be hostile to doctors. In a discussion with another GP, I was told that 'GPs hate [*sic*] patients who come to see them with more than one or two problems at a time'. This was in response to a comment from me that I usually saved up my minor ailments and queries so that when I went to the doctor I would not waste their or my own time.

The lesson I learn from experiences like these, and from more systematic studies of health care professionals' attitudes (Annandale, n.d.), is that health care professionals have as much to learn about users as the latter do about the former if user–professional partnership is to become a reality. This finding is echoed by the director of the Long-term Medical Conditions Alliance:

> Member organisations . . . have . . . reported that patriarchal attitudes continue to exist among healthcare professionals. Although there have been changes . . . the lack of appropriate training in how to work in partnership with patients still prevents the appropriate use of patients' expertise and wisdom. (Wilson, 1999: 773)

This judgement is also valid at managerial and policy-making levels. Clearly, there are exceptions that prove the rule and professional 'bashing' through stereotyping condemnation is unlikely to make things any better. However, it would be wrong to minimize the size of the problem here.

Resources

User involvement and participation is demanding and complex; it needs a good deal of thought, energy, determination, clarity, skill and goodwill on all sides. To overcome the barriers described above, time and money must be expended. Often these are in short supply. Unfortunately, effective consultation and participation 'does not come cheap' (Coote, 1993: 41). Unless sufficient resources are made available, it may not be worth undertaking at all. Indeed, it might be argued that money and effort expended upon this activity when it is not carefully thought through and executed is wasteful of public resources – resources that the public might think (if consulted) should be put into service provision. User involvement and participation have emotional, time and financial costs. Sometimes, the costs may not be worth paying if no consensus can be arrived at, necessary decisions are delayed, or efficiency is put at risk

(New, 1999: 48f.). There can be a wasteful democratic 'surfeit' that may be expensive in terms of decisions unmade or wrongly made.

CONCLUSION: IS REAL USER PARTICIPATION AND INVOLVEMENT POSSIBLE?

Meaningful, imaginative user participation within the NHS is possible. There is a long way to go before it will become a generalized reality rather than an article of faith. Involvement and partnership are riven with complexities that defy simple solutions. In the short term, like rationing, it is more likely to be a matter of 'muddling through elegantly' (Hunter, 1997: 8), and in a variety of ways, rather than of finding a universal solution.

Amidst uncertainty and complexity I am certain of two things. First, effective, appropriate, useful user participation and involvement require adequate expenditure of financial and other resources. Secondly, there will be no useful user involvement and participation without more people (politicians, clinicians, managers and users) really wanting it to occur (Wilson, 1999: 773). Fifteen years ago, assessing the possibilities for a consumer focus in public services, Clarke and Stewart wrote: 'The problem is not *how* to get close to the customer but to want to do so' (Clarke and Stewart, 1985: 7).

REFERENCES

Adams, L. and Barnes, M. (1998) *In The Public Interest*. Wetherby: Department of Health.

Annandale, E. (n.d.) *Working on the Front Line: Risk Culture and Decision-Making in the New NHS*. York: ESRC Risk and Human Behaviour Programme.

Audit Commission (1999) *Listen Up! Effective Community Consultation*. London: The Audit Commission.

Clarke, M. and Stewart, J. (1985) *Local Government and the Public Service Orientation*. Luton: Local Government Training Board.

Cooper, L., Coote, A., Davies, A. and Jackson, C. (1995) *Voices Off: Tackling the Democratic Deficit in Health*. London: Institute for Public Policy Research.

Coote, A. (1993) 'Public participation in decisions about health care', *Critical Public Health*, 4 (1): 36–49.

Coote, A. and Hunter, D. (1996) *New Agenda for Health*. London: Institute for Public Policy Research.

Coulter, A. (1999) 'Paternalism or partnership?', *British Medical Journal*, 319: 19–20.

Crepaz-Keay, D. (1996) 'Who do *you* represent?' in J. Read and J. Reynolds (eds), *Speaking Our Minds*. Basingstoke: Macmillan.

Gabriel, Y. and Lang, T. (1995) *The Unmanageable Consumer*. London: Sage.

Garcia Maza, G. (1996) 'Structuring effective user involvement', in T. Heller, J. Reynolds, R. Gomm, R. Muston and S. Pattison (eds), *Mental Health Matters*. Basingstoke: Macmillan.

Hunter, D. (1997) *Desperately Seeking Solutions*. London: Longman.

Johnson, M. (1977) 'Patients: receivers or participants?' in K. Barnard and K. Lee (eds), *Conflicts in the National Health Service*. London: Croom Helm.

Lamont, S. (1999) 'Patient participation cannot guarantee empowerment', *British Medical Journal*, 319: 783.

Malby, B. and Pattison, S. (1999) *Living Values in the NHS*. London: The King's Fund.

New, B. (1999) *A Good-Enough Service*. London: Institute for Public Policy Research.

NHS Management Executive (1992) *Local Voices: Involving the Local Community in Purchasing Solutions*. Leeds: NHS Executive.

Pattison, S. (1997) *The Faith of the Manager's: When Management Becomes Religion*. London: Cassell.

Seale, C. (1993) 'The consumer voice', in B. Davey and J. Popay (eds), *Dilemmas in Health Care*. Buckingham: Open University Press. pp. 64–80.

Secretary of State for Health (1992) *The Health of the Nation*. London: HMSO (Cm 1986).

Wilson, J. (1999) 'Acknowledging the expertise of patients and their organizations', *British Medical Journal*, 319: 771–4.

Winkler, F. (1995) 'Transferring power in health care', in B. Davey, A. Gray and C. Seale (eds), *Health and Disease: A Reader*. Buckingham: Open University Press.

21

Quality Comes Home

Donald M. Berwick

Never before in the recent history of health care in North America has common sense been so uncommon. I sometimes feel as if I am watching an ant hill on which some passing hoof has trodden. So much scurrying. But to what end? Deming (1986) made 'constancy of purpose' the first and most crucial of his famous 'Fourteen Points for Top Leaders'. Today, 'constancy' seems furthest from our minds.

I was reminded recently with unwelcome vividness what constancy we really need – what, behind the chaos of mergers and acquisitions, downsizing and layoffs, budget cuts and price slashing, integrating and competing, is worth the trouble. It involved my father.

My father was a retired physician in rural Connecticut. For 42 years, he provided care as a general practitioner in the tiny town in which I grew up. Then he retired and found himself no longer giving care but receiving it. I do not know what he thought of health care reform. By the time the national issue became popular, my father was mentally unable to comprehend the debate. I don't think he knew what TQM stands for, and he probably would have defined 'reengineering' as changing the person who drives a freight train.

Of course, he did know quality. He was the guy who got up in the middle of the night because Jimmy had a high fever, or Mr Bernstein had a heart attack, or an awful car accident occurred at the drawbridge. I heard him speak rudely to patients sometimes, but I never saw him unconcerned. And, when I attended my 30th high school reunion in 1994, I was still Dr Berwick's boy. People could not wait to remind me of the time my father delivered their baby or themselves, or sewed a wound, or answered a tough question. They called him a great doctor. He was always there, they said. You could count on him.

My father retired in 1984 and not long afterward began developing symptoms of Parkinson's disease and mild dementia from small, multiple strokes. He remained alert but became progressively weaker until he fell at home and broke his hip in June of 1994. His housekeeper found him and called the ambulance.

First published in *Annals of Internal Medicine*, 125 (10), 15 November 1996: 839–43.

One of my brothers, who lives an hour from our father's home, rushed to the local hospital to meet him in the emergency department. He was told – in error – that our father was not there. Panicked telephone calls followed as my brother searched anxiously for our father's whereabouts until, finally, someone told him that our father was there, after all, and was about to be wheeled into the operating room.

After surgery, my father lay sedated on a special mattress containing sections that alternately inflated and deflated. Within a week, he had a deep pressure ulcer on his right heel. It was painful and interrupted his early ambulation therapy. He became restricted to a wheelchair for most of the day and gradually refused to walk at all. Unable to return home, my father needed to go to a rehabilitation facility, and my brothers and I searched hard for the best one. The signs pointed to a facility 20 miles from his home.

I visited him there on the morning after his admission. He was lying stuporous in the bed, on his back, with his ulcerated heel pressing into the sheets. His mouth was hanging open, and his eyes were rolled back into his head. I asked the nurse for an explanation. 'We sedated him,' she said. 'He was combative. He hit a staff member.' For 10 years, my father had had severe Parkinson's disease, and for most of that time he had been unable to voluntarily extend his own arm, much less throw a roundhouse punch. My father had undoubtedly been angry, yes. But a punch . . . no. I demanded that the sedation be stopped.

Not that it mattered much. For reasons that never became clear, the medication he took for Parkinson's disease, meticulously adjusted for two years by his physician at home, was summarily stopped when he was admitted to the rehabilitation facility. This resulted in a two-week siege of spasm and much decreased mobility. Not that that mattered much, either. By then, the pressure sore on his right heel had opened again, causing pain that prevented him from walking or even spending much time in a wheelchair.

Not that it mattered, because when my brothers and I asked that our father be placed in a wheelchair whenever possible, the nurses on the weekend shift told us that no wheelchairs could be found. They asked that we bring in his rickety old wheelchair from home. They eventually did find a wheelchair, but it was missing the footrest plate that would have protected his injured heel from bruising.

My father spent six weeks in the rehabilitation facility and then gave up, as did the staff. He returned home to a hospital bed and around-the-clock housekeeper coverage. Two weeks after he returned home – almost entirely bedridden and almost certainly never to walk again – a wheelchair finally came: the latest model, with postural supports, custom back rests, and hand controls he could never use. It was beautiful. The price: $6,000. It sat proudly and nearly totally unused in the corner of his bedroom.

It is very hard to convey the special sense of helplessness I felt as a participant in this. In a journal article (Berwick, 1994), I proposed 11 aims for clinical leadership of change that would really matter. 'Aim 5' called for more appropriate use of pharmaceutical agents, especially in the elderly, but I found my own father heavily oversedated with sleeping pills he did not need and dramatically undermedicated with the anti-Parkinson agents that he did need. 'Aim 8' was for the appropriate use of technology, especially in the last stages of life, but I found an excessively complex and nearly useless $6,000 wheelchair freighted to my father's home; a far simpler one could not be found during the week in which it would have made a real difference. 'Aim 7' asked that we decrease the amount of time spent waiting, but my brother sat uninformed and confused for too long in the waiting area of an emergency department. 'Aim 2' involved prevention, including prevention of injuries, but my own father, inevitably, fell at home. And, inevitably, he acquired a debilitating and totally preventable pressure ulcer that interrupted his rehabilitation irreversibly. I felt helpless. So did he.

SOME SUCCESS STORIES

Yet, behind my father's story, and beyond the anger, I now feel a sense of possibility. In the course of my work, I am privileged to see good news as well as bad. In place after place, I see throughout the health care systems of the United States and Canada an ever-increasing collection of glowing successes that rivet my attention. Some examples follow.

My father was oversedated; it did not need to be that way. At Intermountain Health Care's LDS Hospital in Salt Lake City, Utah, the director of critical care medicine, Dr Terry Clemmer, the nurse manager of that unit, Vicki Jensen Spuhler, and their colleagues worked for two years on safe sedation, substituting for new, expensive drugs a class of older, safer and less costly agents. Total savings for Intermountain Health Care have been $209,000, and far safer levels of sedation have been achieved for the patients in the intensive care unit

Dr Ken Petersen and his colleagues in paediatrics at the Alaska Native Medical Center in Anchorage have been working on improving sedation in children having computed tomography. As a result of their efforts, the rate of rescheduling procedures because of ineffective sedation decreased from 40 per cent in May 1993 to less than 1 per cent in September 1994.

Improvement in medication has been a goal of the infectious disease group at LDS Hospital since the mid-1980s. Through the group's work during the past eight years, antibiotic costs are down almost $50,000 per year and have decreased from 46 per cent to 13 per cent of the pharmacy budget. Duration of therapy has been shortened, and outcomes from infections have improved (Pestotnik et al., 1993, 1996).

My father was never successfully rehabilitated from his hip fracture because the rehabilitation system failed him at crucial points. It didn't need to be that way. Dr Bill Nugent, chair of cardiovascular surgery at Dartmouth Medical School, Lebanon, New Hampshire, and his team have reduced the median length of hospital stay after surgery and mortality rates from heart surgery by carefully preparing patients for postoperative care and rehabilitation.

Drs Michael Morris and Peter Mandt, orthopaedic surgeons at Virginia Mason Medical Center's Sports Medicine Clinic in Seattle, Washington, redesigned their repairs of anterior cruciate ligaments tears. Between 1993 and 1995, they reduced actual costs of care by $1,500 per patient, from $4,278 to $2,777, while sustaining clinical success rates of 93 per cent and a rate of returning to work at one year of 100 per cent.

My father's rehabilitation was permanently stalled by a pressure ulcer on his foot. It did not need to be that way. Prevention of pressure ulcers has been the subject of a major guideline by the Agency for Health Care Policy and Research. This guideline was studied and used by a team at LDS Hospital under the leadership of Carol Ashton. The team celebrated a decrease in ulcer rates on the medicine service – from 24 per cent in July to December 1992 to 2 per cent in July to December 1993. For the patients at highest risk, the rate of ulcers in that period decreased from 37 per cent to less than 10 per cent (Horn et al., 1994).

For my brother, the emergency department was a place to wait, questions unanswered, misinformed, anxious, but it didn't need to be that way. Carolyn Jackson and Dr Andrew Greene at Bethany-EHS Hospital near Chicago converted their emergency care for adults with asthma into the first step in a carefully designed sequence of patient and family education, evaluation and support. Between 1992 and 1994, returns to the emergency department decreased from 11.6 patients per month to 2.3 patients per month; rehospitalization rates were cut by 60 per cent; and inpatient length of stay decreased by 30 per cent. In Terry Clemmer's intensive care unit, careful work on improving communications with families over three years increased the rate of orientation of families within 24 hours of a patient's admission to the intensive care unit from 30 per cent to 98 per cent.

Through systematic improvement efforts, committed persons have achieved stunning success in areas ripe for clinical breakthrough. I have suggested that we can, if we wish, safely reduce the rate of Caesarean section in the United States from the current 24 per cent to less than 10 per cent (Berwick, 1994). Many health care professionals have doubted that this is possible, citing threats of malpractice suits and patient expectations. However, Drs Robert DeMott and Herbert Sandmire from Green Bay, Wisconsin, reduced the community-wide rate of Caesarean sections from 16.3 per cent in 1986 to 10.4 per cent in 1993 (Sandmire and DeMott, 1994). Dr Charles Guise, from the obstetrics services at the US Air Force Academy Hospital, reports that the rate of this procedure decreased from 17 per cent in 1989 to 6 per cent in 1993; during the same interval, the rate of vaginal birth after Caesarean section increased from 30 per cent to 85 per cent.

STEPS TO IMPROVEMENT

Improvement is within our reach. Not marginal improvement, but fundamental, breakthrough-level changes that are better for patients, families, clinicians and payers. My father need not have fallen, suffered, lain in bed, and never walked again. What will it take? As a start, I suggest five changes.

1. Change our focus from integrating structures to integrating experiences

I have serious doubts as to whether the current wave of mergers, acquisitions and reorganizations now sweeping into almost every large market in health care in 1996 will matter at all to persons like my father unless the leaders so engaged build on their new structures by asking themselves a simple question: 'Why should the people of this community – those who are sick or those who may become sick – care that this change in structure or ownership has occurred?' The answer, if it is honest, must relate to improving the experiences of care. As structures, our new 'integrated delivery systems' should not be end points in themselves. They matter in the long run only as foundations for redesigning the processes of care so that patients get better help. In my father's transition among facilities – from hospital to nursing home to rehabilitation facility to his home – he was in the care of five different teams of physical therapists. Five different evaluation forms were completed, with five different recommendations for five separate fees. The only evident transfer of evaluation documents occurred when I drove to the hospital, picked up a copy of the evaluation, and took it to the nursing home. There I was told, 'We never use outside evaluations.'

By contrast, integrating appointment processes in one portion of one region of Kaiser Permanente has reduced the waiting list for healthy-adult appointments from 2,000 to 0 in 3 months, while the total clinical staff required to supply those appointments decreased by 4 per cent.

2. Learn to use measurement for improvement, not just measurement for judgement

The dominant use of measurement in health care systems is what I call 'measurement for judgement', not 'measurement for improvement'. Report cards, benchmark comparisons, accreditation processes and employer-based performance surveys are all inspection-based systems, seeking data that can be used to make choices. The underlying strategy is to improve through culling, and it is a distant second-best to the real improvement that comes only through continuous effort and pervasive change. I fear the rush to collect information whose main effect will be to quell aspiration and invite dishonesty. Learning begins with curiosity, and curiosity is never totally safe. Public reports on health care performance may help to motivate change, but the responsibility to make changes that will actually help patients cannot be placed outside the system; it is we, inside, who must change.

Contrast reliance on culling with the approach that Bill Nugent describes as a support system for his team's dramatic improvements in cardiac outcomes over the past two years. In a recent letter to me, Nugent wrote,

> By continuously tracking our outcomes, we have found it much easier to organize ourselves. . . . We needed earlier warnings of statistically real problems. . . . We now rely on control charts . . . used to track input variables (e.g., patient demographics), process variables (e.g., intubation and length of stay), and outcome variables (e.g., mortality, morbidity, patient satisfaction, functional health). All this is now reported back in the form of a cardiac surgical instrument panel . . . In sum, I have worked to develop effective ways to collect high-quality clinical data and, more importantly, to use that data to improve outcomes.

3. Move beyond a naive search for 'best practices' to a much healthier mode of learning from each other

I recently asked my 15-year-old daughter, Jessica, an avid horseback rider, whether it would help her to see a video of the Olympic gold medallist in dressage so that she could copy her. 'I'd enjoy it,' said Jessica, 'but it wouldn't help me much.' Why? 'Because what I need to learn right now isn't what she would show me.'

This sensibility – seeing learning as a process, not a goal – characterizes the persons involved in the best improvements in health care. In reducing the rate of pressure sores by 80 per cent at LDS Hospital, Carol Ashton did not begin by seeking the lowest rates in the nation and then simply copying the practices used to achieve these. She began by seeking knowledge, help and insights and by involving her own colleagues in that undertaking. Hers was a step-by-step process, with infinite respect for the imagination and wisdom of the other adults with whom she worked. Members of Ashton's team avidly looked for ideas from outside their own system, but the solutions were inevitably and powerfully their own. And because the solutions were their own, they worked.

4. Shift our thinking from reduction of local cost to reduction of total cost

At Bethany Hospital, the dramatic gains outcomes for adults with asthma were accomplished in a resource-starved institution that treats the poorest of populations. Ask Carolyn Jackson how it was done, and she will begin by describing new initiatives in patient education, testing and information systems. It will at first be impossible to understand how this inner city hospital could possibly find the resources to improve until you hear Jackson make the case, as she did to her own managers and clinicians, on hard facts about total costs and benefits. 'We pay now,' she says, 'or we definitely pay later.' This was the argument, supported by data inside the hospital, that her team developed, but putting it into practice required a leadership that listened and was able to think about now and later at the same time.

I am troubled by the focus on reducing lengths of hospital stay as an end in itself. Deming (1986) warned against numerical goals, and this is one. We need to keep our minds on total costs, and it may even be that an extra day in the hospital is the best investment. We will miss that possibility if we fail to look. Integrated delivery systems may have a better chance at unifying views of cost, but that unifying will require many departures from classic, fragmenting assumptions about how budgets are made and monitored.

5. Compete against disease, not against each other

We have very little to rely on nowadays other than each other. I called a hospital in Houston, Texas, last year to learn about its allegedly successful innovations in pneumonia care and was told that the gains were enormous but that the methods could not be reported in public – excellent pneumonia care offered the hospital local competitive advantage. No wonder people feel confused! The enemy is disease. The competition that matters is against disease, not each other (a phrase I borrow from Dr Paul Batalden of Dartmouth Medical School). The purpose is healing.

On my drive to work, I see billboard after billboard with silly rhymes urging me to join one health maintenance organization or another; many of these organizations are distinguishable only by their logos, and they often use the very same physicians and hospitals. Every dollar of this meaningless, competitive showmanship is waste. Every beautifully printed sales brochure is care denied someone. The greatest confusion in this terribly confused year of market reform is that we think we will succeed by overcoming each other. My father did not care. He was in bed with a pressure sore, staring at a wheelchair he did not need and living with the undeserved memory of insult, delay and medically induced coma.

If we cannot work together on improvements that matter to those who call on us for help, then we have no cause to take pride in our restructuring, our mergers, our integrated systems or our report cards. I propose that we take aim where it matters. Pressure sores are the enemy. Stop them. Errors in drug use are the enemy. Stop them. Fragmentation is the enemy. It creates waste, cost and disrespect. Stop it. It was my father this time, but next time it will be your father, and then you, and then your child. I have heard it said by cynics that the quality of medical care would be far better and the hazards far less if physicians, like pilots, were passengers in their own aeroplanes. We are.

Postscript: My father, Dr Philip Berwick, died at home on 6 November 1995. His physician, Dr Malcolm Gourley, was at his side at the end, as he was so often and so helpfully in my father's final years.

REFERENCES

Berwick, D.M. (1994) 'Eleven worthy aims for clinical leadership of health system reform', *Journal of the American Medical Association*, 272: 797–802.

Deming, W.E. (1986) *Out of the Crisis*. Cambridge, MA: MIT Center for Advanced Engineering Study.

Horn, S.D., Ashton, C. and Tracey, D.M. (1994) 'Prevention and treatment of pressure ulcers by protocol'. in S.D. Horn and D.S. Hopkins, *Clinical Practice Improvement: A New Technology for Developing Cost-Effective Quality Health Care*. New York: Faulkner & Gray. pp. 253–62.

Pestotnik, S.L., Classen D.C., Evans, R.S. and Burke, J.P. (1993) 'Improving antibiotic use: seven-year results of a process-oriented decision-support system' (Abstract), *Proceedings of the 33rd Interscience Conference on Antimicrobial Agents and Chemotherapy*, New Orleans, LA, 17–20 October.

Pestotnik, S.L., Classen, D.C., Evans, R.S. and Burke, J.P. (1996) 'Implementing antibiotic practice guidelines through computer-assisted decision support: clinical and financial outcomes', *Annals of International Medicine*, 124: 884–90.

Sandmire, H.F. and DeMott, R.K. (1994) 'The Green Bay cesarean section study. III. Falling cesarean birth rates without a formal curtailment program', *American Journal of Obstetrics and Gynecology*, 170: 1790–802.

22

Masculinity and the Redundant Male: Explaining the Increasing Incarceration of Young Men

Sarah Payne

Women form the majority of those entering the psychiatric hospital for inpatient treatment. This over-representation of women has been a feature of psychiatric admission statistics since 1850 (Showalter, 1987), and continues in the UK today. However, women's admission rates no longer outnumber those of men to the same degree, and since the 1980s there has been, in some age groups, an over-representation of men in the figures for admission to psychiatric hospital.

This is an interesting phenomenon, giving rise to a number of speculative interpretations. It may be that with decreasing beds, inpatient treatment is linked with ideas about greater need – the 'rationing' of psychiatric beds in favour of men – or greater threat – where young men are seen more frequently as requiring some form of control and removal from society. This chapter explores the idea that from the early 1970s onwards we see a shift in psychiatric discourse with particular significance for young men in which male economic redundancy is related to changing institutional practice in the psychiatric system. However, the chapter also introduces the idea that psychiatric discourse has recently developed in response to the redundancy of young men in the home, where an increasing surveillance of young men is related to what could be described as domestic redundancy.

The primary focus here is the psychiatric system. However, the criminal justice system is also of interest. In particular for young men, in that we might expect to see an association between the two. This may be either where increasing psychiatric admissions amongst young men might be associated with a reduction in the criminalization of young men (Smith et al., 1992), or where a rise in psychiatric admissions might be associated with a rise in imprisonment. Certainly there are connections between the psychiatric system and the criminal justice system, including the suggestion that a significant and increasing proportion of the prison population are mentally disturbed (Gunn et al., 1991).

MADMEN AND MADWOMEN: CHANGES IN PSYCHIATRIC ADMISSION RATES

Over the past 30 years figures for admissions to psychiatric hospital reveal a reduction in the over-representation of women in all age groups (Payne, 1991a, 1995). As Figures 22.1 to 22.3 show, total psychiatric admission rates for men between 20 and 35 have now overtaken those of women, with the fastest fall in the ratio of women to men from the late 1970s onwards.

The last three decades have seen a fundamental alteration in the practice of psychiatry, with the number of inpatient psychiatric beds cut by over 50 per cent between 1959 and 1989 and the closure of larger institutions (Chew, 1992). Mental health policy from the 1960s onwards emphasized an increasing use of small-scale institutions such as the District General Hospital (Pilgrim, 1993; Busfield, 1993). This transfer to the smaller unit not only re-emphasized the institutional territorial base, but also simultaneously increased the legitimacy of psychiatry as a medically based discipline, within the hospital. The movement has not stopped there, however, and the process continues with an increasing emphasis on care outside the walls of the institution in the 'community'.

The question is whether men and women are more exposed to the risk of institutional treatment as a result of these changes? Where psychiatry is located in general practice women pass more easily through what have been termed *filters* for treatment, and are more likely to be seen by a specialist – the psychiatrist – than before (Geddes et al., 1993). However,

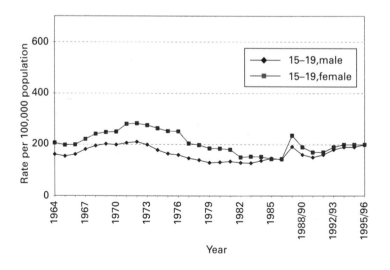

Figure 22.1 *Psychiatric admissions: rate of admission to psychiatric hospital, 1964–95/96: age 15–19*

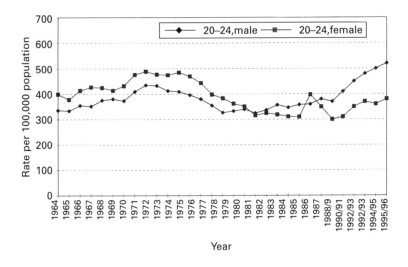

Figure 22.2 *Psychiatric admissions: rate of admission to psychiatric hospital per 100,000 population 1964–95/96, males and females aged 20–24*

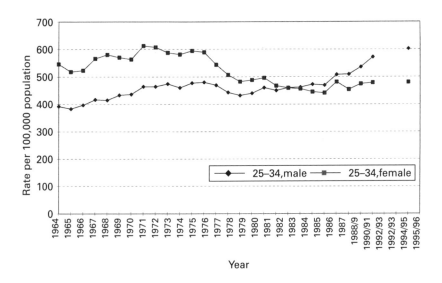

Figure 22.3 *Psychiatric admissions: rate of admission to psychiatric hospital per 100,000 population 1964–95/96: age 25–34*

this means an increase in the proportion of women seen as outpatients, rather than those admitted as inpatients. Men pass more easily through the filters to institutionally based treatment but this is not new – men have always been more likely to be referred 'up' the hierarchy of specialisms (Geddes et al., 1993), and the different experiences of each sex in admissions cannot readily be explained by this shift to community care – other factors are likely to be involved.

THE CRIMINAL MALE AND FEMALE: CHANGES IN THE CRIMINAL JUSTICE SYSTEM

A much greater proportion of young men is drawn into the criminal justice system each year than are admitted to psychiatric hospital. In 1995–96, for example, young men under 20 were more than 30 times as likely to be found guilty or cautioned than to be admitted to psychiatric inpatient treatment, and those aged 20–24 were nearly 10 times as likely to be involved in the criminal justice system. For women, the difference is much smaller, and while those under 30 were more likely to be found guilty or cautioned, after the age of 30 admission to psychiatric hospital is the more likely event (Criminal Statistics [CS], 1993; DoH, 1989, 1997). Young men are also more likely to be imprisoned than admitted to the psychiatric hospital: in 1996 the rate of imprisonment amongst young men was more than four times the rate of hospitalization, while for young women, the reverse is true (CS, 1993; 1997; DoH, 1989, 1997).

Changes in the criminal justice system during the 1970s and 1980s reflect shifts in the psychiatric system in a number of ways, with a reducing role for the institution and an extension of the professional gaze into the wider community, where particular groups are highlighted for special attention. This parallels the mental health system and psychiatric discourse, where amid the rhetoric of closing the institution total admissions to psychiatric hospital actually increased, by more than 100 per cent between 1964 and 1994–95 (DHSS, 1969; DoH, 1989, 1997).

Figures showing the 'admission' of young men into the criminal justice system appear to reflect changes in admission to psychiatric hospital. By the late 1990s, in comparison with earlier years, more young men were pulled into the system: Figure 22.4 shows sharp increases in the rate per 100,000 population found guilty or cautioned among the younger age groups from 1964 to 1996, particularly for young men aged 20, where rates nearly trebled. However, unlike the psychiatric system, there were even more dramatic increases amongst young women, with a rise of 400 per cent for women aged 20 – although total numbers remained small (Criminal Statistics, 1964–97).

GENDER AND REDUNDANCY

In the early 1970s Phylis Chesler sought to explain women's greater susceptibility to psychiatric illness by women's changing status in the domestic arena: 'Many newly useless women are emerging more publicly into insanity' (Chesler, 1974: 33) – the result, in part at least, of the

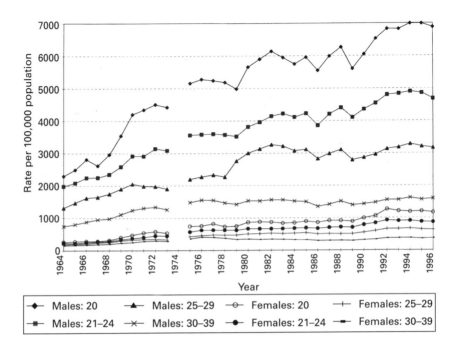

Figure 22.4   *Numbers found guilty or cautioned, 1964–96, England and Wales: ages 20, 21–24, 25–29, 30–39*

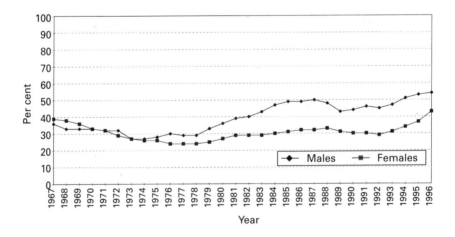

Figure 22.5   *Percentage of those sentenced who receive sentence implying continuing legal control: 1964–83: age 17–20, 1984–96: age 18–20*

increasing 'redundancy' women were suffering as their role within the family diminished or dissolved as a consequence of separation and divorce: 'While women live longer than ever before, and longer than men, there is less and less use, and literally no place, for them, in the only place they "belong" – within the family' (ibid.).

Recently young women have been more successful than men in reducing their risk of admission to psychiatric hospital. Clearly the impact of this shift in the location of treatment is complex: women remain more likely to be prescribed psychotropic medicine, whether inside or outside the institution, and it may be merely the locus of control that has shifted. Psychiatry remains male-dominated and essentially patriarchal (Ussher, 1991; Showalter, 1987). However, in the familial discourse of the institutional setting, the psychiatric hospital, the focus appears to have shifted from the difficult woman to the recalcitrant adolescent son.

Can the increasing risk of admission for young men during the 1980s and 1990s be explained in terms of changes experienced by this age group during this period, and perhaps most obviously, by redundancy? While the most usual understanding of this term – economic redundancy in the public world of paid employment – is undoubtedly significant, given the major increases in unemployment during this same period, we also need to consider redundancy in the private world, that is, to use redundancy for men in the way Chesler used it for women in the context of the private household.

However, it is not only the actual experience of being redundant, in terms of the workplace or 'the family', which is relevant, but also the ways in which a discursive rendering of the redundant male is connected with changes in psychiatry and the criminal justice system. For example, if economic redundancy combined with a declining role in the home has encouraged a more extreme and more public expression of masculinity amongst young men (Campbell, 1993), one result may be an increased risk of being drawn in by the penal system. The other may be an increased risk of being hospitalized in the psychiatric system. Changes in figures for both psychiatric treatment and the rates of criminality for young men need to be viewed in the context of corresponding shifts in psychiatric and penal discourse in which young men are now seen as more of a threat. This is most obvious when they are detached from the world of paid employment and the family. Young men may now be more likely to be seen as in need of inpatient treatment to contain or resolve these difficulties, or to be seen as potential and actual criminals within the criminal justice system.

EXPLAINING MALE EXCESS: THE REDUNDANT MALE IN THE WORKPLACE

In the public world of paid employment, male unemployment increased throughout the 1980s, with particularly marked increases taking place towards the end of the 1970s and in the first years of the 1980s. This is the period in which we also see the most dramatic shift in admission figures for young men (Payne, 1991a).

While unemployment statistics are flawed in a number of ways, there is a general trend of increasing youth unemployment during the late 1970s and the early 1980s: between 1965 and 1984 unemployment increased in the United Kingdom from around 1.5 per cent to nearly 13 per cent overall, but to between 23 and 27 per cent amongst young people under the age of 19 (Jackson, 1985). The sharpest rise came in the early 1980s, when youth unemployment virtually doubled between 1980 and 1981, and when long-term unemployment amongst young people increased (McRae, 1987; Jackson, 1985). By the late 1990s the unemployment rate amongst younger people had begun to level off and decrease again although remaining higher than for older ages (*Social Trends*, 1999).

Economic redundancy was increasing in these age groups in the 1980s, yet the risks were higher for some young people than for others. Unemployment rates amongst younger men and women are very similar, although as age increases the difficulty of measurement also increases, as statistics exclude young women who have responsibility for children. Young women without paid work in the 1980s differed from young men in certain ways: they were more likely to have higher qualifications than were unemployed young men, and to come from less disadvantaged backgrounds (McRae, 1987). However, young unemployed women differ in another way: they are more likely to take on sole responsibility for children during this period of unemployment. One effect of unemployment on young women is 'to advance the timing of motherhood among women from all social backgrounds' (Penhale, 1987:29). There is some debate over the underlying reasons behind this increased likelihood of motherhood – including the question of whether young women use motherhood as a transition to an adult status which is denied young men. A young unemployed man who becomes a father – even where he lives with the mother and child – does not take on such a major change in status as does the mother. Where the mother lives alone, the shift in the father's status and circumstances may be very small indeed.

Unemployment is unevenly distributed in other ways, including in relation to occupational class and ethnicity, with more unemployment amongst young men in lower occupational groups (Bartlett, 1994; Townsend et al., 1992). Unemployment is particularly acute amongst young men from minority ethnic groups (Dex, 1982; *Social Trends*, 1999).

These differences in the distribution of economic redundancy can be placed against similar uneven distributions in both the psychiatric system and the criminal justice system. Admissions to psychiatric inpatient treatment show a higher incidence of psychiatric diagnosis in social classes 4 and 5 (Payne, 1991b). In addition there are higher rates for ethnic minority men and women, with notably high rates amongst young Afro-Caribbean men, and men from the Republic of Ireland (Littlewood and Lipsedge, 1988; Lloyd and Moodley, 1992). Minority ethnic patients – and in particular black men and women – are perceived within psychiatric discourse as more violent, and less compliant with treatment, and are thus treated more coercively than white patients (Lloyd and Moodley, 1992; Payne, 1999).

Both men and women from minority ethnic groups are also more frequently found in the criminal justice system (Sim, 1990; Littlewood and Lipsedge, 1988). In particular, black women and men are disproportionately found in prison, in secure units and high-security psychiatric units such as Broadmoor, and to be administered psychotropic medication while in prison (Sim, 1990).

Thus those groups who suffer higher rates of unemployment also appear more frequently inside the psychiatric and the criminal justice system, and both are disproportionately represented amongst those who are restrained and administered medication without their consent. In this sense, these groups are subject to greater surveillance and control, and appear in prevailing discourse in both systems as more frequently in need of such control (Payne, 1999).

What then is the link between unemployment and increasing control of young men? Unemployment usually means a lack of earned income, the potential for satisfaction from paid work and the opportunities for socializing. As well as this it has also been seen in both psychiatric and penal literature as being outside the external control or regulation of the working day, the factory supervisor and the pay packet. The Parliamentary All-Party Penal Affairs Group (1983), for example, concluded that unemployment amongst young people, and in particular young men, was one of the factors associated with increased crime in this age group.

EXPLAINING MALE EXCESS: THE REDUNDANT MALE AT HOME

In the other site of male redundancy, the family, there is a similar pattern, in which significant numbers of young men have become increasingly less necessary as young women take on the sole responsibility for raising children. In the 1970s and 1980s there were rapid increases in the number of lone mothers, such that by 1995–96 lone mothers represented over 20 per cent of all families with dependent children in Britain (*Social Trends*, 1999). As before with economic redundancy, the notion of redundancy in the familial home is not uniform across all groups: for some young men there may be a greater likelihood of this redundancy. Thus lone motherhood is more usual in minority ethnic groups, with over 40 per cent of all West Indian families being headed by lone mothers, over a quarter of families from African groups, and a third of those described as 'mixed', compared with 13 per cent of white families (Muncie et al., 1994).

I do not intend to argue that being without a family, in which young men can 'father', causes an increase in psychiatric illness. In particular, to suggest that there may be an impact on young men of being excluded from families is calling upon an idealized view of family life. Many men behave appallingly in families, and many women leave men to become lone parents as a result of their experience of male violence and abuse. What I am interested in is the extent to which the detachment of young men from such structures invokes a response which results in the surveillance of young men and an increasing location of young men in other institutions: in particular the psychiatric hospital and criminal justice system.

GENDER AND PSYCHIATRIC DISCOURSE

Psychiatry has tended not to be particularly conscious of the gender of the patient: many investigations of mental illness, including depression, traditionally suffered by women, have failed to consider as relevant the different experiences of each sex (Busfield, 1993). However at another, less overt, level gender has been a significant aspect of the way psychiatry identifies the illness, its cause, and the appropriate cure. Women are seen as more likely to succumb to mental illness, while the model of good mental health is male oriented (Chesler, 1974; Broverman et al., 1971; Ussher, 1991).

Female vulnerability to mental disorder forms an interwoven part of professional discourse: in the emerging scientific discourse of Victorian psychiatry women were mad because of their inferior anatomy, at the mercy of their hormones. Recommended cures were largely 'heroic' (the hero, of course, being the male psychiatrist) and included leeches, ice packs and purgatives applied to various parts of the feminine body (Showalter, 1987; Walkowitz, 1992). Over time the focus gradually shifts from the body to the mind, but the underlying message remains unchanged. By the 1980s there is little evidence that psychiatry had thrown off this perspective on women's mental health (Ussher, 1991; Busfield, 1993).

Male mental health is usually represented by a stereotypical, and unforgiving, array of characteristics – successful, confident, articulate, independent and so on (Broverman et al., 1971). This masculinity may allow psychiatry to see men as unwell when they are not all of these things but cannot take account of the costs of meeting this model, or attempting to and failing. Both economic and domestic redundancy make such characteristics more difficult to attain – unless it is through the kind of public display described by Campbell (1993) which serves to draw young men into the penal, and possibly the psychiatric, system.

The most thoroughly debated risk for unemployed men is suicide (Platt, 1984, 1986), although medical research remains inconclusive (e.g.

Table 23.1 *Characteristics of 'good' and 'poor' parenting*

Good parenting	Poor parenting
Teaching by example	Exposure to deviant models
Providing a secure environment	Inability to provide continuity of care
The mother's presence	Poor supervision
Attachment and bonding	Lack of bonding and attachment
Maturity	Youth of the mother
Affection	Conditional affection
Flexible control	Cruel control
Child centredness	Rejection
Positive affectivity	Negative affectivity
	Unpredictability
	Provocation
	Impairment of health or development
	Harmful or cruel discipline
	Distance
	Hostility
	Intrusion
	Poor mothering
	Ignorance
	Fecklessness
	Lack of empathy for child
	Unrealistic expectations
	Laxity and inconsistency
	Aggression
	Low warmth
	High criticism
	Neglect
	Abandonment

parenting, either poor or good, is difficult to define and to use in research. It is also noticeable that there has been much more focus on poor rather than good parenting. The extremes of good and poor parenting might be relatively easy to identify. The problem, however, is everything else in between. Much of the parenting literature focuses on mothering; fathering is either ignored or its potential importance minimized.

Hoghughi and Speight's discussion (Hoghughi and Speight, 1998) of the components of good enough parenting illustrates these problems of definition; all three of their components would be accepted by most people, but they fail to tackle the problem of a definition, which allows a clear distinction between good enough and not good enough parenting.

'Love, care, and commitment' is their first component. They give appropriate examples of extreme situations in which lack of this component can be assumed, but give no practical definition that could be used by practitioners to distinguish good enough from not good enough levels of love, care, and commitment. Their jokey reference to the need for a measure of 'serum love' is an admission of the difficulties in finding an operational definition of this component.

Crombie, 1989, 1991). Explanations offered focus on the ways life has changed for young men, in terms of reduced expectation of lifelong employment, of family life and opportunities for developing a sense of place within society (Bunting, 1993; Moore, 1995). Accounts of increasing rates of suicide in 'pressured young males' (*Guardian*, November 1993) add to the content of this discourse. Thus within psychiatric discourse the figure of the depressed, suicidal, problematic unemployed man emerges and looms large throughout the 1980s, affecting decisions regarding psychiatric admissions as well as the understanding of mental health itself. At the end of the century the 'problem with boys' is particularly focused on persistently high suicide rates amongst younger men ('Sad culture kills 12 "lads" a week', *Observer*, 17 October 1999), their absence as fathers ('Invisible men', *Guardian*, 17 November 1999), and on social exclusion amongst young men and young women, a prominent aspect of the policies of the Labour government policy after 1997.

The debate has extended from the abandoned delinquent son to the abandoning delinquent father, with the Child Support Act of 1991, which sought to relocate young men in the family – where responsibility rebukes the adolescent male into good behaviour (see for example Murray, 1994). These shifts in masculinity loom large in the early 1990s across wide areas of the policy arena rather than narrowly defined interests of psychiatric and penal discourse: however, in the course of so doing they leave their mark on practice in both psychiatric and penal policy.

By the end of the 1990s, figures show a continuing excess of young men in figures for both institutional psychiatric treatment and legal control in the criminal justice system, whilst public discourse on problem males increasingly centres on high rates of exclusion, criminality and suicide in this age group. Policy solutions have changed over this period, in particular with the introduction of the New Deal, a policy which seeks to relocate young men (and women) in the workplace, in training or in community service, as a means to reducing exclusion and unrest. Masculinity remains a problem, however, as ever increasing proportions of young men absorbed by both psychiatric and legal institutional forms of control demonstrate.

CONCLUSION

We began with the suggestion that increases in male psychiatric admissions might be connected with increased male redundancy. Thus as young men have become more detached from the world of paid work, and from family and paternal responsibilities, they have become more visible in their discontent, and at the same time the need for control of this group has increased and become more visible. In the psychiatric system, the discursive rendering of men shows them to be vulnerable to

Their second component is 'control/consistent limit setting'. The problem here is that control and limit setting are so culturally and socially embedded as to make generalizable measures virtually impossible to devise. For example, can you apply the same rules for 'reasonable boundaries' to the single parent family living on a low income in a high rise flat and the family with a large house set in a large suburban garden where children can safely be left to explore and play? The mother who allows her child out to play in one setting might be regarded as negligent whereas the other would be praised for providing a stimulating environment. Equally, what constitute reasonable boundaries changes rapidly from generation to generation and from culture to culture. Nineteenth-century limits in Victorian Britain would undoubtedly be regarded as punitive and impairing development today. Parents from the Indian subcontinent are likely to view as negligent the normal UK practice of allowing teenage girls the freedom to attend 'discos'.

'Facilitation of development' is the third component listed. This also is deeply embedded in culture and social circumstance. The same yardstick for measuring 'rich and varied stimulation' cannot be applied to families unless realistic account is taken of the material and social resources needed to provide it. In a country such as the UK, with huge differences in family access to economic, social and educational resources, it seems to us bizarre that anyone could discuss this component without reference to these resources.

The components of good enough parenting advanced by Hoghughi and Speight are considered completely outside their social, cultural and historic context and, in each case, the authors conspicuously fail to provide any working, practical definition that professionals could apply.

ACCOUNTING FOR SOCIOECONOMIC STATUS IN PARENTING STUDIES

For the reasons discussed below, socioeconomic status is a significant confounder of the relation between parenting and child health outcomes. It is also a major distal component of the causal pathway to poor outcomes for children of which parenting is a more proximal component. Parenting can be seen as mediating the direct effects on children of material deficits: in some cases, through exceptional personal resources, interpersonal or social supports; in others, personal ill health, trauma or isolation might exacerbate the consequences of these deficits. Focusing on parenting behaviours as though they are the result of deliberate choice, free from external influence, provides ammunition for politicians who wish to reduce all social problems to matters of personal responsibility and morality.

Sociomedical research reflects the dominant paradigm of the societies in which it is undertaken. In the UK and the USA, individual families and parents are seen as responsible for the health and socialization of their children. Individual responsibility in the form of harmful health-related behaviours is given higher priority than societal factors that might be influencing individual behaviours (Logan and Spencer, 1996). In this context, socioeconomic status tends to be either ignored or its effects marginalized. A consequence of this approach is that socio-economic status is inadequately accounted for in many studies that focus on the individual characteristics of parents and their effects on child health outcomes.

The Exeter family study (Cockett and Tripp, 1994) has been influential in persuading politicians and social commentators of the adverse effects on young people of divorce and parental separation. The authors have linked these consequences to parenting (Tripp and Cockett, 1998). Seventy-six children from reordered families and 76 children from intact families were matched on six criteria: age, sex, mother's education, position in family, type of school, and social class group. The authors found significant differences in a range of behavioural, self-esteem and family support outcomes to the detriment of the children in reordered families. However, despite the matching process, the two groups show considerable differences in socioeconomic status. Reordered families were at much higher risk of receipt of state benefits, living in rented accommodation, suffering financial hardship, and having no exclusive use of a car. The authors suggest that some of this might be a con-sequence of a fall in income related to family breakdown. Equally, it cannot be ruled out that these differences predated the family break-down, and consequently behave as potential residual confounders in relation to the child outcomes.

The most widely used measure of the quality and quantity of stimula-tion and support available to a child in the home environment is the 'home observation for measurement of the environment' (HOME) (Caldwell and Bradley, 1984). The measure has been criticized on the grounds that the outcomes are highly correlated with family socio-economic status and, therefore, might be measuring the effects of socio-economic status rather than parenting (Krauss and Jacobs, 1990).

PARENTING AND ECONOMIC HARDSHIP

Hoghughi and Speight acknowledge that wider economic and social issues are involved in parenting but consider none of the evidence supporting this association. There is compelling evidence from USA and UK studies for the role of social factors in parenting.

Socioeconomic factors appear to have a direct effect on parenting behaviour. Economic hardship and heavy income loss in families studied longitudinally in the USA city of Oakland during the depression of the 1930s were associated with more punitive arbitrary and rejecting parenting by fathers (Elder, 1974; Elder et al., 1985). An increase in economic hardship has been linked with a decrease in parental nurturance and an increase in inconsistent discipline by both parents (Lempers et al., 1989). Unemployed fathers display fewer nurturing behaviours than other fathers (Harold-Goldsmith et al., 1988). Low income, in combination with low levels of perceived social support, has been associated with a higher probability of punitive behaviour by the parent towards the child (Hashima and Amato, 1995). Unemployment and low income are strongly associated with child abuse referrals (Baldwin and Spencer, 1993; Gilham et al., 1998).

The socioemotional functioning of children living in poor families seems to be mediated by the psychological functioning of parents and the level of distress in family interaction patterns (McLoyd and Flanagan, 1990). Maternal rejection of early adolescents is closely correlated to the occupational status of the family (Felner et al., 1995).

These direct effects of economic hardship and material disadvantage on parenting are partially mediated by marital stresses. The psychological well-being of adults in the household is affected by economic hardship (Rosenblatt and Keller, 1983), as is the marital relationship (Johnson and Booth, 1990). Disagreement and conflict over the use of the limited money available (Larson, 1984), and loss of warmth and affection and mutual parental respect (Conger et al., 1990), have been shown to be associated with economic hardship. The role change associated with the loss of the father's job and the increased importance accruing to the mother in family decision-making might weaken family unity and increase marital tension (Wilhelm and Ridley, 1988). Stress-related changes in parent–child interactions lead to increasingly coercive parenting, with a resultant increase in childhood behavioural problems and future delinquency (Patterson and Stouthamer-Loeber, 1984).

A study of almost 6,000 members of the 1958 national childhood development study cohort who had become parents (Ferri and Smith, 1996) confirmed the stresses on parents imposed by financial hardship and unemployment. Marital happiness and life satisfaction were significantly lower in families with no earner and these families also tended to show more aggressive parenting strategies.

Parenting is a proximal variable in the causal pathway to adverse outcomes in childhood and adolescence, of which material disadvantage and economic hardship are distal variables (Conger et al., 1992). Behavioural problems and temper tantrums among young children have been shown to increase as a result of parenting changes associated with economic hardship (Elder et al., 1984). Economic deprivation has also been associated with decreased respect for the father and increased dependence on peer group for adolescent boys, and lowered feelings of self-adequacy and reduced goal aspirations for adolescent girls (Krauss

Schorr, L.B. (1988) *Within Our Reach: Breaking the Cycle of Deprivation*. New York: Doubleday.

Smith, D. and Nicholson, M. (1992) 'Poverty and ill health: controversies past and present', *Proceedings of the Royal College of Physicians (Edinburgh)*, 22: 190–9.

Spence, J., Walton, W.S., Miller, F.J.W. and Court, S.D.M. (1954) *A Thousand Families in Newcastle-upon-Tyne*. London: Oxford University Press.

Spencer, N.J. (1996) *Poverty and Child Health*. Oxford: Radcliffe Medical Press.

The Acheson Report (1998) *Independent Inquiry into Inequalities in Health*. London: The Stationery Office.

Tripp, J.H. and Cockett, M. (1998) 'Parents, parenting and family breakdown', *Arch Dis Child*, 78: 104–8.

Webster, C. (ed.) (1993) *Caring for Health: History and Diversity*. Buckinghamshire: Open University Press.

Wilhelm, M.S. and Ridley, C.A. (1988) 'Stress and unemployment in rural nonfarm couples: a study of hardships and coping resources', *Family Relations*, 37: 50–4.

Wilkinson, R.G. (1996) *Unhealthy Societies: The Afflictions of Inequality*. Routledge, London.

Woodruffe, C., Glickman, M., Barker, M. and Power, C. (1993) *Children, Teenagers and Health: The Key Data*. Milton Keynes: Open University Press.

24

Communicating the Implications of Genetic Disease

Aamra R. Darr

In the history of medicine, genetics is a relatively recent development. Whereas the general public is usually aware of the link between germs and disease, the link between their own genes and disease is not so familiar. A family diagnosed as being at-risk for a genetic condition comes face to face with a situation in which they have little knowledge of what this new genetic information means or what implications it has for them and their family. In this context there is a particular responsibility on health professionals to guide the individual or family towards a situation where they understand the information given and receive support during their decision-making process and with coping.

In the context of genetic conditions the 'patient' is not just the individual, but the whole family who are blood relatives. The detection of an individual affected by or at-risk for a genetic disorder is the signpost to a family whose other members may also be at-risk for the same condition, and who need to be informed of the implications of that genetic risk and supported in dealing with those implications.

A family's ability to make informed choices is determined by the effective communication of genetic information by health professionals and the offer of appropriate support in utilizing it: good communication is the cornerstone of effective genetic counselling; misinformation is the main hindrance. In a multicultural society, such as Britain, health professionals need to examine whether the information they are giving is understood by families whose first language is not English; and whether it is useful to families whose family and cultural dynamics may require a modification of standard support.

A person's knowledge of their genetic risk may come about in a variety of ways. It may be through the diagnosis of a genetic condition in childhood or adulthood, or through routine screening. However the knowledge is arrived at, the paramount needs of individuals and families are for a speedy and accurate diagnosis; for information which enables them to make informed choices and for support in dealing with their new situation.

DIAGNOSIS

Prior to diagnosis families tend to have very little information about genetic conditions. Quite often, particularly with very rare conditions, GPs are also faced with a disorder they know little about. The admission of lack of knowledge and an expression of interest in resolving the situation and attending to the family's needs is viewed as a highly positive step. A lack of effort on the part of the GP at this initial stage can be deeply upsetting and frustrating for families:

> I went to my GP, with my husband, and asked for a double appointment to try and talk to him, and he was not at all interested, and showed me the pile of literature he got every day to read, and that we should go to the hospital, there was nothing more he could do for us and he reduced me to tears, I was incredibly angry. He said that it was very rare, and that the chance was he would not come across it again. (Trent Steering Group on Genetics, 1998)

Bad rapport at this initial stage can create alienation between the GP and the family, at a point when they are at their most vulnerable, and when they will be needing to rely on their GP in the future: 'Sometimes it makes me very bitter, but I can't just say turn round and blame the doctor. I still need him a lot and I can't say outright' (Burton, 1975).

It is at this crucial stage that a speedy diagnosis is needed; the correct information should be given sympathetically and referral made to specialist and ancillary support services. An effort made by a GP is highly appreciated:

> when I had one of my miscarriages, one of the GPs had just had a miscarriage, and I'd gone to see her for a check-up afterwards and she was literally back that week, and she spent literally three quarters of an hour at the end of the surgery talking about what could be done. I went back to her for my postnatal check, and have been for smears, and she's just great. And it's not just Ben, it's looking after me, am I getting on all right with whatever's going on. (Trent Steering Group on Genetics, 1998)

Effective communication and collaboration between health professionals is essential and can result in very positive outcomes for patients on emotional and practical levels:

> The main consultant . . . was very good and he was keen to get together with the community nurse that used to come and see us, and my own GP and my health visitor and get together and have little conflabs about . . . what his needs were at the time, which was really very good and they were always coming. One day there was all four of them in our house asking what we wanted and how we felt. Instead of being kept in the background, they were also asking us. (Trent Steering Group on Genetics, 1998)

For a family, getting an accurate diagnosis is extremely important. To be told that a GP or hospital doctor cannot diagnose what is wrong leaves families isolated and struggling to understand the symptoms of a disorder. Knowing the name of a disorder gives reality to a condition, provides an explanation for how it has come about, and makes it possible to calculate the chances of it happening again. It also allows people to link up to others with the same condition for mutual support.

INFORMATION

After a diagnosis has been made a family needs accurate information on many aspects of the genetic condition, in order to make informed choices about the treatment, genetic testing and its implications and, where relevant, future reproduction. All professionals giving genetic information should be confident that their information is accurate, up to date and comprehensive.

Subsequent to receiving a diagnosis, the need for information that families can understand continues to be acute. If information is not forthcoming from health professionals, families are likely to struggle through the maze of other avenues, where information may be inaccurate or out of date: 'I went to the library in Matlock, and the next day I couldn't really find anything, so I went to the Reference Library in Sheffield the following day, because he told us nothing about it' (Trent Steering Group on Genetics, 1998).

Language

Communicating genetic information to families whose first language is not English poses a particular challenge to health professionals; not being fluent in the language used by professionals places a family in a vulnerable situation. The need to transmit accurate information is as acute, as with any other family, but the potential for misunderstandings is greater, sometimes with serious consequences. An example is of Mr A.: not fluent in English, he understood the term 'genes' to mean 'germs', when an English-speaking doctor was trying to explain genetic inheritance to him. Not having grasped the genetic nature of the condition or the details of the treatment, he thought that if the condition is caused by germs, then with the present state of medicine there must be a cure, somewhere. Against the advice of their paediatrician, Mr and Mrs A. returned with their two thalassaemic children to Pakistan, where they hoped to find an alternative cure for thalassaemia major. During that period, one of their children died, as technically he was difficult to transfuse. Distressed, they returned to England with their other child. It was only when the couple spoke to a counsellor who explained the condition to them accurately in their mother tongue, that Mr A. recounted his experience and was able to contextualize his own reactions and the paediatrician's advice (Darr, 1990).

- reproductive alternatives such as contraception, assisted reproduction, pre-implantation diagnosis or adoption, and how to obtain these;
- in the case of people at possible risk of late-onset conditions, options for testing or preventative action and the implications for themselves and their families;
- options for, and implications of carrier status. (Genetic Interest Group, 1998)

Siblings and genetic testing

A GP may be the first point of contact for parents who are concerned about their unaffected children. The siblings of an affected family member can experience feelings of being undervalued in their role as co-carers with their parents if their brother/sister's condition demands a lot of caring from the family. The extra demands of having a caring role thrust upon them can affect other spheres of siblings' lives such as schoolwork or leisure time. There can also be conflicting feelings to deal with, such as protectiveness towards an affected sibling, alongside resentment and jealousy due to the extra time and attention afforded to the affected child by parents. There may be unvoiced concerns of 'Have I got it, too?' or 'Will I get it?'

Parents often find themselves having to deal with these issues, particularly during adolescence, and need support in dealing with them. An added concern at this time for parents is the realization that their children have reached an age when they need to be aware of their genetic status and any implications for future reproduction. Again, a GP may be the first person families contact to discuss these.

People often find genetic and diagnostic testing stressful, and information can help them to tolerate what can sometimes be a difficult and lengthy process. When a genetic test is being considered, people will have a number of concerns:

- whether the test will give a diagnosis or simply provide information about risk;
- whether other tests might then be done to provide further information;
- what a test will *not* show – such as a possibility of other conditions or other mutations of the same condition not tested for;
- any possible implications for insurance or employment, especially in relation to late-onset conditions;
- what a test will entail – for example, will it be unpleasant or painful?
- what subsequent use will be made of any sample. For example, will it be stored for future testing? used for research? disposed of? (Genetic Interest Group 1998)

SUPPORT

Ensuring that families get a speedy diagnosis and provision of genetic information that they understand and are able to utilize in making informed choices, is the first form of support that GPs can offer. The second is to make available information about support groups. These groups are valuable for families:

> Things are getting better because I thought I was the only one in the world who's got this terrible thing, but now I've found there's lots of people suffering from it. (Trent Steering Group on Genetics, 1998)

People need to know how they can contact a support group if and when they wish to – which may be some time after diagnosis. If there is no support group, families should be given the opportunity to contact others in a similar position, for example, through Contact a Family (020 7383 3555) or through other links with users of the genetic service, haemoglobinopathy counsellors or specialist genetic workers. The Genetic Interest Group (020 7704 3141) also provides information on a range of genetic issues to families.

CONCLUSION

As knowledge of genetics increases, it is likely that GPs will increasingly be required to take genetic factors into consideration. Inevitably, they will also be required to provide more information and support in collaboration with genetic and specialist services. As GPs are usually the first port of call for families, in the initial stages at least, family experience of a genetic disorder may be dependent on their GP's knowledge and the sensitivity with which it is communicated.

REFERENCES

Atkin, K. and Ahmad, W.I.U. (1998) 'Genetic screening and haemoglobinopathies: ethics, politics and practice', *Social Science and Medicine*, 46 (3): 445–58.

Bundey, S. and Roberts, D.F. (eds) (1988) 'Health and consanguinity in immigrant populations in Britain', *Biology and Society*, 5: 12–37.

Burton, L. (1975) *The Family Life of Sick Children*. London: Routledge & Kegan Paul.

Darr, A.R. (1990) 'The social aspects of thalassaemia major among Muslims of Pakistani origin in England: family experience and service delivery', Ph.D thesis, University College, London.

Darr, A.R. (1997) 'Consanguineous marriage and genetics: a positive relationship', in A. Clarke and E. Parsons (eds), *Culture, Kinship and Genes*. London: Macmillan Press.

Genetic Interest Group (1998) *Guidelines for Genetic Services*. London: Genetic Interest Group.

Trent Steering Group on Genetics (1998) 'NHS Executive Trent' (unpublished report).

25

The Physiology of Stressful Life Experiences

Gonneke Willemsen and Cathy Lloyd

Despite anecdotal evidence throughout the centuries, the concept of psychosocial experiences having an effect on physical illness has not received much scientific attention until very recently. Initially, the belief that the brain was the seat of the soul prevented scientists from studying the central nervous system, as the Church forbade this on pain of excommunication, imprisonment and even execution. Later, the many scientific breakthroughs in medicine led to the general belief that disease was a product of specific pathogens, and that for every disease a specific antidote could be found. The discovery of vaccines and the improvement in environmental circumstances eliminated a large number of diseases which used to kill substantial numbers of people. However, we know now that the traditional biomedical model falls short of explaining all the factors involved in modern-life illnesses, such as cardiovascular disease and cancer. It is increasingly clear that these illnesses are determined by a variety of factors, including psychosocial factors, such as the way people behave and their social and psychological environment. In addition, there is now substantial evidence which shows the interactions of body and brain, which has led researchers to develop a 'psycho-biological' model of illness and disease.

PSYCHOLOGICAL STRESS AND PHYSIOLOGICAL EFFECTS

One psychological factor, which has received a lot of attention, is stress. Defining the concept of stress has proved difficult and consequently many different definitions have been utilized. One widely used definition has been developed by Lazarus and Folkman (1984: 205), who describe stress as 'a particular relationship between the person and the environment that is appraised by the person as taxing or exceeding his or her resources and endangering his or her well-being'. This strongly emphasizes the appraisal of the situation by a person. Any stressful event is judged by people in different ways, based upon factors such as prior experience, psychological factors and social influences. An event that is seen by one individual as very threatening might be seen as totally harmless by another individual. However, when a situation is such factors, although the precise nature of these complex interactions still remains to be determined (Maier and Watkins, 1998). A review revealed that stress influences both circulating cell numbers and the function of immune cells (Herbert and Cohen, 1993).

In summary the direct influence of the hypothalamus on organs, the autonomic nervous system, the neuroendocrine system and the immune system all prepare the body for action. Muscles are provided with the energy needed, non-essential functions such as digestion are suppressed and the immune system is prepared to deal with wounds efficiently. This stress response is part of an evolutionary adaptation to life as hunters and gatherers, and is adaptive under conditions of threat requiring a physical response. However, in modern life, this stress response is often elicited in circumstances when physical action is prohibited and it is possible that frequent or prolonged periods of stress exposure may lead to a maladaptive sustained activation. This may subsequently result in the development of disease.

Stressful life experiences and the effects on health and illness

In exploring the effects of stressful life events on physiological processes, a helpful classification is suggested by Lazarus and Cohen (1977). They divide life stressors into three categories, which vary in magnitude and duration and in the number of people influenced: cataclysmic events (e.g. earthquakes), personal stressors (e.g. negative life events) and daily hassles (e.g. job strain).

Cataclysmic events   Natural disasters such as hurricanes, earthquakes and man-made disasters such as war or nuclear accidents are powerful stressors affecting large numbers of individuals simultaneously. Although cataclysmic events are often relatively short-lasting and community support may reduce the impact of the stressor, such events may still have far-reaching effects for the individuals involved. Several studies have now shown that disasters can alter physiological variables, and affect mortality and morbidity for this additional reason. A good example of the effects of man-made disaster is the nuclear accident which occurred in March 1982 on Three Mile Island. Although the amount of radiation released was not significant, local inhabitants were strongly affected by the events. A follow-up six years later showed that individuals living within a six-mile radius of the plant had increased blood pressure and heart rate, higher levels of adrenaline, noradrenaline and cortisol and reductions in the number of immune cells circulating in the blood compared to those living further away (Baum, 1990). Similar effects have been found for naturally occurring disasters. For instance, after hurricane Andrew struck South Florida in August 1992, those living in damaged areas showed changes in their immune system (compared to those living in unaffected areas), up to four months after the event (Ironson et al., 1997).

Personal stressors Personal stressors may be thought of as events such as the death of a loved one or the loss of a job. These are often called negative life events. The stressor itself is usually short-lived, although there may be a build-up to the event, and there may be a long aftermath. However, the experience of personal stressors is specific to each individual, and, although most of us will experience these stressors, few people at a time are affected by one. The impact of events varies widely, depending on the individual's situation (e.g. relation to the deceased, support network, or financial consequences). The effects of such events can be substantial; losses and separations are associated with increased mortality and illness. Following the death of a loved one, changes in the immune system can be seen and in some individuals can persist up to one year later (Calabrese et al., 1987).

Daily hassles Although daily hassles are not as powerful as disasters or negative life events, they occur frequently, can be persistent, and as chronic stressors can be harmful. One form of daily hassle is work stress, which has been consistently related to physical well-being and the development of disease. In particular, jobs with high demand and low control have been related to the development of conditions such as myocardial infarction (Karasek et al., 1988). Disruptions in one's career such as conflicts with other workers, and increased responsibility, have also been related to myocardial infarction (Falger and Schouten, 1992). In addition, daily hassles have been linked to the onset and exacerbation of headaches and asthma (Brantley and Jones, 1993). A different source of daily hassles which has received much attention is caring for a partner with Alzheimer's disease. Compared to non-carers, the immune function of carers has been shown to be decreased and wound healing found to be impaired (Cacioppo et al., 1998).

Overall, there is sufficient evidence to suggest that psychosocial stress has a direct influence on physiological processes which can result in the development of disease. However, it is important to realize that stress also influences health in a different way, by having an effect on health behaviour and illness perception. Psychological stress has been shown to increase the incidence of unhealthy behaviours such as cigarette smoking and excessive alcohol consumption, and to decrease healthy behaviours such as exercise. Many different factors are thought to influence whether or not stressful experiences lead to ill health, including age, gender and genetic factors (Adler and Matthews, 1994). However, whilst the relationship between stress and disease has become more accepted by those working in health care provision, the exact nature of the links remain to be clarified.

REFERENCES

Adler, N. and Matthews, K.A. (1994) 'Health psychology: why do some people get sick and some stay well?', *Annual Reviews of Psychology*, 45: 229–59.

Baum, A. (1990) 'Stress, intrusive imagery, and chronic distress', *Health Psychology*, 9: 653–75.

Brantley, P.J. and Jones, N.J. (1993) 'Daily stress and stress-related disorders', *Annals of Behavioral Medicine*, 15: 17–25.

Buckingham, J.C., Cowell, A.-M., Gillies, G.E., Herbison, A.E. and Steel, J.H. (1997) 'The neuroendocriene system: anatomy, physiology, and responses to stress', in J.C. Buckingham, G.E. Gillies and A.-M. Cowell (eds), *Stress, Stress Hormones and the Immune System*. Chichester: John Wiley & Sons.

Cacioppo, J.T., Poehlmann, K.M., Burleson, M.H., Kiecolt-Glaser, J.K., Malarkey, W.B., Berntson, G.G. and Glaser, R. (1998) 'Cellular immune responses to acute stress in female caregivers of dementia patients and matched controls', *Health Psychology*, 17: 182–9.

Calabrese, J.R., Kling, M.A. and Gold, P.W. (1987) 'Alterations in immunocompetence during stress, bereavement, and depression: focus on neuroendocrine regulation', *American Journal of Psychiatry*, 9: 1123–34.

Falger, P.R.J. and Schouten, E.G.W. (1992) 'Exhaustion, psychological stressors in the work environment, and acute myocardial infarction in adult men', *Journal of Psychosomatic Research*, 36: 777–86.

Herbert, T.B. and Cohen, S. (1993) 'Stress and immunity in humans: a meta-analytic review', *Psychosomatic Medicine*, 55: 364–79.

Ironson, G., Wynings, C., Schneiderman, N., Baum, A., Rodriguez, M., Greenwood, D., Benight, C., Antoni, M., Laperriere, A., Huang, H.-S., Klimas, N. and Fletcher, M.A. (1997) 'Posttraumatic stress symptoms, intrusive thoughts, loss, and immune function after Hurricane Andrew', *Psychosomatic Medicine*, 59: 128–41.

Karasek, R.A., Theorell, T., Schwartz, J.E., Schnall, P.L., Pieper, C.F. and Michela, J.L. (1988) 'Job characteristics in relation to prevalence of myocardial infarction in the US Health Examination Survey (HES) and the Health and Nutrition Examination Survey (HANES)', *American Journal of Public Health*, 78: 910–18.

Lazarus, R.S. and Cohen, J.B. (1977) 'Environmental stress', in I. Attman and J.F. Wohlwill (eds), *Human Behavior and the Environment: Current Theory and Research*. New York: Plenum Press.

Lazarus, R.S. and Folkman, R. (1984) *Stress, Appraisal, and Coping*. New York: Springer.

Lovallo, W.R. (1997) *Stress and Health: Biological and Psychological Interactions*. London: Sage Publications.

Maier, S.F. and Watkins, L.R. (1998) 'Cytokines for psychologists: implications of bidirectional immune-to-brain communications for understanding behavior, mood, and cognition', *Psychological Review*, 105: 83–107.

Staines, N., Brostoff, J. and James, K. (1994) *Introducing Immunology*, 2nd edition. St. Louis: Mosby.

PART V

CARING AND CURING

The chapters in this part of the reader consider whether health can be understood by the *absence* of health (disease), and through people's attempts to care for and cure themselves and each other. The notion of 'working for health' is particularly relevant in this section and many lay and professional issues of health work are explored. It may often take an overt effort to cope with disease, or to attempt to restore health, and the selected papers in Part V reflect some of the 'work' that can be involved for people as individuals and for those concerned with the provision of services.

Moyra Sidell (Chapter 26: 'Understanding Chronic Illness') takes us through many of the stages that may be involved for individuals when their health is removed. Using various examples of chronic threats to health, the chapter describes and catalogues the impact that long-standing or irreversible illness may have on people. The chapter is based on detailed research, and describes the 'search for meaning' at various levels which can only be understood when the inquiry goes beyond biomedical understanding of disease mechanisms or pathological explanations based on the 'medical model'.

Christine Webb (Chapter 27: 'Caring, Curing and Coping') turns the spotlight on nursing and others charged with looking after people when they are ill. The chapter laments that 'patients' and their lay attendants are rarely mentioned as carers or curers in professional literature. 'Lay' or 'informal' carers, and the patients themselves, often have very different hopes, fears and expectations of the work done by professional carers, than the members of those professional groups themselves. Research is quoted which showed that patients wanted technical competence from their nurses, while the nurses themselves wanted to focus on the emotional and expressive components of care.

Some of the complexity of providing care with both physical and emotional components is the subject of the chapter by Jocalyn Lawler (Chapter 28: 'Sexuality, the Body and Nursing'). This chapter tackles subjects which are commonly thought about but infrequently researched or discussed, even during professional training. Nurses have contact with the naked human body, perhaps more than any other profession. They are vulnerable to problems associated with sexuality, and may have to contend with unwanted or unwarranted sexual exposure during the course of their professional duties. The feelings and coping mechanisms that this engenders are discussed and explored.

Stephen Pattison and Tom Heller (Chapter 29: 'Swimming in the Sea of Ethics and Values') continue the theme of complexity in caring and curing relationships, describing the way that an ethicist views the work of a general medical practitioner, and the ethical and value systems that seem to be involved in their everyday tasks. The ensuing dialogue between ethicist and practitioner exposes some of the different ways of viewing the world that these two disciplines employ. There is, however, general agreement that 'ethical spectacles' can help the day-to-day work of practitioners, precisely because of the different perspective they throw upon apparently simple or everyday occurrences and relationships involved in care.

Mavis J. Kirkham (Chapter 30: 'Stories and Childbirth') looks for meaning and coherence in the work of midwives and the experiences of women by examining 'individual and collective birth stories and fiction concerning birth'. This is a rich source of material which serves many important functions for all women, as well as specifically for midwives. For women, the recalling and recounting of stories places their personal values within a wider context and reinforces positive meanings of the transition to motherhood. For midwives, stories can be the means of passing down practical guidance and affirmative experiences of care-giving. However, Kirkham warns us to beware of the contagious nature of some stories relating to previous disasters, which may serve to act as 'conservative pressure on current practice'.

Mike Fitter (Chapter 31: 'Research in Holistic Medicine') describes some of the ways in which sensitive research can illuminate aspects of caring and curing and demonstrate what is useful and what is not. Although the focus of this chapter is on research in holistic, complementary or alternative medicine, the message holds good for all those who want to reflect on their own effectiveness in providing care, or when attempting to cure disease. Research can have either an 'inner focus', the need to improve oneself, or an 'outer focus', which is usually the requirement to prove effectiveness to external observers. In either situation the move away from 'reducing everything to its component parts' will eventually demonstrate that 'research into holistic medicine has the potential to influence the development of conventional medical research'.

Julia Johnson and Bill Bytheway (Chapter 32: 'The use of medicines bought in pharmacies and other retail outlets') expands the boundaries of care and cure away from professional realms, to look into the intimate world of older people and the ways that they may use self-help remedies, specifically over-the-counter (OTC) medicines. Johnson and Bytheway's research clearly demonstrates the quest by some older people for control and autonomy, which makes OTC medication more attractive than medicines supplied by, and therefore controlled by, doctors. Although this form of control is available only to those with sufficient financial resources, the older people in the study showed considerable initiative in remaining proactive with regard to the treatment of disease and the maintenance of their own health.

Charlotte Humphrey and Jill Russell (Chapter 33: 'Private Medicine') explore a further area where a proportion of individuals express control and self-determination – that of private health care. Their chapter looks at the factors which have influenced the development of private medical care. The authors raise questions about the quality of care received within the private sector, and they examine some of the other costs and benefits of its existence on the structure and functioning of statutory health care provision.

current thinking on the aetiology of particular chronic illnesses may be interwoven in the narrative but also discarded if it does not help to make sense of personal experience. This narrative reconstruction is not a once and for all account. The uncertain trajectory of chronic illness and its unpredictability require constant reconstructions of the narrative if chaos is to be kept at bay.

THE ASSAULT ON THE SELF

Kathy Charmaz from her qualitative study of 57 chronically ill persons concluded that the suffering involved in chronic illness not only entailed great physical pain and psychological distress but also a fundamental 'loss of self'. She found that ill individuals frequently experienced 'a crumbling away of their former self images without simultaneous development of equally valued new ones' (Charmaz, 1983: 168). Bury's term 'disrupted biography' also describes this assault on the self 'where the structures of everyday life and forms of knowledge which underpin them are disrupted' (1982: 169). This is a consequence of the loss of meaning discussed above where taken for granted assumptions and behaviours are disrupted and common sense no longer makes sense.

Ironically with chronic illness it is the inability to separate the disease from the self which renders the self so vulnerable. Bury (1982) draws our attention to this more positive aspect of the biomedical model of health which objectifies the disease and separates it from the self. He sees this as a powerful cultural resource, one which legitimizes illness behaviour and abdicates responsibility for the condition. But the nature of chronic illness makes this separation virtually impossible in that it pervades all aspects of the person's life. Added to this the failure of modern medicine to treat and cure chronic illness puts the onus back on the sufferer to manage the condition.

The individual with a chronic illness has not only to reconstruct the past to find meaning but also has to re-recognize him/herself and reconstruct a present biography and viable everyday life as well as re-examine future hopes and plans. This process of reconstruction has to take place within a context of uncertainty and unpredictability where the sufferer cannot count on his/her body to do the things which it was accustomed to do but where also even these limitations are constantly fluctuating. Anxiety, loss of self-confidence and loss of self-esteem are the frequent attendants of chronic illness (Bury, 1982, 1988; Charmaz, 1983, 2000) making the reconstruction of a valued self a daunting task. Charmaz identified four ways in which the self is under assault because of chronic illness: by having to lead a restricted life, by being discredited, by social isolation and by becoming a burden to others.

Leading a restricted life

The terms impairment, disability and handicap imply that everyday life is restricted and limited and the normal activities that a person expects to be able to perform are no longer possible. Scales have been constructed such as the GHQ (General Health Questionnaire) and the Barthel Index of ADL (Activities of Daily Living) (Mahoney and Barthel, 1965) which aim to test the severity of the disability and measure handicap. These scales record the person's ability to perform the tasks of daily living such as the ability to wash, bath, or dress oneself, cut one's toenails or other taken for granted personal tasks. But these scales do not measure the impact on the self of not being able to perform these tasks and the loss of self-confidence and self-esteem which can result from these incompetencies. Nor do they take account of the loss of freedom, pleasure and enjoyment from not being able to carry out previously valued activities. But the threat to self-confidence and self-esteem is compounded by the high cultural value that is placed on competence, independence and individualism. The Protestant ethic is at the core of many people's beliefs and attitudes to health and illness. This was identified by Williams and others. It can lead to ill individuals blaming themselves for their chronic illness, as Charmaz points out:

> many ill persons themselves hold ideologies about living with chronic illness, which reveal residuals of the Protestant ethic . . . . Chronic illness becomes the arena in which these values are played out. Maintaining a 'normal' life or returning to one becomes the symbol of a valued self. Under these conditions, chronically ill persons not only view dependency as negative, but also often blame themselves for it. (Charmaz, 1983: 169)

In her reworking of some of her earlier research data Blaxter (1993) explores the issue of why the victims blame themselves. She was particularly interested in how the working-class grandmothers in that sample dealt with the notion of class inequalities in health because, although acknowledged by sociologists and social commentators, this was not an explanation for ill health which they used. She concludes that they acknowledged deprivations in the past but they believed that these indeed were 'a thing of the past' and that people were now much better off and had little to complain about. She explains:

> They were perfectly capable of holding in equilibrium ideas which might seem opposed: the ultimate cause, in the story of the deprived past, of their current ill health, but at the same time their own responsibility for 'who they were'; the inevitability of ill health, given their biographies, but at the same time guilt if they were forced to 'give in' to illness. With this emphasis on selfhood and self-responsibility, and their knowledge of greatly improved general social circumstances, a rejection of ideas about (contemporary) 'inequality' was understandable. (Blaxter, 1993: 141)

Nor do they question the 'normality' of ablebodiedness. Social life is organized on the expectation of ablebodiedness and only in the last two decades has this been challenged by those who are disabled. They have exposed the disabling nature of our society (Finkelstein, 1993; Oliver, 1990). Those whose chronic illness and disabilities creep up on them in later life, who have identified and valued themselves as ablebodied, are not part of what has become a supportive network of disabled people. They do not question the restrictive structures of society and so in many ways contribute to their own restrictions (Charmaz, 1983: 174). But the handicap and disability which accompanies many chronic illnesses is difficult to adapt to precisely because it is so unpredictable. We have already discussed the limits of medical knowledge and the trial and error nature of treatment which contributes to this uncertainty. Added to this many chronic illnesses have long periods of remission when hopes and expectations are raised only to be dashed when the symptoms return. Sufferers also experience 'good and bad days' but the lack of reliability in the body means that people restrict their lives sometimes unnecessarily and find it hard to adopt appropriate behaviour in such changing circumstances. Restrictions on activities imposed by society and by the sufferer are a threat to the well-being, self-confidence and self-esteem of ill individuals, but perhaps an even greater threat to the self comes from the discrediting of chronically ill individuals.

Discrediting

Discrediting can arise from interactions with others as well as from within the individual who is frustrated and disappointed with him/herself because of the inability to function in ways that she/he would like. The stigma attached to visible impairments was identified by Goffman in his classic work on the management of spoiled identity (1963). He was operating within an interactionist framework and was interested in the ways visibly impaired individuals managed their interactions with others. Charmaz (1983, 1995) found that many of her respondents who had visible bodily changes due to arthritis restricted their activities rather than risk being discredited. Others limited their trips out and had to gear themselves up to face going out. But it was not only those with visible impairments who faced being discredited. Lack of competence and the loss of independence gave rise also to discrediting which could result in the individual being discounted. Although public awareness has been raised on this issue and most people are aware of the pitfalls of ignoring a person in a wheelchair and the 'does he take sugar' syndrome, Charmaz found many subtle ways in which her respondents felt discounted. This was particularly the case when their movements were slow or they had speech difficulties. Others would discount them by doing things for them or speaking for them.

Although all discounting and discrediting is hurtful to the self-image and damages self-esteem the significance of the discreditor is clearly important. Children in the street calling names is unpleasant but when valued colleagues, friends or intimates begin to devalue the chronically ill person then the threat to the self is much greater and further fuels the self-discrediting to which chronically ill individuals are prone. Conversely the continued support and affirmation of self-worth provided by intimates can help maintain the self-esteem of chronically ill persons. Personal relationships are very vulnerable to the strains imposed by chronic illness, however, and social isolation is a reality for many chronically ill persons.

Maintaining social relationships

A supportive social network is vital to the well-being of chronic illness sufferers, but chronic illness can test even the best of relationships. Bury (1988) discusses how sufferers are wary and anxious about the effect the news of their chronic illness will have on those close to them. From his study of arthritis sufferers he found that this anxiety was greatest in the home. He describes how people would tell friends more readily about their condition, to test out reactions and gauge the effect of the news on their relationship. Whilst not minimizing the importance of maintaining friendships he found that with family the stakes are much higher. The sufferer is placing demands upon other family members and does not know what the limits of their tolerance will be. He found that rarely did spouses and other family members make a clear, open response to these demands and that the anxiety of both sufferer and supporters about the setting of precedents was high. The disruption chronic illness brings to the reciprocity in social relationships requires the renegotiation of pre-illness roles. People will be brought 'face to face with the character of their relationships' (Bury, 1982: 169). Chronic illness alters the lives not only of the sufferers but also of those close to them. Significant others are intimately involved in the chaos of chronic illness and their lives are likely to be restricted too (Anderson, 1988).

Social isolation is a recurring theme in the literature on chronic illness and although those living with a supporter do at least have some interaction with another person, couples can be equally isolated. Withdrawal from social life because of immobility, lack of energy, embarrassment or preoccupation with the illness and its treatment is evident among sufferers (Strauss, 1975; Bury, 1982; Charmaz, 1983, 2000; Anderson, 1988) and this invariably involves the supporters, thus putting great strain on the relationship. Ruth Pinder from her study of people suffering from Parkinson's disease describes how couples are doubly isolated when friends and other family members do not visit because they find the proximity of chronic illness discomfiting. She quotes one woman who was looking after her husband:

describes the concept as a 'style of adjustment' made within the terms of both social and bodily constraints (Radley, 1989). Two somewhat polarized 'styles of adjustment' were found by Radley (1989) which to some extent parallel normalization and the reorganization of everyday life. 'Active-denial' was very much a style of carrying on as normal whereas 'accommodation' was more akin to readjusting personal and social life. Radley believes that the options open to people in terms of the style they can adopt are much less to do with the chronic condition and more to do with the social situation and the discourses available to people.

Normalization and the reconstruction of everyday life are two main ways of coping identified in the literature. Numerous commentators on chronic illness have described how sufferers strive to maintain their normal everyday functioning (Strauss, 1975; Wiener, 1975; Pinder, 1988; Charmaz, 1983, 1995, 2000). They do this by minimizing their difficulties and disguising their symptoms or by making superhuman efforts to overcome their handicap and carrying on as usual. When this is no longer possible they reorganize their everyday lives and reconstruct the taken for granted in an attempt to renormalize or construct a new normality (Anderson and Bury, 1988; Pinder, 1988).

The way people cope, the strategies and style they adopt do not occur in a social vacuum and clearly are, to a degree, dependent on the economic and social resources available to them.

REFERENCES

Anderson, R. (1988) 'The quality of life of stroke patients and their carers', in R. Anderson and M. Bury (eds), *Living with Chronic Illness: The Experience of Patients and Their Families*. London: Unwin Hyman. pp. 14–42.

Anderson, R. and Bury, M. (eds) (1988) *Living with Chronic Illness: The Experience of Patients and Their Families*. London: Unwin Hyman.

Bhalla, A. and Blakemore, K. (1981) *Elders of the Ethnic Minority Groups*. Birmingham: AFFOR (All Faiths for One Race).

Blaxter, M. (1993) 'Why do the victims blame themselves?' in A. Radley (ed.), *Worlds of Illness*. London: Routledge. pp. 124–42.

Bury, M. (1982) 'Chronic illness as biographical disruption', *Sociology of Health and Illness*, 4: 167–82.

Bury, M. (1988) 'Meanings at risk: the experience of arthritis', in R. Anderson and M. Bury (eds), *Living with Chronic Illness: The Experience of Patients and Their Families*. London: Unwin Hyman. pp. 89–116.

Bury, M. (1991) 'The sociology of chronic illness: a review of research and prospects', *Sociology of Health and Illness*, 13 (4): 451–67.

Charmaz, K. (1983) 'Loss of self: a fundamental form of suffering in the chronically ill', *Sociology of Health and Illness*, 5: 168–95.

Charmaz, K. (1990) 'Discovering chronic illness: using grounded theory', *Social Science and Medicine*, 30 (11): 1161–72.

Charmaz, K. (1995) 'The body, identity and self: adapting to impairment', *Sociological Quarterly*, 36: 657–80.

Charmaz, K. (2000) 'Experiencing chronic illness', in G.L. Albrecht, R. Fitzpatrick and S.C. Scrimshaw (eds), *The Handbook of Social Studies in Health and Medicine*. London: Sage. pp. 277–93.

Ebrahim, S. (1992) 'Health of elderly Asian women', in J. George and S. Ebrahim (eds), *Health Care for Older Women*. Oxford: Oxford University Press. pp. 168–78.

Fennell, G., Emerson, A.R., Sidell, M. and Hague, A. (1981) *Day Centres for the Elderly in East Anglia*. Norwich: Centre for East Anglia Studies.

Finkelstein, V. (1993) 'Disability: a social challenge or an administrative responsibility?' in J. Swain, V. Finkelstein, S. French and M. Oliver (eds), *Disabling Barriers – Enabling Environments*. London: Sage.

Goffman, E. (1963) *Stigma: Notes on the Management of Spoiled Identity*. Harmondsworth: Penguin.

Gunaratnam, Y. (1993) 'Breaking the silence: Asian carers in Britain', in J. Bornat, C. Pereira, D. Pilgrim, and F. Williams (eds), *Community Care: A Reader*. London, Macmillan. pp. 114–23.

Kasl, S. (1983) 'Social and psychological factors affecting the course of a disease: an epidemiological perspective', in D. Mechanic (ed.), *Handbook of Health, Health Care and the Health Professions*. New York: Free Press. pp. 683–708.

Mahoney, F.I. and Barthel, D.W. (1965) 'Functional evaluation: the Barthel Index', *Maryland State Medical Journal*, 14: 61–5.

Oliver, M. (1990) *The Politics of Disablement*. London: Macmillan.

Pinder, R. (1988) 'Striking balances: living with Parkinson's disease', in R. Anderson and M. Bury (eds), *Living with Chronic Illness: The Experience of Patients and Their Families*. London: Unwin Hyman. pp. 67–88.

Radley, A. (1989) 'Style, discourse and constraint in adjustment to chronic illness', *Sociology of Health and Illness*, 11: 231–52.

Radley, A. (ed.) (1993) *Worlds of Illness*. New York: Routledge.

Sidell, M. (1986) 'Coping with confusion: the experience of sixty elderly people and their carers'. PhD thesis, Norwich, University of East Anglia.

Sidell, M. (1991) *Gender Differences in the Health of Older People*. Research report, Department of Health and Social Welfare, Milton Keynes, Open University.

Strauss, A. (1975) *Chronic Illness and the Quality of Life*. St Louis: Mosby.

Wiener, C. (1975) The burden of rheumatoid arthritis: tolerating the uncertainty. In A. Strauss (ed.) *Chronic Illness and the Quality of Life*. St Louis: Mosby.

Williams, G. (1984) 'The genesis of chronic illness: narrative reconstruction', *Sociology of Health and Illness*, 6: 174–200.

Katz also attributes medical authoritarianism to a thwarted need for certainty: 'Professional uncertainty is carefully camouflaged and substituted with an infallible air of professional certainty' (Katz, 1986). When treatment is unsuccessful, doctors feel anxiety and guilt, and this becomes expressed in authoritarianism, so that if control over disease is not achieved at least domination of the decision-making process is secured.

Nuland is also concerned about 'abandonment' of those who are dying, and particularly abandonment by doctors. In a discussion which has parallels with Eliot Freidson's concept of 'the clinical mind' (Freidson, 1975), Nuland describes doctors as 'people who succeed', as evidenced by their achievement of medical qualifications and posts obtained in strong competition. As a result: 'to be unsuccessful is to endure a blow to self-image that is poorly tolerated by members of this most egocentric of professions' (Nuland, 1993).

Referring back to the case of Miss Welch, Nuland (1993) recognizes that it is easy for doctors to convince themselves that they know better than their patients, to give only that amount of information which they think appropriate, and thus influence patients' decision-making. Once this possibility of control is lost, as for example with patients who are dying of cancer, doctors tend to abandon them in an 'abrogation of responsibility'.

Modern medicine has become 'an exercise in applied science' (Nuland, 1993). To counteract these tendencies, Nuland emphasizes the importance of empathy:

> I say these things not to condemn high-tech doctors. I have been one of them, and I have shared the excitement of last-ditch fights for life and the supreme satisfaction that comes when they are won. But more than a few of my victories have been Pyrrhic . . . I also believe that had I been able to project myself into the place of the family and the patient, I would have been less often certain that the desperate struggle should be undertaken. (Nuland, 1993)

The writers quoted so far seem to imply that cure is inadequate unless it is accompanied by care, although they do not explicitly use this terminology. As we go on to consider some of the literature on care, we shall rapidly realize the difficulties and dilemmas associated with this concept too.

CARE: WHAT IS IT?

To say that there is lack of consensus about the definition of care is a major understatement. A selection of the defining characteristics of care found in the literature reviewed are listed (in random order) in Table 27.1. Thus, confusion and ambiguity permeate attempts to define care and caring.

Table 27.1   *Some characteristics of care*

Honesty	Feeling	Actualizing	Reciprocity
Patience	Mattering	Involvement	Engrossment
Courage	Autonomy	Relationships	Respect
Sensitivity	Trust	Dignity	Spirituality
Dedication	Assistive	Being with	Supportive
Commitment	Facilitative	Love	Satisfaction
Knowledge	Tenderness	Compassion	Integrity
Skills	Growing	Empathy	Closeness

Dunlop (1986) asks, 'Is a science of caring possible?', and this question will be familiar to those who have studied 'nursing theory'. Dunlop first notes that there is a distinct and 'emergent' sense of the word 'caring' which has both linkages with and differences from historical uses of the term. According to Bevis (1981) it is possible to trace both common origins for the words 'care' and 'cure' and to find separate derivations, with 'care' being an old English term and 'cure' coming from Latin via French. She concludes that if there is to be a science of caring (she has no problem with the notion of science *for* caring), it cannot be a science in the traditional sense, for this involves concepts of control, domination and measurement that are in contradiction with the notion of care put forward by nurse theorists.

Another source of ambiguity is the definition of nursing itself. Dunlop (1986) states that:

If nursing is caring then the term 'nursing care' is tautologous. Caring is an interactive process which requires the carer to be responsive to the needs of the person cared for, the resources available and the context in which care occurs. This involves skilled assessment, planning, action and evaluation of the implications and nuances of all of these factors. Nurses already have a word for this process – it is called 'nursing'.

Hill (1991) also claims that nursing has 'something special' to offer and that the 'something' is care. She reports superior outcomes in a group of patients treated by rheumatology nurse practitioners (RNPs) in comparison with a group treated by a physician. Among the outcome measures showing better performance were increased articular function, less pain, reduced anxiety and depression, and increased patient knowledge and satisfaction. Hill (1991) attributes the differences to 'dissimilarities in nursing and medical attitudes to care, that is "care v cure" ', the RNPs offering more 'holistic' care. Similar claims are made in North American literature on nurse practitioners (see for example Linn, 1984). Holden and Littlewood (1991) challenge the distinction between caring and curing by asking whether this separation means that:

caring is not curative or that curing is not carative? Does this mean that nurses do not cure and that doctors do not care? When confronted with the implications of this statement one begins to realize how ridiculous it actually is. (Holden and Littlewood, 1991)

Engelhardt (1985) similarly can see 'no essential or conceptually significant differences between the professions of nursing and medicine in their caring for patients'.

Leininger (1977) also suggests that caring and curing are intimately related when she writes that:

> caring acts and decisions make the crucial difference in effective curing consequences. Therefore, it is caring that is the most essential and critical ingredient to any curative process.

What, if anything, then, is distinctive about the nursing–caring link which marks it off from the medicine–curing relationship? Despite the multiple definitions illustrated earlier, there is wide agreement that it is the interpersonal relationships aspect that is distinctive to nursing and caring. Not to acknowledge this element in nursing is to deny the patient's and nurse's subjectivity, according to Gadow (1985). Without this intersubjectivity, both patient and nurse are reduced to objects, their personal dignity is lost, and the 'coherent wholeness from which parts of the self' are made up is thereby excluded. Further, in Fry's (1988) view nurses and patients need 'ample time to connect' in order to achieve the 'reciprocity and mutuality' that are essential to the ethic of caring.

LOGOCENTRIC CARING?

Some writers believe that the interpersonal aspects of the nurse–patient relationship achieve spiritual dimensions. This approach, which could be termed the 'Woody Allen' or logocentric (Dunlop, 1986) version of the caring relationship, is as heavily attacked and defended among nursing theorists as is the psychotherapeutic perspective from which it derives. Some defend it with an almost religious fervour which matches its own terminology.

Watson's work is an example of the genre. She states that:

> Nursing within a transpersonal caring perspective attends to the human center of both the one caring and the one being cared for; it embraces a spiritual, even metaphysical dimension of the caring process. (Watson, 1988)

Krysl, a follower of Watson, writes in a way which might make one question whether it is really the nurse–patient relationship that is being described:

> When two of us enter into each other in this way, willingly and receptively, transformation takes place. The gestalt of our separate beings loosens and

vibrates. . . . And we are filled with energy; a living material, palpable, substantial. (Krysl, 1988, cited in Watson, 1988)

Writing of her work as a midwife and using a poetic format, Krysl says of the third stage of labour

And when it comes I examine the placenta
I'm sorting the particles and waves in the spectrum of light
And when my work is finished and I go from the place of birth
I walk out across the fields of the planets into the spaces between the furthest stars. (ibid.)

Others, including Phillips (1993) and Dunlop (1986), criticize this 'over-psychologization' of nursing. Dunlop is concerned that this 'dematerializing tendency' towards 'disembodied caring', which nurses are adopting in order to separate nursing from the 'physicality' of medicine and establish it as an autonomous profession, militates against the very 'holism' that nurses are seeking.

Salvage, too, is sceptical about what she calls 'new nursing', with its emphasis on a 'quasi-psychotherapeutic' relationship drawing on humanistic psychology and psychoanalysis. She believes that while:

psychotherapy aims to help the client solve emotional problems . . . general hospital patients are seeking help for physical disorders, albeit with an affective component. Their immediate concern is likely to be relief from pain and discomfort, rather than a meaningful relationship. (Salvage, 1990)

DIFFERENT CARE SETTINGS

This leads us on to the idea that what constitutes care and cure and an appropriate balance between the two are likely to vary in different settings. Reed and Bond (1991), for example, report on a study comparing nursing practice in long-term and acute care wards for elderly patients. They found that in both settings the concept of cure was the 'yardstick' by which nurses evaluated their work. For those on acute care wards:

cure and subsequent discharge was the raison d'etre . . . and their efforts were directed towards this . . . nurses revealed that they felt that they achieved this and derived satisfaction from this achievement. Scientific assessment in line with the policy and objectives for hospital geriatric care was therefore important as a basis for planning nursing care.

The authors comment that: 'This kind of *care* was as effective in curing their elderly patients as those in any other type of general acute care ward' (Reed and Bond 1991; my emphasis).

On the long-stay wards, cure was also a reference point, but its 'seeming inappropriateness' led nurses to seek:

satisfaction primarily from giving 'good geriatric care' which was achievable within their own terms of reference. This involved investment in the speedy and efficient completion of ward routines, which precluded assessment of individual patients' problems . . . this espoused professionalism precluded addressing the needs of individual patients. (Reed and Bond, 1991)

It seems that in this example, care which was strongly focused on cure matched more closely the characteristics of care discussed earlier than care which recognized that cure was unrealistic and that nursing was more appropriate.

Gates (1991) compared hospital and hospice settings as caring environments 'grappling with care and cure phenomena'. She found similarities in the two settings in terms of 'caring as closeness', staff needing to care for each other, and 'caring as solidarity' between staff, patents and families. However, there were differences too, in perhaps expected directions. In the hospital a cure orientation was more prevalent, whereas in the hospice 'cure of symptoms' was seen as more important. The hospital was more hierarchically organized, and it was not easy to be flexible over rules. 'Symbolism and ritual activities' associated with dying were more in evidence in the hospice.

These writers, as well as both Nuland (1993) and Salvage (1990), whose work has already been discussed, suggest that a different care:cure balance is appropriate in different settings, including surgical work, care of the dying and care of mentally ill people.

LAY AND PROFESSIONAL CARING

A final issue in relation to nursing and caring is whether there is any difference between caring when it is performed by family and friends as lay carers or when it is carried out by professionally qualified nurses. Kitson (1987) addresses this question, and defines the lay caring relationship as one based on trust by the recipient of care, the commitment of the caregiver, the recipient's belief that this will promote her best interests and respect her integrity, and the carer having the necessary knowledge and skills. In summary: 'The whole interaction is given shape and direction by the close personal relationship existing between the two' (Kitson, 1987).

In a professional caring relationship, these elements should also be present but the contractual nature of the arrangement makes it more complex (Melia, 1981). Patients and nurses come from different backgrounds, do not know each other personally and may not share the same expectations. This can lead the nurse to fail to see the patient as an individual. Because of this complexity, for Kitson (1987) it is 'of vital importance' that professional carers are able to 'assess the effectiveness of the service they are providing' and:

> Where lay caring and professional care differ is in the extent to which
> professional carers set themselves up as a specialist service meeting the care
> needs of those who are either unable to care for themselves or others in an
> acceptable manner. (ibid.)

Once again, then, there is an emphasis on the interpersonal aspects of
care, whether it is given by lay or professional nursing carers.

Having reviewed a variety of contributions to the care:cure debate, one
does not necessarily feel that the essence of caring has been defined.
However, one crucial perspective, that of patients, has not so far been
considered. It is to this that I shall now turn.

PATIENTS, CARE AND CURE

It is only relatively recently that patients' views have been sought using
research methods that allow patients themselves to express what is
important to them and to choose which topics they wish to comment
upon. Previously work in this area tended to fall under the heading of
'patient satisfaction' surveys and the most common research tool was a
structured questionnaire in which patients were asked to respond to
items considered important by nurses and/or managers. This has been
dubbed the 'charm school and better wallpaper' approach (Cooke, 1994).

Limited though this approach is, in a number of instances researchers
have identified disparate views between patients and nurses about what
are the most important aspects of care or what are patients' greatest
concerns (Allanach and Golden, 1988). For example, Johnston (1982)
found greater similarity between the views of fellow patients than
between patients and nurses with regard to patients' worries. These
findings should alert us to the possibility that what nurses consider to be
the defining characteristics of care are not those which patients themselves would identify.

A more recent research approach has been the Q-sort. Q methodology
was designed to allow study participants 'opportunities to express their
viewpoints or beliefs or "versions of reality" by the way in which they
sort a number of items' (Rogers, 1991). The researcher supplies a set of
statements, normally derived from the literature or preparatory research,
and usually on cards, which 'reflect the broad range of ideas, statements
and arguments about the topic in question' (ibid.). Participants are asked
to sort the cards into piles according to their degree of agreement or
disagreement with the statements printed on them. They may also be
asked to explain the reasoning behind the ways in which they arrange
the cards or items.

One of the most common uses of Q methodology in the nursing
literature is the CARE-Q, a 50-item instrument designed by Larson
(1984). The tool has been used to compare patients' and nurses' views
about caring behaviours in oncology and other settings.

In Larson's own study (Larson, 1981) and a replication by Mayer (1987) comparing oncology nurses' and cancer patients' views, nurses more frequently judged expressive, i.e. emotional, aspects of care as important while patients ranked instrumental or physical/technical care as most important. In a further replication by Gooding et al. (1993), patients again focused on technical care as 'most important in making them feel cared for'. The five highest ranking items for patients were:

1 Knows how to give shots, IVs, etc.
2 Gives a quick response to patient's call.
3 Gives the patient's treatments and medications on time.
4 Knows when to call the doctor.
5 Is perceptive of patient's needs and plans and acts accordingly (e.g. gives anti-nausea medication when patient is receiving medication that will probably induce nausea).

As in the original research, nurses 'did not rank the clinical caring subscale highly' (Gooding et al. 1993). Their five highest ranked items were:

1 Listens to the patient.
2 Allows the patient to express his feelings and his/her disease and treatment fully and treats the information confidentially.
3 Realizes that the patient knows himself best and whenever possible includes the patient in planning and management of his/her disease.
4 Is perceptive of patient's needs and plans and acts accordingly.
5 Gets to know the patient as a person.

The authors suggest that nurses 'took clinical competence for granted' and therefore did not rank it highly, while patients could not focus on other aspects of care until their physical needs had been met.

Similar findings emerged in a study by Brown (1986). Using a critical incident technique, 50 patients were asked to describe an experience during their hospitalization when they felt cared for by a nurse. Analysis of these tape-recorded interviews yielded a four-part process of care. These parts were: patient perception of a need or wish that the patient cannot satisfy; recognition and acknowledgement by the nurse of the patient's need; action taken to satisfy the need; and the way in which the nursing action is performed. Brown (1986) reports that:

> Patients speak clearly to the importance of the nurse meeting their treatment needs (instrumental activities) and doing this in a way that protects and enhances the unique identity of the individual (expressive activities). . . . Fundamental to the experience of care is the patient's confidence in the ability of the nurse to provide the necessary physical care and treatment. As this professional competency is demonstrated, the more expressive activities become important.

Von Essen and Sjödén (1991) used a Swedish version of the CARE-Q and a questionnaire to tap patient and nurse perceptions of caring for medical and surgical patients in both a 'community' and 'university' hospital. 'Knowing how to give shots' was again ranked highly (second) by patients.

Nurses in this study ranked listening to the patient, touching the patient, putting the patient first, talking in understandable language, and being calm as the five most important caring behaviours.

Von Essen & Sjödén (1991) note that their study:

> reconfirms evidence that patients and staff have different perceptions of the most important caring behaviours. The results should provide staff with a cautionary note not to assume that intended caring is always perceived as such by the patient.

Medical and surgical patients and staff, and those in the different locations studied, did not differ in their judgements of the relative importance of the caring behaviours. Remarking that staff tend to overestimate patients' emotional needs, the authors suggest that this implies that: 'in their own judgement, staff can never provide enough support and encouragement to patients which may contribute to staff stress and burnout' (Von Essen & Sjödén, 1991).

Uncaring

Burnout has been much discussed in the nursing literature (see for example Llewelyn, 1984). Noddings (1984) defines caring in terms of 'engrossment' of the carer in the caring role and the relationship with the one cared for. When tasks are done in a perfunctory or grudging way, then this cannot be called 'care', and this may arise as a result of burnout. Harrison (1990) is concerned that resource constraints may lead to burnout when nurses are not able to give care in the way they wish and therefore cannot receive the emotional rewards that are part of the reciprocity and mutuality of the caring relationship. 'Uncaring' may then replace caring.

A consensus about care?

A consensus seems to emerge from the empirical studies discussed that patients are most concerned about the physical/technical aspects of care. They have presented for treatment in order to be treated for an illness or condition and it is only when they see this being efficiently and effectively dealt with that they begin to be concerned with more affective or expressive aspects. Nurses, probably influenced by recent theorists of nursing, may misjudge patients' priorities by placing too much emphasis on the psychological aspects of care. That these findings hold good for cancer patients, for whom a strong emotional component might be expected, as well as for medical and surgical patients, adds to their importance for nurses.

REFERENCES

Allanach, E.J. and Golden, B.M. (1988) 'Patients' expectation and values clarification: a service audit', *Nursing Administration Quarterly,* 1 (3): 17–22.
Bevis, E.O. (1981) 'Caring: a life force', in M. Leininger (ed.), *Caring: An Essential Human Need.* Thorofare, NJ: Charles B. Slack. pp. 49–59.
Brown, L. (1986) 'The experience of care: patient perspectives', *Topics in Clinical Nursing,* 8 (2): 56–62.
Cooke, H. (1994) 'The role of the patient in standard setting and audit', *British Journal of Nursing,* 3 (22): 1182–8.
Dunlop, M.J. (1986) 'Is a science of caring possible?' *Journal of Advanced Nursing,* 11: 661–70.
Elias, N. (1985) *The Loneliness of the Dying.* Oxford: Basil Blackwell.
Engelhardt, H.T. (1985) 'Physicians, patients, health care institutions – and the people in between: nurses', in A.H. Bishop and J.R. Scudder (eds), *Caring, Curing, Coping.* Alabama: University of Alabama Press. pp. 142–59.
Freidson, E. (1975) *Profession of Medicine.* New York: Dodd, Mead.
Fry, S.T. (1988) 'The ethic of caring: can it survive in nursing?' *Nursing Outlook,* 36 (1): 48.
Gadow, S. (1985) 'Nurse and patient: the caring relationship', in A.H. Bishop and J.R. Scudder (eds), *Caring, Curing, Coping.* Alabama: University of Alabama Press. pp. 31–43.
Gates, M.F. (1991) 'Transcultural comparison of hospital and hospice as caring environments for dying patients', *Journal of Transcultural Nursing,* 2 (2): 3–15.
Gilligan, C. (1982) 'In a different voice. Women's conceptions of self and of morality', *Harvard Educational Review,* 47 (4): 481–517.
Gooding, B.A., Sloan, M. and Gagnon, L. (1993) 'Important nurse caring behaviours: perceptions of oncology patients and nurses', *Canadian Journal of Nursing Research,* 25 (3): 65–76.
Harrison, L.L. (1990) 'Maintaining the ethic of caring in nursing'. Guest editorial, *Journal of Advanced Nursing,* 15: 125–7.
Hill, J. (1991) 'In defence of Cartesian dualism and the hermeneutic horizon', *Journal of Advanced Nursing,* 16: 1375–81.
Holden, P. and Littlewood, J. (1991) *Anthropology and Nursing.* London: Routledge.
Johnston, M. (1982) 'Recognition of patients' worries by nurses and by other patients', *British Journal of Clinical Psychology,* 21: 255–61.
Katz, J. (1986) *The Silent World of Doctor and Patient.* New York: Free Press.
Kitson, A.L. (1987) 'A comparative analysis of lay-caring and professional (nursing) caring relationships', *International Journal of Nursing Studies,* 24 (2): 155–65.
Krysl, M. (1988) *Midwife: Poetry on Caring.* New York: National League for Nursing.
Larson, P. (1981) 'Oncology patients' and professional nurses' perception of important caring behaviours'. PhD dissertation, University of California, San Francisco.

Larson, P. (1984) 'Important nurse caring behaviours perceived by patients with cancer', *Oncology Nurses Forum*, 11: 46–50.

Leininger, M. (1977) *Caring: The Essence and Central Focus of Nursing*. American Nurses' Foundation (Nursing Research Report) 12 (2): 2–14.

Linn, L. (1984) 'Care vs. cure: how the nurse practitioner views the patient', *Nursing Outlook*, 22: 641–4.

Llewelyn, S.P. (1984) 'The cost of giving: emotional growth and emotional stress', in S. Skerington (ed.), *Understanding Nurses*. Chichester: John Wiley.

Mayer, D.K. (1987) 'Oncology nurses' versus cancer patients' perceptions of nurse caring behaviours: a replication study', *Oncology Nurses Forum*, 14 (3): 48–52.

Melia, M. (1981) 'Student nurses' accounts of their work and training'. PhD thesis, University of Edinburgh, Edinburgh.

Nightingale, F. (1980) *Notes on Nursing. What It Is, and What It Is Not*. London: Churchill Livingstone.

Noddings, N. (1984) *Caring – A Feminine Approach to Ethics and Moral Education*. Berkeley: University of California Press.

Nuland, S.B. (1993) *How We Die*. London: Chatto & Windus

Phillips, P. (1993) 'A deconstruction of caring', *Journal of Advanced Nursing*, 18: 1554–8.

Reed, J. and Bond, S. (1991) 'Nurses' assessment of elderly patients in hospital', *International Journal of Nursing Studies*, 28 (1): 55–64.

Rogers, W.S. (1991) *Explaining Health and Illness. An Exploration of Diversity*. New York: Harvester Wheatsheaf.

Salvage, J. (1990) 'The theory and practice of the "new nursing" ', *Nursing Times*, 86 (4): 42–5.

Tripp, R. (1970) *The Penguin International Thesaurus of Quotations*. Harmondsworth, Middlesex: Penguin.

Von Essen, L. and Sjödén, P. (1991) 'Patient and staff perceptions of caring: review and replication', *Journal of Advanced Nursing*, 16: 1363–74.

Watson, J. (1988) 'New dimensions of human caring theory', *Nursing Science Quarterly*, 1 (4): 175–81.

Webb, C. (1985) *Sexuality, Nursing and Health*. Chichester: Wiley.

28

Sexuality, the Body and Nursing

Jocalyn Lawler

This chapter outlines how nurses maintain the fragile context of nursing practice when they perform body care for others – acts which break many normal social rules about touch, body exposure, sexuality and sexual behaviour. The discussion is based on my own research on how nurses deal with situations which could potentially have sexual meaning, why male sexuality is a particular issue for nursing practice, the ways in which nurses manage when patients define a situation sexually, and sexual harassment by patients.

The relationship between sexuality and the body is a central consideration of everyday practice for nurses for two interrelated reasons, both of which are derived from our constructions of sexuality and sexualized embodiment. First, male sexuality and masculinity are genital and physical constructs to a greater extent than is the case for female sexuality and femininity. Second, the genitalia are not normally exposed or touched in social life except in sexual encounters, but nurses are required to touch and handle these areas of the body as part of their work. Furthermore, we live and work in a patriarchal society in which some types of work, such as nursing, are constructed on notions of 'normal' female roles and femaleness.

Skill is required by the nurse to construct a context in which it is permissible to see other people's nakedness and genitalia, to undress others, and to handle other people's bodies. The difficulties lie in the sensitive construction of a context in which such actions are performed, in managing situations to exclude or minimize the possibility that the patient may define the context sexually, and in managing situations where such sexual definitions are made by patients.

SEXUALITY AND THE CONTEXT OF NURSING

It is often a very delicate matter to attend to patients' need for comfort and physical care in such a way that it is not sexually defined. As one

First published in *Behind the Screens: Nursing, Somology and the Problem of the Body.* Edinburgh: Churchill Livingstone, 1991, pp. 195–213.

interviewee said, patients have 'got to realize some needs cannot be met by the nurse!' Nurses take purposeful measures to manage such situations. First, there is the expectation by nurses that what they do as nursing care ought not be defined by patients as a sexual experience.

> I found it most difficult to cope with . . . the men who drew sexual inferences as you did what you had to do. That made it *very* difficult. If you had somebody who played the game and went along with you it made it a lot easier. If you had someone who laid back there and leered at you and made comments about how enjoyable it was, that made it *much* more difficult.

Secondly, much nursing care is sensual in nature, it is designed for physical comfort, and it necessarily involves touching the bodies of others in soothing and relaxing ways. Sensuality, however, is an aspect of human experience which is continuous with, and part of, many other experiences including sexual arousal, relaxation, comfort and trust – and relaxation, comfort and trust are component parts of an ambiance of mutual sexual expression.

Patients sometimes become sexually aroused as a result of nursing care procedures and with male patients this is patently signified by an erect penis. While female patients may have similar sensual and sexual experiences during nursing care, it is not as obvious as it is with males. Patients can be embarrassed and confused as a result of that arousal for various reasons. They may not have had the experience of being cared for physically during adult life, the context is inappropriate for a sexual encounter, and, as the literature suggests, they have most likely not had many areas of the body touched outside a sexual context. This (lack of) experience can affect situations in which the patient receives care from a nurse.

Thirdly, nurses deliberately construct context by 'the manner' and other contextors when they approach the patient for a procedure which involves sexualized parts of the body.

> *I:* Well that can depend on your attitude also, and how *you* handle them, and 'handle' them also. [*Laughter*].
> *R:* Can you give me an example?
> *I:* Well if you're washing a young virile male you're certainly not going to give him the come-on while you're washing his penis are you? [*Laughter*] Then he might read things into it that aren't there at all.
> *R:* So there is a way for nurses to go about their business that is quite distinctly business.
> *I:* Yes!

Context construction in potentially sexual situations is crucial and methods which nurses employ generally are especially important when sexually invasive procedures are concerned. The following account describes how that is done.

I think it's managed by a very matter-of-fact approach. For example, coming into the room and . . . turning on the fluorescent lights making it a very clinical atmosphere, and the matter-of-fact approach, doing things with . . . two people [nurses present]. . . . Rather than if I was in bed and someone was rubbing my back it would hopefully be with a glass of champagne and dim lights. You know, it's the atmosphere, and . . . if you watch the way that nurses rub backs . . . there would be a lot for whom it would not be a sexual act. Some [nurses] can be fairly rough.

Nursing care as a sexual experience

For some nurses, the potential for nursing care to be sensual and sexually arousing is perceived as a continuum which depends on how ill the patient is. There is a point in the patient's illness when sensuality and sexuality are not issues to be considered because the patient is too ill for those things to be relevant. It is like embarrassment – if the patient is very ill, experiences of a sexual or embarrassing nature are overtaken by the seriousness of the patient's condition. However, patient responses to nursing care which are potentially embarrassing or sexually sensitive can indicate location on a recovery trajectory and in that sense a sexual response can be a recovery marker.

> I: Sometimes there is a difference . . . in how ill the person is, whether it [nursing care of the body] is pleasurable or something that has to be done. It might make them feel better, but they gain no sexual gratification. . . .
> R: But there's a continuous line between the sensual and the sexual?
> I: Yes, and to my way of thinking they move between it according to how ill they are, and certainly as they recover it moves more toward the sexual. . . . Look, for example, at the person who is in hospital with a fractured femur. They are not really ill, they are just inconvenienced. That sort of situation is very heavily . . . toward the end of the continuum of sensual-sexual, but the person who comes in with multiple trauma . . . is beyond sex. . . . There's a line and as they move through from the illness through to the wellness type thing that moves them . . . through the sensual-sexual type thing.

There appears to be a high level of tolerance and acceptance among nurses that much of what they do as nursing care of the body is a sensual experience and that it therefore has the potential to be sexually arousing for the patient. However, situations where the patient defines nursing care of the body as *primarily* sexual threatens the nurse's construction of nursing practice.

> Just to make them [patients] a bit more comfortable, even though some are up and around, you give them a back rub. But some men get to the point – they're up and about, they're showering, they don't really need back rubs but they'll ask you for a back rub and I think then it's only because of their little ego trip, or thrill they're getting out of it. . . . After a while I don't offer it.

Nurses accept that sexuality is part of human life and they expect some sexual expression on the patient's part, although within taken-for-granted social norms and the contexts of hospitalization and nursing care. Sometimes nurses create opportunities for patients to have a sexual experience while in hospital, although such situations are uncommon and when they do occur they are usually not publicized.

> I remember the night [X] let the woman into bed with her husband and Dr [Y] came in the next day and . . . went crook. . . . He said 'you know sex is the most exhausting thing and I told you to keep him quiet'. And [X] said 'I was looking after other parts! This fellow's in plaster'.

The major difficulty, for the (female) nurse, in dealing with the potentially sexual aspects of nursing care, arises in situations where she is the object of sexual expression, and which she may (or may not) call sexual harassment, for example where the patient's behaviour breaks the taken-for-granted rules, particularly the modesty rule. This is most likely to occur at times when nursing care involves the genitalia, in particular the male genitalia. There is an assumed rule among nurses that 'good' patients do not embarrass the nurse by deliberately behaving sexually during nursing care.

THE MALE GENITALIA AND NURSING

The body's genital regions are heavily invested with meaning about the nature of sexuality and gender and male body, particularly the penis, is especially invested with symbolism about the power of men. The penis is the central anatomical feature which illustrates male power and consequently nursing acts involving the penis require careful social management. Further, the sexualized construction of the body and our cultural prohibitions on touching the genitals of another person present the nurse with several socially delicate areas of practice.

> Obviously the big toe is not as difficult as dealing with someone's bowel, or vagina, or penis, or whatever.

Where nursing practice is concerned, however, such taboos must be broken, and this is one of the earliest things nurses learn through experience. Despite that experience, the male genitalia continue to be problematic, and nurses do not easily overcome a primary socialization which proscribes touching other people's genitals. While nurses may become more comfortable about their own feelings, they constantly encounter people who are hospitalized for the first time and require nursing assistance with body care. We live in a clothed society and that means we are not accustomed to seeing or touching other people's genitals or genital regions, nor allowing them to be seen or touched by other people.

Nurses' access to the unclothed body of the patient is usually only a socially awkward problem when it necessitates exposing and/or handling the genitalia, or when the patient is exceedingly modest.

Touching the penis

Situations when nurses must handle genitalia, especially the penis, must be carefully managed because embarrassment can be acute and the social environment can become very awkward and fragile. Handling such areas of the body can be especially embarrassing when nurses are inexperienced and still learning to overcome their primary socialization which incorporates notions about the private nature of the body and some body functions. The account below outlines how one nurse was given advice by her colleagues (in the 1960s) about how to socially manage catheterizing a man.

> I was told 'for God's sake, whatever you do, don't touch it, make sure you use a sterile towel or something and don't dare touch it' . . . because that was just too embarrassing for both you and the person and it might cause an erection. . . . And the other piece of advice from a fairly humorous person was that she dealt with it by piling a stack of pillows on the man's abdomen so . . . you couldn't actually see each other's faces.

Nurses will use a number of techniques, for example wearing gloves, to avoid touching the penis, particularly with their bare hands, and they also use social methods to help them manage. It is a persistently awkward area of nursing and one which is the subject of much informal education and discussion among nurses. One nurse, who is now very experienced, described how she and her colleagues washed male bodies and the genitalia, in particular, when they first started their careers.

> I: You never washed it [the genitalia]. You washed down as far as it and you came up as far as it, and then you gave them the soapy washer if they were able to and then you always had to go and get something.
> R: And what if people weren't able to wash it?
> I: You washed it – as quickly as you could! And talked! While you did it – about anything that came into your head. [*Laughter*]

With experience, however, nurses become less embarrassed by having to handle male genitalia, although they recognize that the patient may be very embarrassed in requiring such assistance, and they become less impressed by the apparent power of masculinity vested in the penis. Acute embarrassment on the part of the patient, however, is a problem for the nurse, and it seems that men in their sixties and older can be especially prone to very acute embarrassment.

> I: Old farmers who've always done for themselves . . . are highly embarrassed and say 'you shouldn't have to do this sort of thing for me', or [they are]

protective or unwilling to have the sheet removed . . . and they do not like young girls, and that could be anyone from me [in my 40s] to a young girl, having to do for them.

R: But it's alright to clean their teeth?

I: Yes!

Accidental erections

One of the major difficulties in dealing with male genitalia is the possibility that the penis will become erect as it sometimes does during nursing care. Such situations require particularly sensitive social management on the nurse's part in order to continue to define the situation as a nursing event and not a sexual event. If the patient is perceived to be embarrassed and the erection is perceived as 'accidental', the nurse will interpret the situation as one in which the patient did not intend 'anything to happen'. There is, therefore, no intentional rule-breaking. However, if the patient appears to be interpreting the situation as a sexual encounter, or to be enjoying the event, the nurse may feel professionally compromised and/or harassed and respond accordingly.

Unintended erections are usually managed sympathetically and sensitively by the nurse using a variety of strategies. These include taking time out, using their learned lack of affect to define the situation as manageable and unremarkable, or ignoring the fact that the patient is having an erection.

Occasionally . . . a man has had an erection. . . . That isn't pleasant for us and he's embarrassed too. . . . Put a towel over it and come back later. . . . Sometimes discretion is probably better than making an issue of it.

Nurses who are male also find it necessary to manage situations when a patient has an erection during body care. This situation can be embarrassing and disturbing for the patient and the nurse. The following account illustrates how one registered nurse, who identifies himself as homosexual, manages such situations.

I: I've never commented, that's one thing. I have never laughed, and sometimes I could have laughed. What I've done is go on as though it [the erection] wasn't there.

R: What have you been doing at the time?

I: Usually washing there. And by the time the erection is at full mast I've nearly finished and you can roll them over and do [wash] their backs. . . . I mean it must be fairly embarrassing. . . . The only time it's ever happened to me was with a gay patient. I've never had it happen with a patient who was presumably heterosexual, but mostly with quite overt, open, gay men.

The other three men in this study did not identify sexual behaviour (of male or female patients) as problematic for them, except in situations where the patient was exposing himself or herself deliberately. Like their female colleagues, male nurses do not tolerate such exposure. It is outside the boundaries of socially acceptable body exposure in public. Sexual arousal, however, of the kind outlined above, which is presumed by the nurse to be unintended, and which embarrasses the patient, is managed as a relatively routine part of nurses' work in stark contrast to sexual behaviour which is perceived to be deliberately directed at the nurse.

OVERT SEXUAL BEHAVIOUR, BODY EXPOSURE AND HARASSMENT

Overt sexual behaviour by patients (directed toward nurses) is not tolerated among nurses unless the patient has impaired judgement from illness or injury. For example, patients who suffer brain damage are usually treated with tolerance and understanding, but unnecessary body exposure, particularly exposure of the genitalia, including female breasts, and sexually suggestive talk are violations of the modesty rule at least. They can also violate another rule that nurses take for granted, that is, that the patient should not exploit nursing situations or nursing care, and may well be seen by the nurse as a form of sexual harassment. The data reported here illustrate how nurses deal with rule-breaking situations in which the patient is sexually explicit.

Sexual actions directed toward female nurses almost invariably involve male patients, although two incidents were related in this study where female patients made sexually explicit advances to some male nurses, but one of those incidents involved a patient who was psychiatrically disturbed at the time, and the other was a post-partum woman (which is often an emotionally labile time). Another incident involving male harassment of a male nurse is also reported, but it concerned verbal abuse rather than a sexual advance. Advances where the female approaches the male generally take the form where the female makes known her willingness to participate in sexual activity. It is an indication of availability rather than an overt invitation or request, which characterizes male advances to female nurses, and in that sense these incidents are in keeping with notions that females are passive and receptive (rather than proactive) sexually. Situations in which patients make advances to nurses would also seem to be exclusively heterosexual and some nurses perceive this as a form of sexual harassment.

Situations in which patients expose their genitalia to nurses in sexually suggestive ways reflect a belief that nurses tolerate such behaviour, and/or that their work involves sexual favours for the patient. In this sense, therefore, it is not simply a reflection of social attitudes of men toward women, but also a reflection of a specific stereotype of nurses. The following account, which is very explicit and possibly an extreme example, illustrates how one patient's perception of what nurses do in their work influenced his approach to the nurse.

> *I:* Oh this [incident] was horrific. I was a second year nurse. A fellow came in with burns to his hands and trunk. [I was] sponging him, he was a little older than us – 21, 22, and he said 'my friend told me a nurse would help me out', and I said, 'yeah, what's your problem?' [And he said] 'you know', and I said 'do you want a bottle?'. 'No, my friend told me you'd help me out' [he said] and suddenly . . . it just suddenly clicked what he meant. I just picked up the bowl and ran out and did not want to go back in that room.
> *R:* In his head nurses perform the functions of prostitutes?
> *I:* Yes.

On a less extreme level patients are sexually suggestive toward nurses and expose themselves without being as direct as the patient in the account above.

> I know with one patient . . . it [erections and sexually suggestive behaviour] used to happen quite often. And I know one day he just got to me so I threw a towel at him and walked away until things cooled down and he'd settled down, and then I came back and started showering him again. . . . He wasn't embarrassed, he started being crude.

Overt sexual behaviour directed at the nurse is a common feature of nurses' work environment and one which they manage with a variety of methods. Some nurses respond to patients' sexually explicit behaviour by using jokes and humour, and they use a form of trivialization. One experienced nurse related her account of the first time a patient ever showed her his erect penis and she also describes how nurses will trivialize male patients' attempts to make the nurse the object of their sexual advances.

> He sort of lifted the bedclothes and said 'what do you think of this?' [*Laughter*] My mother had been a nurse and she had told funny stories about this sort of thing and how to react, and her answer was 'I've never seen a good looking one yet', which was guaranteed to deflate the occasion. And I can remember not even remembering to try that – just sort of beating a hasty retreat [*laughter*] from the room and bursting into gales of laughter in the pan room with another nurse who was there. Now I think at [age] 40 plus, after 23 years [of nursing] sometimes it can be a little flattering in its own funny way [*laughter*] that they even think you're worth the effort [*laughter*]. But the people who respond now are getting older [*laughter*]. It's not the young ones any more. We had a funny instant the other week. A young fellow asked one of the nurses, who is the same age group as me, where the young pretty sexy nurses were this particular evening. She said 'I'll go and get one for you', and came and got me [*laughter*] and I told him he was much better off with an experienced person [*laughter*]. He didn't catch the joke, but the man in the next bed, who was about 52–53, thought it was a scream [*laughter*].

Other methods to manage situations' where patients break the rules with explicit sexual behaviour, include making their intolerance known to the patient, trivializing what the patient does, and indicating to the patient that nurses' work does not include sexual favours. Generally, but not always, such incidents are dealt with by nurses in a way that defines them as relatively harmless sexual advances rather than as sexual harassment, and a direct approach to the patient is usually used.

If the behaviour is persistent the patient's reputation is spread rapidly among the staff, who then employ mechanisms to protect each other. For example, nurses will not tend to the patient alone, and they will spend the minimum amount of time necessary to do nursing care, and, if there is a male colleague on the staff, they may ask him to help with any body care that is required for that patient. Irrespective of the methods used, the aim in these circumstances is to provide only the care which is essential. Nurses will maintain a vigilant and distant approach to the patient, particularly if his behaviour is persistent and perceived by the nurse to be sexual harassment. As well as being protective of nurses, these strategies are also designed for avoidance, and to minimize opportunities for the patient to exploit the nurse sexually. If the patient continues to be sexually explicit, the situation can be very difficult to manage, and often it is relieved only when the patient is discharged.

However, the point at which this sort of behaviour is perceived as harassment, if it is perceived that way at all by nurses, is difficult to establish. Persistent sexual approaches from the patient are difficult to manage in nursing because of the need for someone to continue to have a professional nursing responsibility for the care provided. It seems as though sexually explicit verbal advances from patients are more easily managed than physical harassment, for example, touch and stroking the nurse's leg, when she turns a patient over in bed.

When is overt sexual behaviour harassment?

The term 'sexual harassment' did not come into common usage until the 1970s and since that time we have become more aware of it as a phenomenon to be named and understood. Much of what has been reported in this chapter can alternatively be viewed as sexual harassment – it is a way of looking at a situation, a way of defining what is happening. Much of what happens to nurses in their daily work can be constructed as sexual harassment, if the person doing the perceiving chooses to see things in that way. If we are to name aspects of nursing care as sexual harassment, we will subject much of nurses' work to analyses through a sexual lens – a process which may make people (including nurses) uncomfortable. Nurses, like most women, have not readily discussed or named or made sexual exploitation explicit. In nursing there are some salient points which may indicate why this is so, and one of them is that overt sexual behaviour by patients towards nurses has been incorporated into their working lives to point where it is institutionalized as part of the job.

Nurses do not see sexual harassment as a major problem. Rather, it is perceived as an aspect of their work which they must manage from time to time, and many have become accustomed to it – and that raises other issues. As an occupational group, nurses have always encountered a level of overt sexual attention from patients and from the public. Nursing has not only been a highly sex-typed occupation, but also a highly sexualized one. The difficulty for the researcher in matters of this kind seems to lie in nurses having seen the sexualized nature of their work as part of the job, taken it for granted, and never having explicitly identified it as a topic for research, debate or discussion. It has not been problematized within the context of an occupation particularly prone to sexual exploitation, at least not in so far as patients are concerned.

It is also possible that sexual harassment of nurses by patients is a taboo topic among some nurses, and that they, therefore, do not want it researched. Despite such attempts to protect the image of nursing, nurses continue to encounter men who see them only as women (and not as professionals providing care) and behave toward them accordingly. Such men stereotype nurses as members of a particular occupational group that is highly tolerant of overt sexual behaviour or even invites and welcomes it.

> I think that people think that we're used to that sort of thing. My boyfriend thinks I am. He says 'you're used to that sort of thing by now'. I think that's the general public . . . image of the nurse . . . – that because we're so used to it . . . seeing the naked body and accept it, [we] think nothing of it, whereas the general public doesn't and if they see a naked body they take a double look.

Sexual harassment and nursing ideology

Where nursing practice is concerned, nurses do not necessarily identify overt sexual advances from patients as sexual harassment. Nurses have preferred to call such actions things other than sexual harassment, for example, 'seductive behaviour' (Assey and Herbert, 1983), they have located them in the context of the care the nurse *should* give the patient, and they have discussed the issue in moralistic tones.

It is possible that sexual harassment has been kept hidden, not only because it may tarnish nurses' image, but also because nursing ideology closely resembles Christian doctrine in many ways. Nursing has many of its roots in religious orders, and many of its professional ideals reflect that history. The ideal that a nurse should not make critical remarks about any patient, and the strong emphasis on nurses' responsibility to care, have been accompanied by an ideological stance that locates the patient beyond criticism and places a heavy burden on the nurse to tolerate harassment. A study such as mine, therefore, helps to remove the silence surrounding this issue and makes it a problem to be named and discussed, especially when the research topic concerns the intimate nature of the work which nurses do. Sexual harassment, or a sexual encounter of any kind, is an action designed for intimacy and my work is very much about intimacy among people, how that intimacy is managed and made possible, and how it is integrated into our social system.

Nurses have not systematically challenged the professional (religious) notion that one must be able to care, irrespective of the patient, the patients' behaviour, or the circumstances. To challenge the care ethic would be heretical, yet this ethic contributes to a practice environment in which sexual harassment is not openly and officially discussed, although everyone knows it occurs. There is a moral quality to this ideology which suppresses formal talk about the sexually harassing patient. It is not considered appropriate for nurses to make derogatory remarks about patients – at least officially. As an area of discourse in nursing, and one so closely related to the body and the intimacy which surrounds body care, sexual harassment and the sexual aspects of nursing have been absent or highly censored.

Assey and Herbert (1983) provide a good illustration of this pervasive ideological stance. They define 'seductive behaviour' (read sexual harass-ment) as behaviour which 'the nurse *perceives* as an intention to attract her, usually for the purpose of sexual activity' (Assey and Herbert, 1983: 531). They further claim that this sort of behaviour on the part of patients may only indicate 'a need to receive friendliness or warmth from their caregivers' or that they feel 'isolated and lonely' and may touch the nurse only for the purpose of establishing a relationship (ibid.). They also assert that the nurse should strive to understand such patients in order to better meet their needs, and the nurse is urged to see seductive behaviour as a normal response to hospitalization (Assey and Herbert, 1983). These authors also admit, however, that seductive behaviour is one method that patients use to 'demonstrate anger toward a nurse who is considered aloof or condescending' (Assey and Herbert, 1983: 531). The clear message in this stance is that the nurse should tolerate this behaviour because the nurse's primary role is to satisfy the needs of patients, and there is a moral imperative that she (not he) should be a 'good' nurse by understanding the patients' needs. What Assey and Herbert call 'seductive behaviour' is what others have called sexual harassment, in that it is unwelcome, uninvited, gender based, and a manifestation of the power of men over women. These authors do not see 'seductive behaviour' as problematic, and neither do they see it as essentially about male power over women. Rather, their emphasis is on what the nurse should do to minimize it, and they also claim that nurses, without realizing it, may invite seductive behaviour by 'sending signals the patient perceives as seductive' (1983: 532). They continue:

> Nurses often straighten their posture when approaching a patient. This straightening involves tightening the abdominal muscles and putting the

shoulders back, which may make the breast protrude. It is also not unusual for a nurse to place her hand on her hip or cock her head to one side while talking with the patient.

Likewise, because of the intimate nature of patient care, it is common for the nurse and patient to be in a situation that has characteristics of the stage of positioning [for courtship]. (ibid.)

The Assey and Herbert position takes male sexuality to be unproblematic. Sexual harassment (or 'seductive behaviour' as they call it) is a problem for which the nurse should find a solution, and it may well be a problem of her making. They also see it as exclusively a male-to-female heterosexual matter. This approach appears to promote the same ideas which support the myths surrounding rape – that women who are raped invite it by wearing particular clothes or walking along the street alone at night. It also leaves three important notions unquestioned – that male sexuality is relatively uncontrollable; that women can be seen as essentially carnal creatures; that the social construction of nursing roles provides ideal opportunities for patients to be sexually expressive toward their caregivers.

Other papers about sexual harassment of nurses by patients have not regarded either male sexuality or the intimate nature of nurses' work as notions worthy of question and exploration. Jordheim (1986), for example, refers to male patients' needs to express themselves sexually, and suggests that hospitalized patients may have stronger sexual feelings because they have nothing to do all day. In similar fashion to Assey and Herbert (1983), Jordheim emphasizes how nurses can learn to cope with sexual harassment and suggests that with more understanding of human sexuality, nurses will find it easier to deal with sexual harassment. She admits, however, that there is a greater potential for men to misinterpret nursing actions as sexual, particularly with the recent trends toward greater emphasis on touch and therapeutic touch.

SEXUAL HARASSMENT OF NURSES BY PATIENTS

The nurses I interviewed for this study tended to see sexual harassment as irritating and annoying, and disruptive to their clinical functions, but not necessarily problematic because they have effective ways of dealing with it. One of the interviewees described it in these terms:

I guess it depends on your interpretation of what's prudish and what's overreacting. . . . They're [the patients] not considering how we feel . . . – that we might be embarrassed. . . . To me that's harassment if a fellow exposes himself. They're not considering the nurse at all.

Generally, the nurses I interviewed find it intolerable that patients should touch the nurse in sexual ways, for example, touching her breasts or leg, or that they should verbally harass the nurse. Touching the nurse is seen in a different way from situations in which patients expose themselves, probably because touch is a more invasive and intimate act. They also acknowledge that much harassment remains hidden, invisible, unidentified as harassment and unofficial.

> I think a lot probably goes on that goes unreported because nurses are afraid that they might be thought to be encouraging it or something. . . . Nurses do not appreciate being mauled. . . . It shouldn't be that we're expected to put up with it.

Orthopaedic patients: sexual harassment as sport

Orthopaedic patients are particularly prone to becoming sexual harassers. Young male orthopaedic patients were singled out by the majority of interviewees as particularly prone to the initiation of sexually difficult situations. They are hospitalized for long periods, though for most of that time they are not sick, they begin to feel 'at home' in the hospital environment, and they behave as 'normal' men (whatever that means), except that they are not very mobile. They are stereotypically sexual harassers of nurses.

> You've got these young guys, strung up in traction for 3 or 4 months at a time. They get a bit frustrated. . . . If somebody did it [sexually harassed] once, they would never do it twice to me, whereas some other people they would pick on. But that's because you tolerate it once. You wouldn't tolerate it again. But if they're a head injury they do all those peculiar things anyway, so they really don't know what they're doing, so you've got to accept that. But if he's just a young fellow with a broken leg who makes sexual connotations all the time you just tell him, you know, 'grow up'. You usually do find they grow up, or they might pick on someone else.

Orthopaedic patients provide a good illustration of the extent to which male sexuality is competitive and similar to sport. Where orthopaedic patients are located together in groups (of four, for example) this is especially apparent, and sexual harassment is one manifestation of that. It may, in fact, be the only sport available to them, because they are immobilized and virtually captive in a small environment. Orthopaedic wards can resemble other male-dominated situations where sex-as-sport forms part of the local culture, for example hotels, building sites and cricket fields. Considerable attention is paid to the female form and to females' responses to sexual innuendo. Patients make sexually explicit and suggestive comments to each other when one patient is receiving attention from a nurse behind drawn screens.

Not all harassment, however, is directed at female nurses. One male nurse reported being the target of considerable verbal derision from male orthopaedic patients, who called him 'a poofter' and refused to receive any nursing from him. While this is not sexual harassment in the usual sense, it is, nevertheless, interpreted by this registered nurse as such. He believes that such actions not only reveal homophobia, but that they also sex-type nursing practice in a way that can be regarded as sexual harassment, especially when patients make their bias known. In this sense, therefore, harassment is the use of male (sexual) power in a patriarchal system to impose compulsory heterosexuality and to impose sexual metaphors on work.

SEXUALITY AND NURSING PRACTICE: A SUMMARY

Sexual harassment of nurses by patients highlights many of the sensitive and intimate aspects of nursing practice and it indicates how sexuality is constructed in our culture. Nursing practice incorporates kindness, a caring approach, warmth, gentleness and friendliness to the patient – all of which can be perceived as sexual availability if not sexual invitation, and all of which are part of the traditional caring roles of women. Nurses are meant to practise in a way which emphasizes that patients' needs matter. However, as women, they can become the object of sexual advances from patients, and some stereotypes of nurses promote this image of nurses and the work that they do.

The data reported here should assist in opening up the debate on the sexualized nature of embodiment and the extent to which nursing must take account of the sexualized body. That patients should at some times take advantage of nurses should not be surprising, but what is an issue to be considered is the extent to which sexual harassment and the management of the sexualized body have not been explicitly addressed as topics for nursing research. If the body is as sexualized as I have argued, then it seems only sensible that nursing should take up this issue as a central one; however, the risk here is in opening up a debate which hovers uncomfortably close to the margins of respectability. It is one thing to research embodiment in illness experience – it is another matter entirely to initiate a dialogue about sexual matters as they impact on nursing practice, particularly because nurses have tried to overthrow their heavily sexualized public image.

Nurses are stereotyped as sex objects, among other things, as the considerable literature on their image indicates. Nurses make special provisions to manage that image, their work and the stereotypes that people have of them, because a very considerable amount of nurses' work overlaps with behaviours which in other contexts would have elements of traditional female roles – mothering, housekeeping, catering and cleaning – all of which are service oriented and which incorporate elements of social life where women serve men (and others).

In many ways, nursing practice mirrors the way(s) men relate to women in patriarchal society, and in 'civilized' society where the body and sexuality have been privatized. Sexual harassment of nurses by patients is a reflection of the sexual exploitation of women generally.

In nursing, sexual harassment is an essentially heterosexual matter. Even though there are allegedly large numbers of homosexual nurses, and I interviewed some for this study, (homo)sexual harassment in which sexual invitations or advances are made between nurses and patients of the same sex is (reportedly) extremely rare. One interviewee explained this in terms of a dominant heterosexual ideology thesis.

There are important differences in the way homosexuals and heterosexuals define sexual contexts. In heterosexual life, sexuality is a pervasive aspect of social life and almost any situation is a potential occasion for sexual expression. For the homosexual, however, there are particular and specific places when it is acceptable to be sexually expressive and active. Those places and contexts are learned within the homosexual subculture. The heterosexual, however, has a more ill-defined set of surroundings in which it is acceptable to be sexually expressive and almost any behaviour is open to a sexual interpretation. The high level of mutual recognition among homosexuals and the more proscribed contexts for sexual expression in the homosexual subculture would seem to minimize the potential for a homosexual to harass a nurse.

The difficulty for nursing, however, which differentiates it from other forms of women's work, is the extent to which nurses' work brings them into such sustained and intimate contact with bodies and the privatized aspects of social life, including sexuality. They see life 'in the raw', so to speak. Much of nurses' work is, therefore, open to misinterpretation, like so much of women's lives.

REFERENCES

Assey, J.L. and Herbert, J.M. (1983) 'Who is the seductive patient?' *American Journal of Nursing*, April: 530–2.

Jordheim, A.E. (1986) 'What's the best way to handle a sexually aggressive patient?' *Journal of Practical Nursing*, 36 (4): 30–3.

29

Swimming in the Sea of Ethics and Values

Stephen Pattison and Tom Heller

Ethics and values are often perceived as being necessary to consider only when issues of life and death, such as abortion or euthanasia, are in the spotlight. In this chapter, by contrast, we want to suggest that ethical and value issues thread their way through the totality of ordinary, everyday health care practice. Health care workers and users effectively 'swim' in a 'sea' of ethical values and issues (Pattison, 1994). They mostly may not notice this, precisely *because* there is nothing unusual happening. Like choosing the left-hand side of the road to drive on every day, people using and providing health care generally follow rules and habits automatically. Thus they help both to create and to maintain an organizational ethos in which certain values, actions and attitudes are regarded as normal and implicitly desirable, while others come to be regarded as unacceptable.

Working within a context where ethical and value issues are not explicitly raised all the time does not imply that people are necessarily unthinking or immoral. On the contrary. It would be exhausting and dysfunctional if, at every moment of the day, individuals had to make conscious decisions about which values to promote or how they should behave. However, sometimes the assumed habits, attitudes and behaviours of a lifetime may benefit from a little self-conscious criticism.

In this chapter, we aim to expose something of the nature of everyday ethics and values and the way these thread themselves fundamentally, but almost unnoticed, through health care practice. This is done in the form of a correspondence between the authors resulting from observational visits that Stephen Pattison, an ethicist, paid to Tom Heller, a general practitioner, in the latter's surgery. Stephen observed Tom at work with colleagues and patients on two separate days in 1997. In his first letter to Tom, he outlines some of the issues that he thinks arise in Tom's ordinary practice. Tom responds to Stephen's comments in a second letter, and the correspondence is concluded with Stephen's final thoughts.

The chapter is written as a dialogue. This seems appropriate here. First, recognizing ethical and value issues in everyday life and practice is a matter of interpretation, and more than one interpretation is possible.

Secondly, this dialogue on paper reflects the kind of conversation or dialogue that we would like to promote amongst practitioners and others in health care.

LETTER 1

Dear Tom,

For you, probably the days I was with you seemed normal and unexceptional. For me, however, it was a privilege to enter a world I do not normally see. It was brave of you to let me observe you in action and I hope you will be interested in some of the things that I saw that I think raise ethically related issues and questions.

I think you were a bit sceptical about whether anything of ethical interest arose in the course of your everyday work. If by ethical one means dilemmas, hard choices and issues of life and death, I would concur. As far as I could tell, there were only two cases in which 'classic' moral dilemmas might have arisen. One was referring a woman for an abortion, something you seemed to find relatively unproblematic, presumably because you already have a thought-through general position on this kind of case. The other related to a man whose sight was deteriorating and who wanted to continue to drive his car. In this instance you referred him for sight tests, but did not immediately inform the Driver Vehicle Licensing Authority.

However, beyond these cases, I was fascinated to see how rich a tapestry of ethics and value-related issues underlies your work at almost every point. Here are just a few of the things that I observed with my personal reflections upon them.

Inevitably, you quite often give people physical examinations. You almost always said, 'Well done' to the patient when you had finished your examination. I was intrigued by this response. It seemed to me that this was rather a parental thing to say to adults. I wondered whether this might indicate a somewhat paternalistic attitude to people indicating a kind of superior–inferior attitude in a relationship where power in terms of status and class is quite an important underlying issue (Waitzkin, 1991). I was quite clear that you were trying to be kind and reassuring and I think this was appreciated. However, it seems to me that underlying this spontaneous habitual response of yours there might be issues of paternalism, responsibility, and respect for people that you might want to think about. Along the same lines I wondered if your calling patients 'love', as you often did, embodied a mutually respectful attitude. This suspicion was somewhat allayed by the fact that they seemed quite happy to call you 'love' too! So maybe I am mountain-building here.

A number of the patients who came to visit you appeared to be drug addicts. It seemed to me that you were often rather sharp with these people and a bit inclined to lecture them as to how they should behave. It may be that this is a deliberate therapeutic strategy that you use with a particular group of people. However, I wondered if you were maybe a bit over-directive and parental in these cases. As a lay person I was a bit concerned that perhaps these people did not command much respect from you and that you felt somewhat frustrated by them. Here again, issues of paternalism, respect for autonomy and really seeking to be of use to people (beneficence) might be a relevant thing to think about (Beauchamp and Childress, 1994; Boyd et al., 1997).

By contrast, it seemed that with other kinds of patients you were very willing to accept their own evaluation of their needs and to give them what they asked for, e.g. a prescription, if they asked for it. This meant that most people did not go away empty-handed. Various questions arose for me here. Who should define the patient's needs? How should these needs be defined or negotiated between doctor and patient? Should the professional expertise of the doctor take proper precedence over the self-perception of the patient? Is there a danger of not taking enough professional responsibility in prescribing? All these are issues concerning the doctor–patient relationship and involving autonomy, power, respect and responsibility. Beyond this, there are wider issues of justice and equity.

This brings me to the wider context of your practice. While you never mentioned money or resources to individual patients it seemed to preoccupy you and your colleagues a good deal. It was apparent, for example, that some patients were obviously very 'expensive' to manage because of the amount of time and treatment they needed. I was particularly struck with the way in which you had to think about how to pay and employ people in the practice and have regard to their well-being as well as that of the patients and community. Clearly, financial pressures about prescribing, time allocation, immunization targets etc. do have an important effect upon morale, the numbers and kinds of staff available, the kinds of patients that practices might take on, and even to some extent upon treatment decisions in particular cases. This raises all sorts of very practical ethical issues about prioritizing, use of resources, and dealing fairly with stakeholders in your practice who are not simply patients (Hunter, 1997).

Even though I have only highlighted a few issues and questions here, I hope I have given you enough to think about. I have to say that I rather admire the way that you were able to pass through a web of ethical and value issues during a day weighing alternatives and maintaining basic trust with both patients and colleagues.

Yours,

Stephen

LETTER 2

Dear Stephen,
Thank you for spending time with me at my work and for the thought
and analysis which you have shared in your letter.

I agree with your general premise that ethical and value issues
surround all health care workers and that this was evident from our time
together. Just having you next to me made me aware of my own
'performance'. This sharpening was valuable at the time and additionally absorbing now that we have a chance to reflect and analyse some of
the things that took place. The exercise has helped me to understand
more about what an ethicist is trained to think about, and quite a lot
about my personal and professional dynamics.

I will try not to be too defensive in my responses to the specific
observations that you made, or to your interpretations of those interactions. The word 'practice' is interesting for me in this respect. If I now
plead that the things that you saw and felt were just artefacts, and that
really what you observed was not typical of my usual working practices
then I would be missing this opportunity to learn from your astute
comments.

The two 'classic' moral dimensions you observed (the abortion request
and the person worried about driving with deteriorating vision) illustrate very much the core work of general practice. I have an active debate
going on in my own mind about the issue of abortion, often with vivid
images involved. At the same time I have come to an externalized
rationale for the way that I behave when trying to help someone
requesting an abortion. My own internal doubts and unease are covered
up as an essential part of the routine. There is a sort of cascade of
priorities going on, and I act only in response to what I consider to be the
most dominant one, viz. that I believe in the woman's own right to
choose in these circumstances. What happens to my own underlying
thoughts and feelings?

The dilemma about the man's driving ability taps into a rich seam of
problems that I also wrestle with regularly. My predominant notion is
that I am working as an *advocate* for any person who comes to consult
with me. Often this can become adversarial against other official or
professional agencies. For example, it might involve putting forward the
best case for someone who is applying for additional benefits, or for a
change of housing. I usually have no problems with bending the truth
as much as it takes to get the family an extra bedroom, or egging the
pudding when describing someone else's mobility problems. In the case
you observed, my duty as an individual advocate was certainly tem-
pered with a wider responsibility. What if he causes a terrible accident
because of his visual impairment? Sending him for further testing could
be defended because of the importance of the decision for him as an

individual . . . or was it me not wanting to recognize the limits of my personal advocacy for him and be seen to take the inevitable side of authority?

Which brings me on to one of the more general themes from your observations about paternalism and the use of language. I hadn't realized previously that I call people 'love' all the time, or that I say 'well done' at the end of physical examinations. Your interpretation that this could be a sign of a superior–inferior attitude is important for me to take seriously. I suppose there are instances where the use of 'superior' knowledge, if not of status, may be important. It is inevitable that I have come to know more than many of the people who come to see me about the *technical* side of their medical care, and even of their biological internal workings. What does this do for our relative positions in a social hierarchy? And is this important? Or is it more to do with putative family dynamics? Is it within my inherent make-up that I constantly, but usually sub-consciously, want to be a father figure and that medical practice is the best way to act this out? I suppose that this is where I need help to understand where the boundaries of ethics meet with psychodynamics.

In any event your observations about my general 'style' of working with opiate drug users forces me to think seriously about what is going on here. For a long while I seem to have been personally attracted to work with drug users and I have published various articles about my relationship with drug users (Heller, 1993, 1994, 1998). Is this work a manifestation of my need to exert power over the group of people with the very least possibility of exerting power back over me? The fact that you were able to observe my behaviour in respect to drug users 'as a group' is especially worrying for me. For years I have tried to move away from stereotypical labels for people who find themselves addicted to opiates, and here I am observed actually treating them similarly to each other and differently from others who come for help.

Finally, the points you make about the relationship between health care and budgets and how this may relate to individual episodes of 'care' are very apposite. I do 'confess' that I do take every single decision during my working life in relation to its potential cost. Money is on my mind whenever I order any test, write any prescription or refer anyone to specialist care. Furthermore, since becoming 'executive partner' at the practice, exploring the costs of every wider action within the medical centre is part of my explicit duty. On a regular basis I get reports of how much money I personally, and the practice in total, have spent on medication, laboratory tests, staff, referrals, etc. Understanding the balance-sheet and accountancy reports has become as much part of my working life as trying to interpret pathology reports, X-rays or letters from the hospital. For me this is another 'subtext' of reality, playing as a constant theme in my mind as the face to face work with individual people continues.

You can tell from my response that your visits to the surgery and your report have stimulated me in several ways. The report has made me observe again many elements of my practice and resolve to try to understand and improve my actions and reactions. I have been goaded to see my professional life through 'ethical spectacles' and I feel that some of my usual practices have been disturbed.

Yours,

Tom Heller

LETTER 3

Dear Tom,

I think it is very necessary for ethicists and practitioners to have mutual trust, respect and a willingness to learn from each other if a constructive and critical dialogue is to be possible. If people are just confronted with 'what you are doing wrong', as they often are in the blame culture that may easily seep into the NHS (Malby and Pattison, 1999), they are understandably likely to retreat, become defensive, and to learn nothing.

I was pleased that you had thought through your responses to issues of abortion and protecting people from harming themselves and the public. I guess some people would disagree strongly with your stances on both issues, but at least you seem to know what you think and why you do what you do in these cases. Your response here confirms my view that where issues of life, death and danger are concerned, many health workers have thought a lot about the issues. This is not necessarily the same with less obviously significant issues such as the ones I mentioned to you, a fact that you recognize in your response.

One point you mention is that your behaviour and attitudes in particular situations depends on your overall vision of your role as a doctor. You see yourself as an advocate. I would be interested if other practitioners saw themselves in the same way. Perhaps one of the things that confuses lay people is that they do not really understand how health care professionals conceive their roles and aims. This could have quite an impact on how they are treated by different individual professionals. It suggests that the traditional ethical 'virtue' of creating good communication that allows people to make and sustain relationships of trust and respect might be indicated here (Campbell, 1975). It is very important that health care professionals and users should understand that the overall character and purposes of the moral agent, e.g. the doctor, may have an important effect upon what sort of relationships, values and, ultimately, services might be offered (Pence, 1991). Practitioners are whole people with their own self-understandings, goals, ambitions and values. They do not leave these at the clinic door, but often, I think, they forget that they bring these things with them into their professional work.

You rightly point out that what I have loosely labelled 'ethical' issues about power, paternalism, justice, etc. are integrally linked to ostensibly 'non-ethical' factors such as social context, personal style and psycho-dynamics, so it can be difficult to separate these things out. I entirely agree. The point is that all the issues you deal with, all the people you deal with, and your own situation and personality are bound up together. Ethical perceptions and analysis are just part of the picture and sometimes it seems arbitrary to tag the word 'ethical' on to what may seem a commonsensical observation. What a more self-consciously analytical 'ethical' or 'value' approach might allow is a larger and perhaps more specific framework of language and understanding which might help to increase vocabulary and concepts in such a way that reflective practice is enhanced. In this way, people might be better able to communicate with each other about what is possible and desirable at all levels, from that of the professional–patient encounter to that of health policy-making.

I once saw a cartoon in which a man was coming out of a psycho-analyst's consulting room. A second person sitting in the waiting room asks, 'What did the psychiatrist do for you?' The first man replies, 'Well it's not that I'm less confused, but I do feel I am confused on a higher level now!' I think this is a good parable for ethical deliberation and education. It does not so much provide straight answers, rules and solutions as pose useful questions that may help people move on to more complex understandings of their situation, which is itself bound to be complex. Hopefully this is an enriching experience even if, as your answers indicate, it can also be a bit uncomfortable for all involved, especially when it means examining fundamental assumptions and values in everyday life and practice.

Yours,

Stephen

REFERENCES

Beauchamp, T. and Childress, J. (1994) *Principles of Biomedical Ethics*, 4th edn. New York: Oxford University Press.

Boyd, K., Higgs, R. and Pinching, A. (1997) *The New Dictionary of Medical Ethics*. London: BMJ Publishing.

Campbell, A. (1975) *Moral Dilemmas in Medicine*, 2nd edn. Edinburgh: Churchill Livingstone.

Heller, T. (1993) 'The real person within', *British Medical Journal*, 307: 1013.

Heller, T. (1994) 'Drug users and the GP', *International Journal of Drug Policy*, 5 (2): 82–89.

Heller, T. (1998) 'Snowballs and acorns: medicine by impact', in M. Allott and M. Robb. (eds), *Understanding Health and Social Care*. London: Sage.

Hunter, D. (1997) *Desperately Seeking Solutions: Rationing Health Care*. London: Longman.

Malby, B. and Pattison, S. (1999) *Living Values in the NHS*. London: The King's
    Fund.
Pattison, S. (1994) 'The value of ethics', *Local Government Studies*, 20 (4): 547–53.
Pence, G. (1991) 'Virtue theory', in P. Singer (ed.), *A Companion to Ethics*. Oxford:
    Blackwell. pp. 249–58.
Waitzkin, H. (1991) *The Politics of Medical Encounters*. New Haven: Yale University
    Press.

30

Stories and Childbirth

Mavis J. Kirkham

> The universe, somebody said, and I know now it is true, is made of stories, not particles; they are the wave functions of our existence. If they constitute the event horizon of our particular black hole they are also our only means of escape. (Brink, 1996)

Our life experience is constructed as a myriad of linked stories. The construction of these stories renders our experience coherent and gives it meaning.

As children we absorb the structures of our social world through stories, and as adults we demonstrate and consolidate our value systems as we build the stories of our lives. Our stories express our selves and in their telling we convey our sense of self and negotiate it with others (Linde, 1993). Most of this is done without conscious consideration of all that is transmitted. Efforts to change values through stories, as in recent writing of feminist fairy stories or Plato's more ambitious plans (*The Republic*, Book 3) serve as tribute to the social power of stories.

A story tells more than its tale. It speaks of context and of values. Listeners absorb the story through the web of their own view of the world and by links with their own stories. The tellers reinforce different aspects of their own values in each unique storytelling. The meanings of stories may be multiple and their embodied social constructs many-layered. This is true in several dimensions. I seek to examine individual and collective birth stories and fiction concerning birth. Cultural values and personal experience pervade all these stories.

Stories reveal important aspects of midwives' work and their careful examination may open up new dimensions in which we can usefully be with women.

> Women's writings about birth do not reveal a common or universal experience, but they often demonstrate a dazzling ability to interweave memory, fantasy, theory, myth, ideology and science, and they may show us a way to turn the reproductive revolution to women's advantage. (Adams, 1994: xi)

First published in M.J. Kirkham and E.R. Perkins, *Reflections on Midwifery*. London: Baillère Tindall, 1997, pp. 183–201.

As midwives our scope is even wider, for we work with the spoken as well as the written story.

STORIES OF BIRTH AND LIFE AS WOMEN

Women who have given birth construct a birth story which they will tell for the rest of their lives though the context of the telling and therefore the significance of the story will change.

Box 30.1

My mother told the story of her first birth to nurses in the hospice shortly before her death. A practical woman, she chose to praise the hospice nurses for their kindness and gentleness by recounting the harshness and hurt she experienced at the hands of midwives:

> . . . and in the morning [after my mother had laboured through the night alone, hearing bombs fall nearby and fearing they fell on her husband] this lady came round. She said 'How are you?' and put her hand on the bedcover. I reached out for her hand and she pulled it away then tapped me on the back of my hand and said, 'I am the Matron'.

This had been told for 50 years as a tale of hurt and humiliation at a time of great vulnerability. When told to the matron of the hospice, who sat by her bed, held her hand and listened, it turned into a song of praise for hospice care. The teller, though vulnerable again as she approached her death, could now smile at the shortcomings of a wartime matron.

The entrance of a new member into a society and a woman's transition to motherhood provide rich material for stories. These stories have a special intensity. In describing the letters she received at the Patients Association, Jean Robinson reported:

> Letters about birth were different. They had an immediacy and clarity of expression which made them leap off the page. Even if the writer was poorly educated descriptions of labour and birth were incredibly vivid. Women had intensity of recall for birth experiences which was different from other memories. (Robinson, 1995)

Stories of birth create bonds between women as they recount their common though unique experiences. Birth is a rite of passage in which much is revealed. A woman recently turned to me after a strong contraction and said, 'Now I know what my mother went through.' It is interesting that 'Women for the most part, undergo initiation through their natural processes' (Lambert, 1993) rather than through constructed rituals. There is much ritual around childbirth but in this society little of that is constructed by childbearing women, which makes women's stories even more important. The sense that an experience is held in common is strengthening. As Sorel wrote in the introduction to her anthology of personal reflections on childbirth: 'Never mind, I told myself – it was the same for Cleopatra, for Maria de Medici, for Anna Magdalena Bach and Sophia Tolstoy and Sophia Loren – and Eve.' (Sorel, 1984). It was also at the same time different, and birth stories can shed light on the similarities and the differences.

Particular common experience can be immensely strengthening, as can be seen in the poignant stories in the newsletters of self-help groups such as the Miscarriage Association. These newsletters give testimony to how common experience makes support possible. Stories with which we may identify can also help us to understand our own situation as individuals and as mothers. In Adams' view, 'the closest we can come to reconstructing our origins is to ask our mothers to tell us their stories' (Adams, 1994). Other women's birth stories can shed light on our own childbearing. They can help prepare pregnant women for labour and motherhood and they can certainly deepen midwives' understanding.

Stories also affect the teller, and birth stories crystallize out as a woman takes on the responsibilities of parenthood; just when she needs support and reinforcement of her ability to cope with such responsibilities. Yet so often women's birth stories have experts as central, active figures and the woman's part in her own story is personally undermining and profoundly disempowering. As a fictional heroine observed, 'They do the doing, I do the suffering (patient means that)' (Bowder, 1983). The tap on the hand embodied in Box 30.1 can go on wounding, more subtle undermining may go on disempowering.

Old wives' tales

Professionals acknowledge the power of the recounted birth story in warning pregnant women against 'old wives' tales'. Bourne's book *Pregnancy* is described on its cover as 'The Pregnancy Bible' and has been in print since 1972. It states:

> The majority of old wives' tales are essentially destructive or demoralising. . . . Probably more is done by wicked women with their malicious lying tongues to harm the confidence and happiness of pregnant women than by any other single factor. (Bourne, 1996)

The language used in early editions of *Active Management of Labour* suggests that O'Driscoll and colleagues saw the recounted experience of multiparous women as a real threat to their view of pregnancy (O'Driscoll and Meagher, 1980). The current edition still sees these women as in need of 'an exercise in rehabilitation' (O'Driscoll and Meagher, 1993), which must be kept separate from antenatal education of first-time mothers who must learn 'correct attitudes' (Bourne, 1996) from medical experts, not from experienced mothers.

Rapid technological and social change together with increasing emphasis on the experts' version of events now inhibits mothers from telling their daughters the story of their birth. It often surprises me in taking antenatal histories how many young women know little about the labour that preceded their own birth.

Thus the voices of women are muted by the voices of experts, though only women experience birth. The derogatory meaning which the term 'old wives' tales' has taken on has hastened this muting process and 'fosters the process of self-silencing' (Astbury, 1996).

MIDWIVES AND STORIES

Midwives bring support and technical skill to women in their care. In recent years the technical skills needed by midwives have greatly increased and the proliferation of technical and organizational tasks has lessened the time and priority given to supporting clients. At the same time, the increase in status which came with identification with medical advances has also led midwives towards medical habits of thought as well as record-keeping. Nevertheless, the midwife's fundamental job remains to provide safe care for mothers and babies. Research (MIDIRS, 1996) as well as government documents (e.g. DoH, 1993) have also stressed the importance of support and the relationship between the childbearing woman and her carer. This can put added stress upon the midwife whose relationship with the narrow technical focus of obstetric practice and with obstetric language may be strained when she seeks to support women in all of the many ways in which support may be needed.

Midwives and birth stories

Midwives are closely linked into all the many strands of 'their' women's childbearing stories. Indeed these stories, and the midwife's own stories of caregiving, are woven into the material with which the midwife works with each successive client. Jordan's research as an anthropologist leads her to state that, in a traditional setting: 'To acquire a store of appropriate stories, and, even more importantly, to know what are appropriate occasions for telling them, is part of what it means to become a midwife' (Jordan, 1993). In such a setting her growing skill in the use of child-bearing stories is important in defining the point at which an apprentice comes to be seen as a midwife. In any culture, as a midwife's own story grows richer, she gains in repertoire and skill in effective storytelling.

A growing wealth of clinical experience as a midwife affects our practice in a number of ways. With real experience we recognize the clues to the unexpected in physiology and in behaviour. Previous

---

Box 30.2

Some years ago I helped Rose arrange a home birth in a situation where this was difficult. She asked me to be with her in labour as her friend. When she rang to say she was in labour I went to her and we spent some time pottering around the house preparing for the birth. Her contractions became stronger and she asked me to examine her, which I did and found her cervix to be 6 cm dilated. We therefore called the community midwife. Shortly afterwards two community midwives and a student midwife arrived, all strangers to Rose, plus her general practitioner and her husband returned with friends. The community midwife examined Rose and found her cervix to be 2 cm dilated. After this she doggedly coped with a long labour and delivered normally at home.

I pondered the change in Rose's cervix for the rest of her labour and many years after. I felt I understood when her divorce revealed the dominance of her husband, whom she feared. She still maintains that her cervix 'shrank when officialdom arrived'.

---

experience alerts us in a way theoretical knowledge cannot. With growing expertise we learn to recognize patterns in increasingly sophisticated ways and the practice of real experts has a subtlety which theoreticians strive in vain to capture.

A community midwife with much experience of home birth without the use of ergometrine (Syntometrine) recently gave me an example of this. 'When the placenta is about to deliver you usually see a little shiver. You can see it in her shoulders, you don't need to be intrusive'. Observation at my next delivery showed this to be the case. Thus a small and practical gift has been added to my body of clinical knowledge.

Sometimes our stories, if we assemble rather than suppress them, challenge our textbook knowledge and can be complex, as shown in Box 30.2.

Thinking about Rose's contracting cervix and other similar circumstances made me aware that the cervix can contract in labour, and less dramatically but more frequently it can fail to dilate, when a woman feels threatened (there may, of course, be other reasons). Often she may feel threatened by someone in the room. Sometimes she may feel threatened by a parallel in her past experience, so a woman's reactions to care in labour may give crucial clues to past trauma such as sexual abuse. The relationship between a woman's past life, her present labour and cervical dilation is complex, as is illustrated in Box 30.2. Midwives' awareness of such parallels in the stories of which we are a part can be one factor in our endeavours to give more sensitive care.

The experienced, independent midwife who told me the story in Box 30.3 said, 'I really don't know what caused the penny to drop.' She

---

Box 30.3

Leah and Gordon came to book and consult with me at 39 weeks. This was their second pregnancy; the first had resulted in the normal birth in hospital of a little boy, James, who died of congenital abnormalities at eight days. They clearly had very bitter memories and felt antagonistic towards the hospital and its staff, though it was known to me as a friendly and progressive establishment. Three days later Leah called me in early labour. They coped well with a slow and tedious labour, unlike the first which had progressed easily. Eventually her cervix was fully dilated; Leah wanted to push, was apparently pushing and the vertex was visible. Half an hour of good contractions passed without progress. She tried hands and knees, my birth stool, left lateral and the supported squat she had used in her first labour without progress. She was finding pushing very painful, but couldn't stop. We changed position again to all fours, more good contractions. I had a good look at the perineum and vulval area and checked the position. It was definitely LOA, well flexed and not a very big baby. As I looked and felt she had a contraction, tried to push and to my surprise I observed the perineal muscles and the introitus in spasm and tightening. I had seen this before but only in women whom I knew, or subsequently discovered, has been sexually abused. Leah had no vaginismus when I examined her and, while one never knows, I thought it unlikely that she had been abused and she had an easy normal birth with the first baby.

I said, 'Are these the position you tried when you had James?'

'Yes,' she yelled, as again she tried to push and screamed with pain.

'I think your body is afraid, and isn't letting you have this baby. You body seems to be remembering what happened last time,' I said. 'I want you to do something totally different . . . on your bed and on your back.' Gordon and I got her onto her bed and onto her back, and helped her hold her legs. She pushed. It was quite different, up came the head. With the next contraction Roger was born, and we all wept.

---

laughingly said she never used the 'trussed chicken' or 'stranded beetle position', but it worked on this occasion. Aware of the dissonance between the favourable factors and the lack of progress, she knew that parallels with previous threatening experience could stop progress and felt that the threat could be the fear of facing again the terrible discovery at James's birth. So she changed the birth position away from that used in the progressive hospital which was so deeply associated, for Leah, with loss and fear of further loss. During the next few days the midwife helped the couple grieve for James as they hugged Roger, and Leah confirmed that, despite all the tests, she had been terrified this baby would be abnormal and could not face the possibility of another loss.

It must be said that not all midwives learn in this way from their past experience, however long they may have been practising. Indeed, the power of medical orthodoxy serves to suppress awareness of dissonance and thus keeps the doors of perception shut. When such knowledge is recounted, it is as stories of past experience with common threads. Some midwives appear particularly skilled in gaining expertise from situated knowledge rather than from theory. It must, however, be said that this is the point where qualitative research and the ability to learn from stories come very close together (Clarke, 1995).

Old professionals' tales

Stories of past experience can act as a conservative pressure on current practice. We all know midwives or doctors whose practice is marked by a past negative experience. The fact that the experience was rare and research evidence shows that it cannot be generalized, does not weigh as heavily with the individual as the scars from one bad personal experience. Thus some practitioners are opposed to home births, vaginal breech births or whatever they generalize from an experience of disaster. Midwives' and doctors are scarred by their pasts, and sometimes I think these scars may be contagious: as stories of past disasters are recounted, they can also slip into institutional policies. Old professionals' tales have a wider and more powerful influence than old wives' tales. The ability to generalize from negative experience is sometimes very great and we all know settings where every suggestion for innovation is met with the response, 'We tried that before and it doesn't work.' These negative aspects of learning from experience merit closer attention. Perhaps they are symptoms of incipient burnout. Perhaps such scars lead to defence mechanisms as a result of a lack of professional support or the absence of opportunities for professional debriefing. Certainly these negative stories go on being told.

The midwife's tale

Before the twentieth century most midwives were illiterate members of the working class or agricultural communities which they served. They could not leave us their story and we inherit descriptions of 'meddlesome midwives' written by male practitioners who were often competing with them for trade. There are notable exceptions such as the diaries of Martha Ballard, a midwife in Maine 1785–1812 (Ulrich, 1991). More recent historical research also gives us insights (e.g. Gelis, 1991; Marland, 1993). In Britain medical dominance was profound, and where the midwife's story is told it is in the context of medical innovation and reforming zeal for the new, as in *The Midwife: Her Book* (Gregory, 1923).

For more recent times, Leap and Hunter's work on the oral history of midwifery brings us something of the stories of ordinary midwives (Leap and Hunter, 1993). Yet this is little compared with the literature on developments in obstetrics, and some books claiming to give a history of midwifery simply recount the achievements of great medical men (e.g. Rhodes, 1995).

Modern midwifery in Britain was very much defined by the more powerful profession of medicine and there is clear evidence that midwives internalized the values of that profession. Midwives therefore fit the definition of an oppressed group (Roberts, 1983) as one 'which is controlled by societal forces that have determined its leadership behaviour'. The analysis of Freire (1972) gives us insight into how, in the process of internalizing the values of the masters, the original characteristics of the subordinate group come to be negatively valued. This creates a situation where the midwife's tale cannot be told except as one that is being transformed by medicine. The insights of the midwife's tale are therefore muted or denied, with damaging effects for those who thereby reject all value in their own identity and tradition. The resulting low self-esteem is highly self-destructive, especially as it is held in counterpoint with submission to the powerful profession. The tension thus produced was seen by Fanon (1963) as released in 'horizontal violence': conflict within the oppressed group especially towards those seen as slightly deviant, which in turn reinforced the status quo. A secondary process is fear of change. How often I have seen both these processes acted out in midwifery.

In countries where midwifery was not 'co-opted' (Weitz and Sullivan, 1985) by medicine, the situation was different for the midwives who practised, often outside the law, were aware of their difference from medical practice and did not internalize its values. American texts for midwives (as distinct from nurse/midwives who had another orthodoxy), such as Elizabeth Davis's *Hearts and Hands* (1983) and Ina May Gaskin's *Spiritual Midwifery* (1977) are structured around women's birth stories and are still eagerly read by student midwives in Britain. The American journal *Midwifery Today* is similarly grounded in the stories of mothers and midwives which are distilled out in its 'tricks of the trade' page. It is significant that the anthology of stories and poems *Life of a Midwife: A Celebration of Midwifery* is published by *Midwifery Today* (1995), and has no equivalent in Britain.

WEAVING THE STORIES TOGETHER: IMPLICATIONS FOR PRACTICE

Before any changes are possible we must listen to each other. Otherwise we cannot cross the 'reality gap' between 'the one-dimensional approach' (Leap, 1996) based on the 'official story' (contained in women's maternity records) and women's experience. Brown et al. (1994) concluded from their research that what women wanted most was the recognition that someone was listening. Sensitive midwives have always known that listening to women is a very clear way of stating that they are worth hearing. Such a demonstration of worth boosts women's self-esteem. This is equally true of midwives.

Significant changes are now taking place. Efforts to increase continuity of carer are strengthening the bond between midwives and mothers. Research evaluating such projects suggests that the midwives involved are experiencing the profound discomfort of a change in primary allegiance from employing institution to clients (Brodie, 1996). Changes in the organization of midwifery care to facilitate such changes in practice could also have profound effects upon allegiances and power structures (e.g. Page, 1995; Warwick, 1996) as power is devolved downwards to the clinical midwife and the mother working together. An increasing attention to support, supervision and relationships amongst midwives (Kirkham, 1996), together with the beginnings of services aimed to meet the emotional needs of women (e.g. Menage, 1996), should make more powerful the relationships between mothers and midwives and their need to hand on their mutually linked stories.

It can be said that in the recent past 'birth was kept a mystery by medical men who sought to control it', whereas: 'Today women are reclaiming their birthing rights, and it is our hope that in sharing their birth stories, women will further understand the process and their individual power to take control' (Wellish and Root, 1987).

This 'individual power' comes in a social context, and 'control' is a word now used, together with 'choice' and 'continuity of care', to describe what the service should offer to the childbearing woman. This implies great political change and it is real progress that we can openly work towards this. To do so we must change the story of midwifery:

> Oppressed people resist by identifying themselves as subjects, by defining their reality, shaping their new identity, naming their history, telling their story. (hooks, 1989)

In such redefining the stories of mothers and midwives come together, as do our needs around storytelling.

The present climate is such that we have a real opportunity for change, but constructive change is deeply political. Tales can be told to different effects. Stories can raise collective consciousness, bring dissonance to light and be a spur for real organizational change. Yet we also have a culture where personal stories are increasingly told as confessions. While such stories make their subjects an issue of public concern: 'it is in the very nature of the self help culture not to make them political. Instead a central organising idea of the therapeutic culture is the individualisation of problems' (Plummer, 1995).

This can easily lead to personal self-blame which weakens individuals and thereby undermines any possibility of collective action. We can learn here from the struggles of black women, where in bell hooks's view 'our collective struggle is often undermined by all that has not been dealt with emotionally' (hooks, 1993). Emotional issues can be addressed in ways that are collectively strengthening, but in doing this control of the emotional story is crucial. We can see this in the medicalization and inevitable personal isolation of postnatal depression, which is now beginning to be retold as postnatal distress (Barclay and Lloyd, 1996), and in research on social aspects of postnatal depression, not least the muting referred to above (Brown et al., 1994).

Within midwifery we repeatedly find that the defence mechanisms we built to enable us to cope with the alienation of the past prevent us from moving into new ways of working. For instance:

> Many senior midwives and medical staff opposed the change [to team mid-wifery] since the need to devolve responsibility, for total care of the woman, down to the team midwife caused them anxiety. (Wraight et al., 1993)

More recently the response of midwives working around new team midwifery schemes has been found in a number of settings to be threatening to those schemes and evidence of a profound wish for them to fail, because the midwives in the core staff themselves felt threatened by such change (Brodie, 1996). It is essential that we address these issues, or the scars we bear from our past will undo our efforts to move forward.

If 'stories can be told when they can be heard' (Plummer, 1995), then the political climate is such that our time has now come, even if ironically a conservative, individualistic political context made this possible. Mid-wives and mothers must plan together how our personal sufferings can become collective participation and how medicalized language can be turned to be empowering for women. There are moves in this direction such as the Listen With Mother conferences (Dodds et al., 1996). For other social groups, 'stories of private pathological pain have become stories of public, political participation' (Plummer, 1995). This must be possible here, for stories of birth affect us all.

REFERENCES

Adams, A.E. (1994) *Reproducing the Womb: Images of Childbirth in Science, Feminist Theory and Literature*. Ithaca: Cornell University Press.

Astbury, J. (1996) *Crazy for You: The Making of Women's Madness*. Oxford: Oxford University Press.

Barclay, L.M. and Lloyd, B. (1996) 'The misery of motherhood: alternative approaches to maternal distress', *Midwifery*, 12 (3): 136–9.

Bourne, G. (1996) *Pregnancy*. London: Pan.

Bowder, C. (1983) *Birth Rites*. Brighton: Harvester.

Brink, A. (1996) *Imaginings of Sand*. London: Secker & Warburg.

Brodie, P. (1996) *Australian Team Midwives in Transition*. International Confederation of Midwives 24th Triennial Congress, Oslo.

Brown, S., Lumley, J., Small, R. and Astbury, J. (1994) *Missing Voices: The Experience of Motherhood*. Oxford: Oxford University Press.

Clarke, L. (1995) 'Nursing research: science, visions and telling stories', *Journal of Advanced Nursing*, 21: 584–93.

Davis, E. (1983) *A Guide to Midwifery: Hearts and Hands*. New York: Bantam.

Dodds, R., Goodman, M. and Tyler, S. (1996) *Listen With Mother: Consulting Users of the Maternity Services*. Hale, Cheshire: Books for Midwives.

DoH: Department of Health (1993) *Changing Childbirth*. Report of the Expert Maternity Group. London: HMSO.

Fanon, F. (1963) *The Wretched of the Earth*. New York: Grove Press.

Freire, P. (1972) *Pedagogy of the Oppressed*. Harmondsworth: Penguin.

Gaskin, I.M. (1977) *Spiritual Midwifery*. Summertown, TN: Book Publishing.

Gelis, J. (1991) *History of Childbirth: Fertility, Pregnancy and Birth in Early Modern Europe*. Cambridge: Polity Press.

Gregory, A, (ed.) (1923) *The Midwife: Her Book*. London: Frowde/Hodder & Stoughton.

hooks, bell (1989) *Talking Back: Thinking Feminist, Thinking Black*. Boston, MA: South End Press.

hooks, bell (1993) *Sisters of the Yam: Black Women and Self Recovery*. Boston, MA: South End Press.

Jordan, B. (1993) *Birth in Four Cultures*, 4th edn. Prospect Heights, IL: Waveland.

Kirkham, M. (ed.) (1996) *Supervision of Midwives*. Hale, Cheshire: Books for Midwives.

Lambert J. (ed.) (1993) *Wise Women of the Dreamtime: Aboriginal Tales of the Ancestral Powers* (collected by K. Langloh Parker). Rochester, VT: Inner Traditions.

Leap, N. (1996) 'A midwifery perspective on pain in labour'. MSc dissertation, South Bank University, London.

Leap, N. and Hunter, B. (1993) *The Midwife's Tale: An Oral History from Handy-woman to Professional Midwife*. London: Scarlett Press.

Linde, C. (1993) *Life Stories: The Creation of Coherence*. Oxford: Oxford University Press.

Marland, H. (ed.) (1993) *The Art of Midwifery: Early Modern Midwives in Europe*. London: Routledge.

Menage, J. (1996) 'Post-traumatic stress disorder following obstetric/gynaeco-logical procedures', *British Journal of Midwifery*, 4 (10): 532–3.

MIDIRS and the NHS Centre for Reviews and Dissemination (1996) *Informed Choice for Professionals: Support in Labour*. Bristol: MIDIRS.

Midwifery Today (1995) *Life of a Midwife: a Celebration of Midwifery*. Eugene, OR: Midwifery Today.

O'Driscoll, K. and Meagher, D. (1980) *Active Management of Labour*. London: WB Saunders.

O'Driscoll, K. and Meagher, D. (1993) *Active Management of Labour*, 3rd edn. London: Mosby.

Page, I. (ed.) (1995) *Effective Group Practice in Midwifery*. Oxford: Blackwell.

Plato (1987) *The Republic*. Harmondsworth: Penguin.

Plummer, K. (1995) *Telling Sexual Stories*. London: Routledge.

Powell, J. (trans.) (1993) *Sappho: A Garland*. New York: Farrar Straus Giroux.

Rhodes, P. (1995) *A Short History of Midwifery*. Hale, Cheshire: Books for Midwives.

Roberts, S.J. (1983) 'Oppressed group behaviour: implications for nursing', *Advances in Nursing Science*, July: 21–30.

Robinson, J. (1995) 'Why mothers fought obstetricians', *British Journal of Midwifery*, 3 (10): 557–8.

Sorel, N.C. (1984) *Ever Since Eve*. London: Michael Joseph.

Ulrich, L.T. (1991) *A Midwife's Tale: The Life of Martha Ballard Based on her Diary 1785–1812*. New York: Vintage Books.

Warwick, C. (1996) 'Leadership in midwifery care', *British Journal of Midwifery*, 4 (5): 229.

Weitz, R. and Sullivan, D. (1985) 'Licensed lay midwifery and the medical model of childbirth', *Sociology of Health and Illness*, 7 (1): 36–54.

Wellish, P. and Root, S. (1987) *Hearts Open Wide: Midwives and Births*. Berkeley, CA: Wingbow.

Wraight, A., Ball, J., Seccombe, I. and Stock, J. (1993) *Mapping Team Midwifery*. A report to the Department of Health. Brighton: Institute of Manpower Studies.

31

Research in Holistic Medicine

Mike Fitter

Many holistic practitioners view research into medicine as deriving from the paradigm of reductionist science, and therefore to be incompatible with the practice of holistic medicine. There is indeed considerable justification for this conclusion. There are many examples of research which has applied reductionist methods with unfortunate and alienating consequences. One study, the reporting of which had a significant impact on me as a researcher working for the Medical Research Council, was the evaluation of the Bristol Cancer Help Centre (Baganal, 1990). The study reported, with much publicity, that women with breast cancer who went to the Bristol Centre were twice as likely to die as women who did not. Even though the findings were later retracted (the data had been analysed inappropriately), the damage had been done. In retrospect, the people who had invited in the medical researchers realized that, because they had so little research experience themselves, they had been forced to trust the researchers blindly.

The lesson from the Bristol experience, for me, is that practitioners need to have an understanding of research and its methods so that they can either conduct their own research as practitioner-researchers or work in equal partnership with professional researchers. A consequence of the Bristol experience for me was to refocus my skills and experience towards working in close collaboration with holistic practitioners, to learn from them what they need from research, and to develop an approach to health care research that could both support the work of holistic practitioners and build bridges with the world of medical science.

Most importantly, I believe that the development of skilled practice ought to have a research focus, because it requires practitioners to be reflective about what it is they do, and thereby learn from experience. Therefore research should be an integral part of holistic medicine – reflection and practice intertwined. Research need not involve a paradigm which does not do justice to holism: holistic practitioners need to reclaim research as a way of developing themselves creatively 'on the

First published in C. Featherstone (ed.), *Medical Marriage*. Findhorn: Findhorn Press, 1998, pp. 614–27.

job' and, as such, research should be integral to 'being professionally alive'.

THE PRESENT SITUATION OF RESEARCH INTO HOLISTIC MEDICINE

In my observation, holistic practitioners who have worked with medical science have experienced a kind of 'cultural imperialism', whereby they have provided the data, while medical researchers have set the agenda (by assuming that they were the experts in research and its methods and that holistic practitioners were usually well intentioned, but uninformed, naive and overly idealistic).

I have concluded that research is seen by some holistic practitioners as a 'necessary evil', which cannot be ignored because people with power are insisting on it, but which must be treated with caution. Others seemed to regard it as an 'outright evil', having nothing to do with it.

Richard Thomas castigated the complementary medicine professions for having so little interest in research (Thomas, 1995). He made a damning attack on osteopathy, acupuncture and homoeopathy in particular. His point is that there will be a take-over of complementary therapies by conventional doctors who, as a profession, are active in research. He sees the very survival of the holistic practice of these therapies as depending on the creation of a substantial research base – and by this he means 'proper' clinical trials. Although I disagree with some of Thomas's specific views on what sort of research is needed, and feel that now is the time to give support, not undermine, his harsh assessment does have some justification.

If it is to survive and to thrive in our culture, holistic medicine needs to develop from within as a process of reflective practice and also to direct its gaze outwards and engage with conventional doctors, with health service purchasers, and with the public. Research has an important role to play in both the 'inner' and the 'outer' directed activities. Clearly identified research activity is the one thing that is currently conspicuously lacking from most holistic medical practice. This needs to change.

OBSTACLES TO CONDUCTING GOOD QUALITY RESEARCH

Historically, holistic practitioners have been reluctant to submit their work for evaluation by people they have regarded as potentially hostile; yet they have not had the skills or resources to scientifically evaluate the therapies themselves. Likewise, doctors and medical researchers in the past have not generally been open to working in collaboration with complementary therapists.

The situation has now changed significantly. Of particular importance, the second BMA report on complementary medicine acknowledged that complementary therapies were now a significant part of many people's health care and therefore recommended that each therapy should be properly regulated; it also argued for good quality research and the setting up of systems of audit (BMA, 1993). This is now beginning to happen. For example, the five major complementary therapies – acupuncture, chiropractice, homoeopathy, medical herbalism and osteopathy – have each established their own research programmes. In a survey of over 1,000 UK acupuncturists registered under the Council for Acupuncture (now the British Acupuncture Council), it was found that there were two main reasons that practitioners were interested in research – to aid their professional learning and development and to demonstrate and promote the benefits of acupuncture (Fitter and Blackwell, 1993). These reasons reflect the 'inner' and the 'outer' focuses identified previously as essential for development.

Another obstacle has been a dispute over appropriate methodology. The orthodox medical view has been that the only truly valid way of evaluating the usefulness of a therapy is to carry out the classic 'randomized controlled trial' (RCT), any other research design being regarded as inferior to this 'gold standard' of research methods. This view has been challenged by holistic practitioners and researchers, in particular because the classic RCT design constrains therapists to practise in a standardized way during a trial, thus preventing them from providing what they would regard as the best treatment for their patients.

However, opinions are beginning to change in mainstream medical research with growing recognition of the need for a variety of research methods, there being no single best method (Fitter and Thomas, 1996).

A third obstacle to good quality research has been lack of funding – 'outer-focused' research can be very time-consuming and expensive. This continues to be a problem. Although there is a significant growth in collaborative studies between medical researchers and holistic practitioners, there is still relatively little funding because the Department of Health and the Medical Research Council do not regard it as a priority area for funding. However, the Labour Party has published a policy document proposing a strategy of research and development linked to support for statutory regulation (Primarolo, 1994).

THE NHS AND EVIDENCE-BASED PURCHASING

An important development, which is refocusing research efforts, is the initiative by the Department of Health to promote evidence-based purchasing. The result is that health authorities in the UK now have a policy requiring scientific evidence of effectiveness before they will fund new forms of treatment. This is clearly relevant to the uptake of complementary/alternative therapies since there is now a new hoop through which these therapies must jump. It is interesting to note that the majority of conventional therapies currently used in the NHS have not passed through this hoop, and there are indications that some would not stand up to the scrutiny of these new guidelines. However, because they are used routinely, their effectiveness is rarely questioned and it is not, for example, generally being suggested that they should be withdrawn until proved effective. Thus, there is a sense of complementary/alternative therapies being introduced on to an unlevel playing field.

However, these new standards are not necessarily undesirable, provided they are applied evenly, because there is considerable confidence amongst holistic practitioners that their therapies are effective, and would be cost effective if compared over the longer term with conventional treatments.

APPROPRIATE RESEARCH METHODS

'Inner' focused research is about self-development and requires the practitioner to be an active participant. 'Outer' focused research has other beneficiaries, 'stakeholders' who stand to benefit from its results, but who do not necessarily actively participate in the action. Research studies may have several different 'stakeholder groups' with an interest in the outcome and may have both an 'inner' and 'outer' focus. It is important that practitioners and researchers are clear about why specific types of research are necessary and who are the 'stakeholders' interested in the results.

For inner-focused research ('improve it'), the reflective practice, the primary stakeholders are the practitioners themselves. Their aim is self-development, improving their professional practice, thus providing a better service to their clients and increasing their own job satisfaction.

For outer-focused research ('prove it'), an important aim is to demonstrate convincingly that the therapy is of value to a population of users and potential users. Thus the stakeholders are the users themselves, the purchasers of the therapy (such as NHS health authority purchasers or insurance company purchasers) and medical practitioners (GPs who need evidence to decide whether to make referrals for specific therapies). The potential value of a therapy has several aspects: it includes the effectiveness for specific clinical conditions, the safety (that is, an assessment of potential risk), the cost of providing the therapy (including negative costs, that is, associated savings that may arise if a treatment is effective), and the users' (client patient) satisfaction with the service.

An important question put by Reilly (1995) is, 'What evidence is necessary to demonstrate benefit to stakeholders?' He argues that there is a need to develop an 'evidence profile' for each therapy. For example the evidence profile for homoeopathy includes:

Is it effective when examined scientifically?
Is it effective when applied clinically?
Is it clinically relevant?
Is it able to be integrated with orthodox approaches?
Is it safe?
Is it cost effective?
Is it in demand by patients?
Is it in demand by doctors?
Is it in demand by purchasers?

He concludes that systematic evidence of a beneficial outcome is most important, with cost-effectiveness and patient satisfaction surfacing as emerging priorities for the medical profession. Personal experience (or the experience of a colleague) is also very influential in doctors' and purchasers' decisions.

How should this evidence be collected? Or, what research strategy is necessary to develop and promote holistic medicine and to maximize the opportunity for it to play a key role in twenty-first century health care? As holistic medicine does not lend itself to the classic RCT, research methods are needed which ensure:

- the holistic principles of the therapy are not compromised by the research method;
- users' (patients') preferences for therapies are taken into account;
- practitioners are free to give treatment, without constraint, individualized to the needs of each patient;
- every opportunity is taken to maximize the quality of the patient–practitioner relationship;
- the assessment of the 'outcome' of treatment takes a broad view of potential benefit and includes changes in lifestyle, health beliefs and quality of life, as well as alleviation of the symptoms of illness.

A key aspect of the research strategy should be to build up, within each complementary medicine profession, a community of practitioner-researchers, that is, practitioners who have training in research methods, who can carry out their own research studies (both 'inner' and 'outer' focused), who can 'hold their own' in dialogue with orthodox medical researchers, and play a full part in collaborative research projects.

CONCLUSION

After a rather slow start for research into holistic therapies, much is now beginning to happen. In approach and method new ground is being broken, fuelled by the passion and commitment to an holistic approach in health care.

My strongest motivation is the belief that research into holistic medicine has the potential to influence the development of conventional medical research in significant and valuable ways. Helping it turn itself around from the direction in which it originally set off, that of understanding the human being by reducing everything to its component parts, towards a recognition that to understand health and healing processes we need to attend to the integration of body, mind and spirit.

REFERENCES

Baganal, F.S. (1990) 'Survival of patients with breast cancer attending Bristol Cancer Help Centre', *The Lancet*, 336: 1185–8.

BMA: British Medical Association (1993) *Complementary Medicine: New Approaches to Good Practice*. London: BMA Publications.

Fitter, M. and Blackwell, R. (1993) 'Are acupuncturists interested in research? A survey of CFA acupuncturists in the UK', *Journal of Oriental Medicine*, 1(2): 44–7.

Fitter, M. and Thomas, K. (1996) 'Evaluating complementary therapies for use in the NHS: horses for courses', *Complementary Therapies in Medicine*.

Primarolo, D. (1994) *Complementary Therapies within the NHS: Facilitation not Prescription*. London: The Labour Party.

Reilly, D. (1995) *Building a New Future for Homoeopathy and Integrated Care: the 1995 Portfolio*. Glasgow Homoeopathic Hospital, Scotland: the Academic Departments.

Thomas, R. (1995) 'The fatal flaw', *International Journal of Alternative and Complementary Medicine*, May: 18–19.

32

The Use of Medicines Bought in Pharmacies and Other Retail Outlets

Julia Johnson and Bill Bytheway

For many people, particularly older people, self-care includes the routine consumption of medicines. One tends to think of this in terms of visiting the doctor and taking prescriptions to the chemist. This, however, is only part, often a very small part, of how some people use pharmaceutical products for health purposes. Virtually every shopping centre has a retail pharmacy where a wide range of medicines can be purchased 'over the counter'. In addition, many medicines can be purchased in super-markets, garages and increasingly through mail order and the internet.

Every five years, member states of the European Union are required to review the legal classification of medicines and, as a result of these reviews, many medicines that were previously only available on pre-scription have become 'deregulated': they are now available for pur-chase. Cranz (1995) has shown that more drugs are being deregulated in the UK than in Germany, Italy, France or Spain. For example, unlike these other countries, Cimetidine and Beclomethasone have been deregu-lated in the UK. The trend towards deregulation has been described as reflecting changes in health care that 'have had both a symbolic sig-nificance and a real and tangible impact' in how people use community pharmacists (Davis, 1997: 59).

It is also important to appreciate that the act of purchasing a medicine may directly follow from a consultation with a GP. Since 1994, GPs have been encouraged by the NHS Management Executive to recommend medicines to their patients that can be purchased from the chemist, 'provided that this is at the request, or with the consent, of the patient' (Tegner, 1999). The OTC Directory (PAGB, 1999) is readily available to GPs and provides them with full details of non-prescription medicines. Tegner, noting that the list of deregulated medicines is 'more compre-hensive' than many doctors may realize, draws their attention to this source of information. The rationale for this development is primarily that of reducing the prescribing costs being met by the NHS (Thomas and Noyce, 1996). But it is also argued that purchasing medicines promotes patient autonomy and the development of shared responsibil-ity. The GP might also point out to patients who are not exempt from prescription charges that it would be cheaper for them if they were to purchase the medicine from the chemist. People over the age of 60, however, receive prescription medicines free of charge and so, in advising them, some GPs may be reluctant to make such a recommendation. Apart from the cost to the patient, the GP could be regarded as being in breach of contract in 'withholding' a prescription for a medicine that the patient needed.

Despite this, it is evident, from any visit to a retail pharmacist, that people over 60 do regularly purchase medicines. Why? Might this reflect patient autonomy, a facet of self-care that is of some significance in later life?

THE MANAGEMENT OF LONG-TERM MEDICATION BY OLDER PEOPLE PROJECT

This chapter is based on the findings of a research project funded by the Department of Health on the management of long-term medication by people aged 75 years or more (Bytheway et al., 2000). The aim was to obtain a broad picture of how older people obtain medicines, how they do rather than don't manage them, and the impact that routine medicine-taking has on their lives.

The study was conducted in South Wales, north London, Sheffield and the Midlands. Through two contrasting general practices in each area, a representative sample was drawn totalling 77 patients. All were aged 75 years or more, were living in their own home, and had been receiving long-term prescribed medication for at least 12 months.

Each was interviewed several times and all their medicines were logged by a fieldworker. These included those prescribed by the GP (or some other doctor) and those purchased 'over the counter' (the 'OTCs'). We specifically instructed the fieldworkers, 'if in doubt, include it,' with the qualifier 'particularly if it is currently being used': dietary supplements, painkillers, cough mixtures and lozenges, copper bracelets, herbal remedies, etc. The only specific exclusion were cosmetic products.

We realized that, in setting out to log all the medicines held by a participant, the fieldworkers were faced, potentially, with a formidable undertaking. For example, they would have limited opportunities to check such private places as bathrooms and bedrooms. In addition, some participants were reluctant to show all their OTCs. For example, one fieldworker commented:

> (Mrs Partridge) was very reticent to discuss her OTCs . . . At times I could not handle the medicines to see what they were, even when I tried to prompt her. . . . There were many old medicines in the house in the bathroom, kitchen and spare room, some of which I was able to log, and others which she would not allow me to hold.

The participants were also asked to keep a two-week semi-structured diary. In this they recorded, amongst other things, their medicine-taking. Predictably we found that what people *say* they do (as noted on the OTC forms) is not always what they *actually* do (as recorded in the diaries). Where this was immediately apparent, the fieldworkers sought explanations. This triangulated information about the use of OTCs is revealing, and it challenges some of the assumptions that are often made about self-care in later life and about the use of OTCs.

RECORDED OTC USAGE

For a variety of reasons, no medicine logs were completed for six of the participants and so this analysis is limited to the remaining 71. Eleven of the 71 said that they did not buy or use OTC products and offered the following reasons for this. Mrs Hyde said that she did not believe in buying things you could obtain from the doctor. Mrs Boden and Mr Garlick both said that they had been instructed by their doctor not to take medicines other than those prescribed. Mr Garlick said he was afraid that, should he use OTCs, the doctor would say 'Well, get your own tablets then.' Two others said that they did not like taking medicines and did not need any OTC products. In contrast, Mr McCormick said he would buy them – but only when needed. At the time of the interview, he had no OTCs in the house but he said he had recently finished a packet of Panadol tablets. Mrs Russell said that she and her husband used to take cod liver oil but had given it up because 'it didn't do any good'. Mrs Boden, despite her doctor's instructions, said that she had recently taken one of her husband's paracetamol tablets. Furthermore, the fieldworker noted Germolene, Vaseline and zinc and castor oil in her bathroom. Thus, although these participants were not current users of OTCs, it is clear that this is an ambiguous classification.

In logging OTCs, the fieldworkers asked how often a particular item was being used. Sometimes, the participant said it was being taken *every day* according to a specific routine, sometimes it was used *only when needed*, and sometimes the participant said it was kept *just in case*. We refer to all these items as 'in current use'. Those that were not being used and which the participant *did not expect to use* in the future are excluded from this analysis. Typically these were either old medicines which they did not like or had found to be ineffective, or medicines they kept for other people to use: visitors or co-residents. In the case of two participants, all the OTC items they showed the fieldworker were excluded in this way. So this left 58 who, between them, were 'currently using' OTC medicines; they showed the fieldworkers an average of 3.6 OTC items. This compares with an average of 8.7 prescribed medicines. Typically they had one to three OTC items each, but there were exceptions. At the extreme, Mrs Moffatt showed the fieldworker 29 items, of which 15 were in current use.

There were a few (but only a few) instances where an item listed as an OTC was not a medicine purchased for the participant's own use. The Difflam cream used by Mr Coupe, for example, had been given to him by a friend of his wife who 'gets it on prescription'. In this way, a prescription medicine for one person can become a non-prescription medicine for another. In a similar way, old prescription medicines are sometimes brought back into use, effectively as non-prescribed treatment.

TYPES OF OTC MEDICINES RECORDED

Using the BNF (British National Formulary) coding scheme, it was possible to classify the 207 OTC items currently being used by the 58 participants. The two most common were treatments for nutrition and blood, and for the skin, closely followed by those for the central nervous system (CNS) and for gastro-intestinal problems.

For most of the 15 BNF categories, the most common source of drug treatment was the prescription (for seven categories, over 90 per cent of all treatment was prescribed). In only two categories were medicines more likely to have been purchased than prescribed: nutrition and blood, and ENT problems (typically for the throat). There were some other categories where OTC products were significant: half of all urinary and stoma appliances, and between a quarter and a third of all treatments for gastro-intestinal, respiratory, CNS, musculoskeletal and skin conditions, were purchased rather than prescribed. So, despite prescribed medicines being free for this age group, it is clear that OTC medicines do play a significant part in the lives of older people.

Regarding the diaries that the participants kept, OTC usage was under-recorded. Some participants had to be reminded to enter OTCs as well as prescription medicines. Only 26 of the 58 made diary entries that recorded OTC usage. These 26 participants showed the fieldworker a total of 130 OTC items in current use, but only 46 of these items appeared in their diaries. The fact that so few of the 207 appeared in the diaries may be due in part to the participants not thinking of them as medicines and not recording their use, but the evidence of the dates when they were purchased indicated that many were old medicines, either no longer in use, or being used only very occasionally.

The diaries indicated that half of these 46 OTC items were taken either daily or on more than half the days in the diary: typically, these were health maintenance products such as vitamins, garlic and in particular cod liver oil. In contrast, items that were recorded in the diaries, but less frequently, were taken to treat symptoms such as coughs, skin problems, indigestion, constipation and, in particular, pain.

THREE CASE STUDIES

Mrs Austin is a retired wages clerk, 78, widowed and has no children. She leads a busy social life, has many visitors, and takes several holidays a year. She loves gardening, rarely goes to bed before midnight and gets up early. She suffers from recurrent skin ulcers and thrombo-phlebitis in her legs, which she says started nearly 50 years ago when she got frostbite in a blizzard.

For health advice, she relies heavily on her neighbours, a retired nurse and her husband, a retired heart surgeon. She checks all her medicines with them. For example the surgeon told her she was 'shrinking' as a result of osteoporosis. Her GP, however, had told that she did not have osteoporosis. What he had prescribed for her were medicines for her circulation (Oxpentifylline), for indigestion (Cimetidine), for dry skin on her legs (Unguentum Merck cream) and for dressings for her ulcers (Inadine).

Mrs Austin says that she is a firm believer in vitamin tablets: 'I take as many as Barbara Cartland . . . You name it, I take it.' She keeps her vitamins in the kitchen. The following seven items were logged:

- Kwai garlic tablets, taken before breakfast 'for her heart, circulation, stomach . . . for everything';
- kelp with calcium tablets, taken before breakfast 'for her bones, to ward off osteoporosis';
- tablets of selenium and vitamins A, C and E, taken before breakfast 'for her heart and to keep arthritis at bay';
- natural vitamin E, taken after breakfast 'for her circulation'. She doubles the dose if her legs 'get a bit puffy'. Her neighbour suggested this many years ago. He said it would be good for the circulation in her legs. She swears by it and says she will only use 'natural' as opposed to 'synthetic' vitamin E;
- vitamin B complex, taken at lunchtime 'for general well-being and for the blood': a lack of vitamin B, she says, could lead to anaemia. She uses complete vitamin B because just taking B6 'causes an imbalance';
- chewable vitamin C: two a day 'for its healing properties';
- Oilatum Bath Formula which she keeps in the bathroom and uses 'for dry and itchy skin'. She says she could get this on prescription but prefers to buy it herself. It was recommended by a friend.

Mrs Austin buys these products variously from the supermarket, the pharmacy or the local health shop. Her diary indicates that she takes the first five items every day, but there is no record in the diary of her taking the vitamin C or using the Oilatum.

Mrs Moffatt is 77 years old and married. Although her husband recently developed a leg ulcer, they regard themselves as healthy and active.

They neither drink for pleasure nor smoke, and they believe in healthy eating. Mrs Moffatt has no time for people who go running to the doctor when 'they only have a headache'. Like other couples in our sample, they have a stock of OTC medicines that either might use. Four years ago there was an unexpected death in the family and, as a result, Mrs Moffatt was prescribed amitriptyline as an antidepressant. She still receives it on a repeat prescription. In addition, she has a repeat prescription for nitrazepam and Gaviscon.

There are 29 items listed on her OTC form, 15 of which she says she uses. The rest are old items or supplies she keeps in her travel bag for when she goes on holiday. Mrs Moffatt keeps three of these items in the kitchen and takes them every day with her breakfast: evening primrose for 'women's things', pure garlic capsules which they both take 'for the heart', and cod liver oil and vitamin A, D and E capsules which are 'good for the skin and general health'. All these she gets through mail order. They were recommended by her daughter, 'who is a home help and knows about these things'.

She showed the fieldworker some old vitamin tablets which she said she used to get on prescription but these were no longer available. In addition, she takes whisky in her tea every morning. She sees this as medicinal and says her mother used to do the same. It is kept in a plastic bottle with the vitamins. The rest of her OTCs she uses only when needed: skin treatments, cough and cold medicines, tablets for pain and headaches, Anusol and Andrews Liver Salts.

According to her diary, the only OTCs she used during the fortnight, other than the three breakfast items, were two Veganin tablets taken for a headache.

Mr Richards is 82 and a retired hospital administrator. He is registered blind and had a stroke about ten years ago. More recently, he has had some serious problems with blood pressure.

He lives with his wife in a semi-detached house about half a mile from the centre of a small affluent market town in rural England. They moved there a few years ago from a nearby village and registered with the practice in the town. They are very satisfied with the service they receive from their local surgery. They are concerned about their health and have health checks every six months. On occasions they have sought the opinion of a second doctor regarding treatments. The diary (which was completed by Mrs Richards) indicates a regular daily routine which includes his wife driving them both into town to shop or visit the surgery.

Each day he takes amlodipine and thyroxine. He thinks that his current dosage of thyroxine should be increased because he is putting on weight. He also has a monthly repeat of Betnovate Scalp Application for psoriasis, a six-weekly prescription of oxytetracycline to control the same condition around his eyes and weekly prescriptions of hypromellose eyedrops, which he uses as needed. He keeps these medicines in a tin beside his bed and uses them when he shaves each morning.

He also has a repeat prescription for low dose aspirin (75 mg). He does not collect this prescription, however. Instead, he purchases his own aspirin (300 mg) because, in his view, the higher dosage will not only treat his circulation problems but also provide him with some relief for the rheumatic pain he suffers at night. As he explained this, his wife commented that one couldn't expect the health service to supply every-thing. Excessive and inappropriate demands she thinks are undermining its purpose.

Mr Richards belongs to the Macular Degeneration Society and through this he has obtained a number of useful aids and other services for blind and partially sighted people. In addition, he is a member of an arthritis society as both he and his wife suffer considerably from rheumatic and arthritic pain. Through its monthly magazine, they pick up a number of health tips: they do not eat red meat or butter and have tried a variety of healthy diets.

They buy a variety of OTC products including garlic tablets, halibut liver oil, vitamin B complex, vitamin C tablets and arnica tablets. These are stored in a shoe-box in the kitchen and are taken with breakfast. They take a second dose of vitamins at bedtime. Mrs Richards also purchases her own potassium tablets even though these are included on her prescription list. This is because the prescribed tablets have to be dissolved in water and made her feel sick, whereas the ones she purchases can be swallowed whole. Several of these OTC products are bought through a mail order firm but they also buy some of them from the local health shop.

All five, Mrs Austin, the Moffatts and the Richards, are taking OTC medicines to sustain health and to ward off illness. They are active consumers in the health market. They appear to be satisfied with, and willing to pay for, products they believe to be good for their health. Each is consuming several OTC products every day. They are willing to exchange recommendations and to take informal advice from those with acknowledged expertise. They prefer not to bother the GP, limiting their use of prescribed medication to long-term conditions.

They may appear to be archetypal middle-class people and they are, of course, people who have the income to cover the costs of OTC medi-cines. However, it is also a fact that, like smoking, the health market is carefully managed. As a result, people living in an impoverished area with high levels of ill health have comparatively greater opportunities to purchase medicines (relative to, say, fresh food), than do those living in a more affluent rural area where the GPs may have established a dispens-ing practice and the nearest OTC medicines are several miles away in a garage or supermarket.

THE USE OF OTC PRODUCTS IN ROUTINE MEDICATION

It is clear from these case studies that the prescribing GP and the retail pharmacy are not mutually exclusive sources. Very often OTC remedies are bought and used *alongside* existing prescription items for the *same* condition. There were 15 other participants who were using both prescription and OTC medicines to treat a particular complaint in this way: typically for arthritic pain, gastro-intestinal problems and respiratory conditions. Here are five examples:

- Mrs Harper prefers the Nurofen she purchases to the paracetamol she is prescribed because she finds it a more effective painkiller.
- Mrs Ankers was being prescribed co-codamol for arthritic pain, but bought Panadol and paracetamol. She frequently takes these as an alternative to the co-codamol, which makes her constipated. For 10 out of the 14 diary days, she took three doses of painkillers a day, only one of which was the co-codamol. Similarly, Bisodol is a medicine she has used for years, and which she uses as an occasional alternative to the prescribed Gaviscon.
- Mrs Sawyer also buys Bisodol which she keeps beside her bed and uses in addition to the Losec tablets that the district nurse put out for her in a Dosett box (a specially designed container intended to help patients organize their tablets).
- Mrs McNeil occasionally uses liquid paraffin BP for constipation as an alternative to her prescribed Regulan which is too powerful at times.
- Mrs Bradley, who has several inhalers on prescription for her chest, buys Benylin which she takes three times a day for the same condition.

There were other participants who were treating health problems with OTC medicines as an *alternative* remedy to consulting the doctor. For example, Mrs Fitchett takes antacid tablets to treat the symptoms of a hiatus hernia. She buys these each week at the supermarket and, although she says she uses them only 'when needed', her diary indicates that she is taking several each day.

In contrast, some have abandoned self-medication and have turned to the doctor. Mrs Thompson, for example, had been using White Embrocation to treat arthritic pain, but had recently been given a prescription for ibuprofen gel. Others gave up using an OTC medicine because they thought it might interact with a newly prescribed medicine for another condition. For example, on the advice of a friend, Mrs Bastock had been taking herbal Tabritis tablets for her arthritis for ten months. These are quite expensive given she is taking six a day and they were costing her £11 for a bottle of 200. Nevertheless, she thought they were better than the prescribed ketoprofen tablets and her leg was a lot more supple.

Temporarily, however, she had stopped taking them, whilst taking prescribed warfarin.

CONCLUSIONS

Many of the people in our sample are managing health problems through a variety of strategies. In addition to consulting their GPs, they seek advice from friends and relatives and act upon their recommendations. They are interested in learning from available evidence and are influenced by advertising and promotional literature. They spend what they can afford on their health, and often prefer to exercise autonomy in the chemist's shop rather than being subject to the control of the doctor.

Overall the data suggest that the purchase of OTC products falls into four categories. First, there are products for *prevention and health maintenance*, taken normally on a daily basis. These products largely fall into the 'nutrition and blood' category. They include vitamins and mineral supplements and, to a lesser extent, aspirin and garlic which are widely believed to be 'good for the blood'. This preventive aspect of health care, we suggest, is one that people regard primarily as their own responsibility, and one that they may be more conscious of as they grow older and more vulnerable to ill health.

Secondly, there are products that are bought to treat symptoms for which self-medication is favoured as an *alternative* to going to the doctor. These are primarily products bought to treat what are perceived to be minor ailments, ailments over which one should not trouble the doctor. Often these medicines are kept in stock 'just in case'. They also include treatments for indigestion, wind, constipation, skin irritations, headaches and sleep problems.

The third category are those medicines that are purchased to treat symptoms that are also being treated by the doctor, *to supplement or replace prescription medicines*. Our findings suggest that these are primarily pain relievers, both oral and topical, but particularly paracetamol. They also include indigestion and constipation remedies for which patients are concurrently receiving prescribed medicines. These tend to be medicines over which the patient is expected to exercise some discretion and, as such, may be used interchangeably with OTC products. They also include, however, items that are being purchased *to counteract the side effects* of prescription medicines. Most notable here are laxatives that are purchased to relieve the constipating effects of some prescribed painkillers.

This last category is important in understanding how people manage their prescription medicines. If the concordance initiative of the Royal Pharmacological Society (1997) is to be successful, doctors need to be aware of patients who are using OTC products to supplement, replace or counteract the medicines they are prescribing. Equally, so do the pharmacists who agree to the sale of the OTC medicines. More generally, what we have found is that older people are proactive in health matters. They do have views about whether or not medicines are effective, damaging or discomforting, and they will tailor their routines and dosages accordingly.

REFERENCES

Bytheway, B., Johnson, J. and Heller, T. (2000) *The Management of Long-Term Medication by Older People*. Report to the Department of Health. Milton Keynes: Open University Press.

Cranz, H. (1995) 'Switching in Europe: prescription to non-prescription status', *Drug Information Journal*, 29: 1117.

Davis, P. (1997) *Managing Medicines*. Buckingham: Open University Press.

PAGB (1999) *The OTC Directory 1999/2000*. London: Proprietary Association of Great Britain.

Royal Pharmacological Society (1997) *From Compliance to Concordance*. London: Royal Pharmacological Society.

Tegner, H. (1999) 'When to recommend an over-the-counter medicine', *Prescriber*, 19 June: 81–7.

Thomas, D.H. and Noyce, P.R. (1996) 'The interface between self medication and the NHS', *British Medical Journal*, 313 (7094): 115–16.

33

Private Medicine

Charlotte Humphrey and Jill Russell

When thinking about health care in the United Kingdom we tend to focus on the NHS, which provides the majority of care for most people. But alongside the NHS runs another important and overlapping system of care, that which is provided by the private sector. We know far less about private health care than we do about the NHS, and policy analysts have traditionally shown little interest in studying this aspect of provision. In part their indifference reflects doubts about the relevance of knowledge about the private sector to the more central and pressing concerns of the NHS. There also appears to have been ideological resistance on the part of both researchers and funding agencies to acknowledging and confronting the significance of private health care and its relationship with the NHS. Salter (1998) describes the 'hegemony of traditional welfare state values' as having imposed a set of 'analytical blinkers' on social policy observers, which have maintained the focus firmly on the public health care system. Consequently, the lack of knowledge about the private sector has, until recently, gone almost unremarked.

We can see this reluctance mirrored in the political arena. Government statements about health care rarely acknowledge the existence or significance of the private sector. If referred to at all, private health care tends to be presented as 'an irrelevant irritation' (Day and Klevi,1999). In 1999, the House of Commons Select Committee on Health, having for the first time in its history devoted an entire inquiry to the independent sector, noted that the latest annual report of the Department of Health made no mention of private health provision, 'despite the fact that it makes a considerable contribution – for better or worse – to the nation's health' (House of Commons, 1999).

However, things may now be changing. In all sectors of national life there is increasing acceptance of the interdependence of public, voluntary and private sector activity and of the relevance across the whole spectrum of service provision of current policy concerns such as quality of care and professional regulation. In this new environment there is growing appreciation of the need to understand the nature of private health care and the practices of those who provide it.

The private sector can be defined as comprising all practitioners, goods and services that are privately owned, produced or financed. By these criteria, the private sector in the UK includes all the self-employed professionals (general practitioners, dentists, pharmacists, complementary therapists) who contract their services to the NHS as well as those who see patients privately; the industries involved in private medical insurance, pharmaceutical production and hospital supplies and services such as catering and laundry where these have been contracted out; and privately financed hospitals and other clinical services. This chapter does not attempt to cover all aspects of the private health care system but focuses specifically on private medical care. We begin by presenting some basic facts and figures about the private sector to give an indication of the nature and scale of its activities and show how these interface with NHS provision. We then explore the influences that have shaped the development of private medicine alongside the NHS over the past 50 years. The chapter ends with discussion of two key questions about private health care – how does its quality compare with that provided by the NHS and what are the costs or benefits of its existence to the NHS and society as a whole? The chapter contains some brief extracts from interviews carried out as part of a study we are currently undertaking of doctors' experience of private practice.

SOME FACTS AND FIGURES

The total value of health services provided by the independent sector in 1997–98 was estimated at £14.5 billion (Laing, 1998). The percentage of total UK health care expenditure financed or provided outside the NHS is currently around 16 per cent, which represents a considerable increase from the 1960s when it was more like 3 per cent (Keen et al., forthcoming). The most recent figures available indicate that almost 15 per cent of all elective treatments in England and Wales (excluding abortion) are purchased privately (Williams et al., 2000). Table 33.1 shows the 10 elective operations and procedures most likely to be funded in this way. Acute care is provided by 230 private hospitals with nearly 10,000 beds. In addition, the private psychiatric sector comprises 64 hospitals with some 2,000 beds (House of Commons, 1999). The great majority of private hospitals are in London and the south-east of England.

The private sector is funded mainly by private medical insurance, which accounts for about 70 per cent of the market (House of Commons, 1999). The proportion of the population covered by such insurance increased dramatically between the 1970s and early 1990s, but levelled off during the last decade. About 11 per cent of the population is currently insured (Laing, 1998). Twenty per cent of acute care is funded by patients paying for themselves, a marked increase from the 12 per

Table 33.1   *Elective operations and procedures (excluding abortion) most likely to be funded privately (residents of England and Wales 1997–98)*

	Total number of procedures undertaken	% privately funded
Gender reassignment	156	70.5
Cosmetic operations	61,481	38.6
Joint endoscopy	114,856	28.8
Total hip replacement	47,601	22.5
Abdominal hernia repair	103,559	20.8
Varicose vein ligation/stripping	63,515	20.8
Coronary artery operations	27,132	20.2
Prolapsed vagina or uterus	27,786	19.7
Partial excision of breast	43,021	17.6

Source: adapted from Williams et al., 2000

cent found by Williams and colleagues in 1992–93 (Williams et al., 2000), and it is suggested that self-payment is now the fastest-growing source of finance for private health care (Keen et al., forthcoming). Five per cent of private treatment is funded by the NHS and 5 per cent by other groups, including patients from overseas (House of Commons, 1999).

These figures give some indication of the size of the private sector. As important, however, is the extent of its interpenetration with the NHS. Figure 33.1 presents a conceptual map of public/private relations in UK health care. The shaded quadrants indicate areas of overlap between the two systems of health care.

The NHS buys a considerable amount of acute care from the private sector (£252 million in 1995–96: Keen and Mays, 1998). For example, in 1997–98 the NHS commissioned some 29,000 elective ordinary admissions and 62,000 day cases from the independent sector to help reduce waiting times (House of Commons, 1999). One key area where the NHS purchases acute care from the private sector is psychiatry. The majority (55 per cent) of the UK's medium- and low-security acute psychiatric beds are now provided privately, reflecting a gradual withdrawal of the

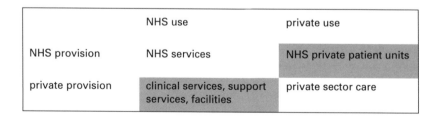

	NHS use	private use
NHS provision	NHS services	NHS private patient units
private provision	clinical services, support services, facilities	private sector care

Figure 33.1   *The interface between NHS and private sector health care (adapted from Keen and Mays, 1998)*

NHS from direct provision of substantial elements of some psychiatric services (House of Commons, 1999).

The NHS also provides acute care for some private patients. At mid-1998 the NHS offered about 3,000 private beds, 1,375 of which were in 75 dedicated private patient units (House of Commons, 1999). The remainder were pay beds on NHS wards. Together, NHS pay beds and private patient units account for nearly one fifth of the total private health care market (Fitzhugh, 1999a). While relatively small in number, private patient units represent a significant form of income for a number of major NHS Trust hospitals. The Royal Marsden Trust in London has the highest income from private patients, accounting for 21 per cent of its core income (Fitzhugh, 1999b).

Many people use both NHS and private sector care on different occasions and patients may also move between the two sectors during episodes of treatment. For example, the private sector is used selectively for treatments (such as cosmetic surgery) or mild conditions (such as moderate back pain) where the desired treatment may be unavailable on the NHS and also for operations known to have long waiting times. Private appointments with NHS consultants enable patients to jump queues for treatment. Patients seen in this capacity may then be placed on a NHS waiting list on the basis of clinical priority, effectively bypassing the waiting list of outpatient appointments. In the reverse direction, patients receiving private treatment are sometimes transferred to NHS hospitals for emergency intensive care or for follow-up care, such as cardiac rehabilitation, after a private operation.

A further important area of overlap is staff working across both sectors. All NHS consultants are legally entitled to undertake private practice. Those on full-time contracts are permitted to earn up to 10 per cent of their gross NHS salary from private practice. A maximum part-time contract (forgoing one-eleventh of the NHS salary) enables unlimited earnings from private practice, provided a consultant devotes substantially the whole of their time to the NHS. In 1992, the Monopolies and Mergers Commission estimated that 71 per cent of NHS consultants undertook some private sector work. The gross mean income from private practice was £33,000; a minority of consultants were earning over £200,000 per year (Monopolies and Mergers Commission, 1993).

I was a full time consultant here, but two years ago I dropped a session because my private practice earnings had reached the point where I could no longer sign the form saying they didn't amount to more than 10 per cent of the total. So I dropped a session, which entitles me to half a day. So I go to X on a Tuesday evening, which doesn't interfere with my NHS work, and operate there on a Friday evening after my NHS list here. And then at the Y I start seeing patients about 2.30 and work through till 7, and then if there are any operations I do them on a Thursday evening after that. (Consultant surgeon, London 1999)

FACTORS THAT HAVE SHAPED THE CURRENT PICTURE

How have we ended up with these two overlapping systems of care in the UK? What are the factors that have shaped the development of private health care? We can identify a whole web of interlocking influences including the self-interest of the medical profession, the political ideologies of governments, public demand and commercial interests. For example, the increased market for private health care was initially generated as much by increasing provision of private health insurance as an employment benefit as by the exercise of individual patient choice. The increased availability of private health insurance as an occupational perk was itself a result of politically motivated tax changes and the rapid growth of the economy during the 1980s. The position presently occupied by the private sector is not the consequence of a rational plan, but rather a product of the interplay of ideological commitment, political pragmatism and financial opportunism. As such it represents a clear example of policy-making as a process of 'muddling through' (Lindblom, 1959).

Professional power

There is no doubt that the introduction of the NHS in 1948 heralded the beginning of a new era in the history of the nation's health care. But its creation involved a long record of 'serious and substantial concessions' to doctors to ensure their willing co-operation (Bevan, 1948). Among other compromises, consultants were permitted to maintain both NHS and private practice and NHS pay beds were created. More than 50 years later, despite enormous changes in the governance and management of health care, the capacity of the medical profession to protect its right to private practice remains as strong as ever. Under the current contract, consultants do not have to specify the number of hours they work outside the NHS or provide any information to their NHS employers about their other commitments. The only requirement is that their NHS work should not be compromised by what they do elsewhere, but what this means in practice has never been defined.

It has been observed that 'the history of the British health service is the history of political power, ministers, civil servants, parliament, accommodating itself to professional power' (Klein, 1973). The battle over pay beds in the 1970s provides a good example of this and also demonstrates the sometimes unintended consequences of political action. The then Secretary of State for Health, Barbara Castle, took on the medical profession and tried to phase out pay beds, which she saw as incompatible with the principles of the NHS. But ultimately she lost because the Labour Prime Minister Harold Wilson would not back her against a 'formidable alliance of the BMA, the hospital consultants' association, the royal colleges and the private insurers' (Pollock, 1999). Subsequently the number of pay beds did diminish, but the unintended, paradoxical effect was to trigger an expansion in private hospital provision.

Political ideology

The influence of New Right thinking on Conservative policies of the 1980s, with its belief in the superiority of the private sector, did a number of things to stimulate the growth of the private health care sector. Tax incentives were provided for the purchase of private health insurance, consultants' contracts were altered to facilitate their private practice, and planning restrictions on private hospital developments were relaxed (Klein, 1995). In the early 1990s, the creation of the internal market in the NHS provided a strong impetus for Trusts to develop private services to maximize their incomes. NHS private patient income rose from £83 million in 1988 to £230 million in 1995 and the NHS share of the private acute health care market from 11.2 per cent to 15.1 per cent over the same period (Laing, 1996). But, equally, the Conservatives knew that outright attempts to privatize the health service would be politically unpopular. In 1982 when partial privatization of NHS services was suggested by a think-tank, the government dissociated itself from the leaked report, reassured the public that the NHS was safe in its hands and Margaret Thatcher restated the principle that 'adequate health care should be provided to all, regardless of the ability to pay' (Thatcher, 1982). Since leaving government, the Conservatives have become less cautious. The present line, as expressed by Shadow Health Secretary Alan Duncan is that 'the NHS cannot do everything' and people should be encouraged to make their own provision for health care as part of a wider private–public partnership to improve universal provision (Warden, 1999).

Active support for the private sector is no longer confined to Conservative governments. While traditionally presenting itself as the party most strongly committed to the welfare principles of the NHS, the present government is keenly promoting policies to develop public–private partnerships in the health sector, particularly financing for capital projects through the private finance initiative (PFI). Keen et al. suggest that the rationale is a pragmatic rather than an ideological one. The government 'wants access to private capital, and also to private sector knowledge and practices in facilities management, because it helps with a particular problem, of trying to square the circle of pressures on public expenditure' (Keen et al., forthcoming). The effect will be a further stimulus for the private sector as PFI hospitals increase the proportion of private beds to generate the income required to meet their new commitments (Pollock et al., 1999).

QUALITY

I go to visit a friend at a private hospital in London and am childishly thrilled that patients can call room service for drinks. The menu is all the treats you'd buy in Marks and Spencer: Italian hams, tomato bread, pasta salad. The room is quiet and spacious, with a big TV, the bathroom is as tasteful as that found in a four star hotel. The last time I'd visited him was in the main ward of an NHS hospital. The paint was peeling and he was less than an elbow from the next bed. (*Luisa Dillner, Guardian, 18 October 1998*)

How good is private health care and how does its quality compare with that provided in the NHS? From the patient's perspective, the main advantages of going private appear to be those associated with speed and convenience and a 'better' experience in terms of hotel facilities (private rooms, quality of environment and food), more courteous care and individual attention from a specific consultant (Cant and Calnan, 1992). It is also suggested that some people choose private care to obtain a more equitable relationship with their doctors (Wiles and Higgins, 1996). But there is little indication that patients who go privately believe that the care they receive will be technically or clinically superior to that available on the NHS.

At present there is no solid evidence about comparative clinical quality in the two systems. There are no data, for example, on rates of readmission of private patients or the number of patients transferred to NHS hospitals. There has been no systematic comparison of the activities of individual consultants in private practice and in the NHS, to establish whether they are applying the same standards of care, and there is no relevant information about health outcomes. There is, however, a growing volume of anecdotal evidence about the provision and experience of private practice. Box 33.1 identifies the clinical issues most consistently identified by patient representative groups in evidence to the Select

---

Box 33.1: Reported sources of additional clinical risk in the independent health care sector

- An increased risk to patients occupying single rooms in that they were less well supervised than those in wards.
- A lack of specialist wards in independent hospitals resulting in less specialized nursing and medical care.
- Little information available to NHS trusts or private providers about the overall working hours of staff, resulting in patients being seen by staff who were exhausted.
- A lack of resuscitation and other emergency back-up facilities.
- Inexperienced resident medical officers.
- A lack of doctors on duty who have taken the Advanced Course in Life Saving Technique.
- An absence of even informal peer review since clinicians in the independent sector tend not to work in teams as they do in the NHS.

Source: House of Commons, 1999: para. 41

Table 33.2 *Probable areas of difference in the care provided in the NHS and private sectors*

	NHS	private sector
Waiting times for treatment	variable	usually short
'Hotel' facilities – rooms, catering, general environment	variable	usually good
Time for consultation	variable	adequate
Continuing individual consultant attention	unlikely	yes
Comprehensive back-up of specialist and junior staff	yes	variable
Comprehensive clinical support facilities	yes	variable
Procedures for audit and clinical governance	yes	variable
Thresholds for intervention	higher	lower

Committee as contributing to additional clinical risk in the independent health care sector (House of Commons, 1999).

Table 33.2 summarizes some probable differences between the NHS and the private sector. However, interpretation of their implications for quality of care is complicated by the fact that some of the apparent benefits of the private sector are not clear cut. Deep-pile carpets and wallpaper can be unhygienic, rich diets may be inappropriate, third floor consulting suites in handsome Georgian houses are not well suited to disabled patients. Some consultants may be set in their ways and out of date, overworking in unsocial hours to make as much money as they can. Lower treatment thresholds may mean inappropriate and unnecessary operations. On the other hand the apparent disadvantages of the private sector do not necessarily apply. For example, in NHS teaching hospital private patient units the full range of NHS back-up services is available for private patients also. In the best private hospitals, protocols and procedures for quality assurance may be more rigorous and highly developed than in the NHS.

What does seem likely is that variation in quality is both greater and more unpredictable in the private sector than the NHS. The private sector contains fewer of the legislative and institutional safeguards and supports that help to minimize adverse effects and reduce patient risk, but it is also freer of the major resource constraints on time, money and manpower that prevent the NHS from providing optimal care. In the absence of these organizational strengths and constraints, the quality of patient care in the private sector is more strongly influenced by the individual consultant and the particular choices they make about where and how to work.

> You get the people at the one extreme, who seem to be spending all their weekends and they're operating from dawn to dusk. And you wonder how they ever have time to spend any of the money they must be getting. And I suppose you try and put yourself somewhere on that spectrum which you feel is a sensible level. But you have to keep control of it because you can let it get out of hand if the opportunities arise. Working in London you've got the *choice*

of the private hospitals and you can either go to all of them, in which case you neglect your NHS practice seriously, or just confine yourself to one or two, in which case you don't earn nearly so much, but you do get to sleep at night. (Consultant surgeon, London, 1999)

BROADER COSTS AND BENEFITS OF THE PRIVATE SECTOR

Intrinsically the National Health Service is a church. It is the nearest thing to the embodiment of the Good Samaritan that we have in any aspect of our public policy. What would we say of a person who argued that he could only serve God properly if he had pay pews in his church? (Barbara Castle, Minister of Health, House of Commons, 27 April 1976)

The two main concerns about the continuing existence of private health care in the UK are that it undermines the egalitarian principles associated with a universal public health service and that it adversely affects the care provided by the NHS.

There is no doubt that those who can afford private care get more and quicker treatment. Data on differential waits for private and NHS patients in NHS hospitals in 1994–95 show that private patients were admitted sooner than others for operations for potentially serious conditions, and much sooner for less urgent procedures (Williams, 1997). At a wider level it has been suggested that access to private health care compounds existing health inequalities between social groups (Acheson, 1998). Private health insurance certainly tends to be the preserve of the relatively well-off, who are also more likely to have such insurance funded by employers (Mulligan, 1998). The private sector has been criticized as parasitic on the NHS, in so far as it uses staff trained in the NHS, takes on only the most 'profitable' types of treatment and relies on the existence of NHS services for back-up when things go wrong. It has also been suggested that private practice takes consultants away from their NHS responsibilities and may actually lead to longer waiting lists (Yates, 1995).

In mitigation, those in favour of private practice contend that, although some consultants do undertake an 'unacceptable' level of private work, for most this does not impinge unduly on their NHS commitments (National Economic Research Associates, 1995). One reason is that use of NHS operating theatres is often severely constrained by shortages of beds and staff, which limits the amount of time that consultants can operate within the NHS. A further argument used to support the private sector is that it increases patient choice, which may be seen as a virtue in its own right and also helps reduce the pressure on the scarce resources of the NHS. Finally it can be suggested that private practice actually supports the NHS, providing income through private patient units and enabling the retention of doctors in the NHS on lower salaries than would otherwise be acceptable. Again, a lack of good evidence leaves many of these issues open to contention. Without the basis for a comprehensive analysis of all potential costs and benefits, the scope for ideologically based assertion remains considerable.

REFERENCES

Acheson, D. (1998) *Independent Inquiry into Inequalities in Health Report*. London: The Stationery Office.

Bevan A. (1948) speaking in House of Commons, 9 February.

Cant, S. and Calnan, M. (1992) 'Using private health insurance. A study of lay decisions to seek professional medical help', *Sociology of Health and Illness*, 14: 39–56.

Day, P. and Klein, R. (1999) 'Privates on parade', *Health Service Journal*, 20–2 (23 September).

Fitzhugh, W. (1999a) *The Fitzhugh Directory of Independent Healthcare and Long-Term Care: Financial Information 1999–2000*. London: Health Care Information Systems.

Fitzhugh, W. (1999b) *The Fitzhugh Directory of NHS Trusts 1999*. London: Health Care Information Systems.

House of Commons Select Committee on Health (1999) *Fifth Report: The Regulation of Private and Other Independent Health Care*. House of Commons 281–1.

Keen, J. and Mays, N. (1998) 'The NHS is not an island', in A. Harrison (ed.), *Health Care UK 1997/98*. London: King's Fund.

Keen, J., Light, D. and Mays, N. (forthcoming) *Public–Private Relations in Health Care*. London: King's Fund.

Klein, R. (1973) *Complaints against Doctors*. London: Knight.

Klein, R. (1995) *The New Politics of the NHS*, 3rd edn. London: Longman.

Laing, W. (1996) *Laing's Review of Private Health Care 1996*. London: Laing & Buisson Publications.

Laing, W. (1998) *Laing's Healthcare Market Review 1998–99*. London: Laing & Buisson Publications.

Lindblom, C. (1959) 'The science of muddling through', *Public Administration Review*, 39: 517–26.

Monopolies and Mergers Commission (1993) *Private Medical Services: a Report on Agreements and Practices Relating to Charges for the Supply of Private Medical Services by NHS Consultants*. London: HMSO.

Mulligan, J. (1998) 'Attitudes towards the NHS and its alternatives, 1983–96', in A. Harrison (ed.), *Health Care UK 1997/98*. London: King's Fund.

National Economic Research Associates (1995) *Are Pay-Beds Profitable? A Report for Norwich Union Healthcare*, London: NERA.

Pollock, L. (1999) 'Can we afford to go private?' *Health Matters*, 38: 12–13.

Pollock, A.M., Dunnigan M.G., Gaffney, D., Price, D. and Shaoul, J. (1999) 'Planning the "new" NHS: downsizing for the 21st century', *British Medical Journal*, 319: 179–84.

Salter, B. (1998) *The Politics of Change in the Health Service*. London: Macmillan.

Thatcher, M. (1982) Speech to Conservative Party Conference, Brighton, 8 October.

Warden, J. (1999) 'NHS "cannot cope" says Tory', *British Medical Journal*, 318: 1028.

Wiles, R. and Higgins, J. (1996) 'Doctor–patient relationships in the private sector: patients' perceptions', *Sociology of Health and Illness*, 18: 34–56.

Williams, B. (1997) 'Utilisation of National Health Service hospitals in England by private patients 1989–95', *Health Trends*, 29: 21–5.

Williams, B., Whatmough, P., McGill, J. and Rushton, L. (2000) 'Private funding of elective hospital treatment in England and Wales, 1997–8: national survey', *British Medical Journal*, 320: 904–5.

Yates, J. (1995) *Private Eye, Heart and Hip*. Edinburgh: Churchill Livingstone.

PART VI

LOOKING TO THE FUTURE

This part of the Reader looks into the future. It is the shortest part of this compilation, containing only four chapters. This is not because there isn't a myriad of health professionals and assorted analysts wanting to give their opinions on the future shape of health, disease and health care, but because these four chapters together give a sufficient view of the way ahead for our purposes. Once again no single discipline can offer us this complete insight (or foresight), so we have chosen four examples which stimulate a diverse view of the future. These will allow room for your own reflection on what the future will hold for you as an individual, and for necessary speculation on the development of the health-related organizations that you relate to.

Part 6 reflects some of the technical and policy related developments that are predicted to come to fruition in the near future. These are concerned with certain technological concepts which are reflected in the language the authors use. We have decided to leave this language unchanged, and even the title of the first chapter in this part, 'Pharmacogenomics', may be an unfamiliar term. But we make no apologies for the introduction of some technical words into the text at this stage. These are terms that everyone will have to understand in the future so that we can all take part in debates and decision-making on the shape of health and health care.

The first two chapters consider different aspects of the *technical* future for medicine and health care: 'pharmacogenomics' (the way that individual genes and our total genetic structure affect the way that medicines will be used in the future), and cybermedicine (the use of the internet for medical or health-related purposes). Wolfgang Sadée (Chapter 34: 'Pharmacogenomics') looks at the way that this emerging discipline is able to tailor specific medicines to the individual genetic make-up of people. This has already led to certain therapeutic advances but has also 'shattered any complacency as it has revealed profound gaps in our knowledge'. Sadée discusses profound changes in the way that medicines will be used in the future and the potential to avert the type of drug toxicity which is genetically determined. In addition the future design and development of new drugs and the prediction of drug efficacy will be considerably improved; in summary: 'this approach has the potential to revolutionize prevention and treatment of disease'.

Gunther Eysenbach et al. (Chapter 35: 'Towards the Millennium of Cybermedicine') also promise us that the developments they describe 'will once again revolutionize the discovery and dissemination of knowledge in medicine'. As well as some of the technological advances which are envisaged, the chapter does introduce discussion of some of the potential problems and social issues involved in access to this 'revolutionary' form of health information.

Julian Pratt et al. (Chapter 36: 'Working Whole Systems') look to the future of health care systems and the way that they might be manipulated so that they have the potential to tackle complex problems in a more cohesive way. Complex problems, such as tackling teenage pregnancy, are unlikely to be satisfactorily dealt with by bureaucratic or inflexible organizations. Pratt and his colleagues describe a way of working within organizations and among several groups of involved agencies with potentially diverse outlooks to bring about realistic social and health-related changes for the future. Whole systems working should help 'people make connections that enable them to find sustainable solutions to complex organizational problems'.

The final chapter in our collection, by Michael Peckham (Chapter 37: 'Future Health Scenarios and Public Policy'), mirrors Chapter 1, by Porter, which took a widespread view of historical health developments. Perhaps it is best to leave the last words of this introduction to Peckham himself while entirely concurring with the sentiments that he expresses: 'Despite the spectacular advances of medicine and the general improvements in health statistics across the world, the gap between our technological sophistication and social primitiveness is stark. Thus, as mankind enters the third millennium, it is capable not only of etching nanocircuits with electrons, or of performing microsurgery on neonates, but also of engaging in ethnic cleansing and the widespread violation of human rights.'

34

Pharmacogenomics

Wolfgang Sadée

We all differ in our response to drug treatment – occasionally with dramatic effects. The era of 'one drug fits all patients' is about to give way to individualized therapy matching the patient's unique genetic make-up with an optimally effective drug (Sadée, 1998). Pharmaco-genetics and pharmacogenomics are the emerging disciplines that are leading the way towards individualized medicine (Weber, 1997; Kleyn and Vesell, 1998). Initially, researchers focused their attention on pharmacogenetics – variations in single candidate genes responsible for variable drug response. Subsequently, studies involving the entire human genome broadened the scope of investigation, giving rise to pharmaco-genomics as one of the 'hottest' fields in biotechnology today.

Box 34.1: Summary points

- Response to drug treatment can vary greatly between patients; genetic factors have a major role in treatment outcome.
- Pharmacogenetics and pharmacogenomics are emerging disciplines that focus on genetic determinants of drug response at the levels of single genes or the entire human genome respectively.
- Technologies involving gene chip arrays can determine thousands of variations in DNA sequences for individual patients; most variants are single nucleotide polymorphisms.
- Pharmacogenomics aims at establishing a signature of DNA sequence variants that are characteristic of individual patients to assess disease susceptibility and select the optimal drug treatment.
- This approach has the potential to revolutionize prevention and treatment of diseases.

PHARMACOGENETICS

Unexpected drug reactions have been noted for some time, but the systematic study of hereditary origins began only in the 1950s. A few

First published in the *British Medical Journal*, 319, 13 November 1999: 1294.

patients developed prolonged respiratory muscular paralysis after being given succinylcholine (suxamethonium), a short-acting muscle relaxant widely used in surgery and electroshock treatment. In the 1970s, a trial with the antihypertensive agent debrisoquine resulted in a precipitous drop of blood pressure and collapse in nearly 10 per cent of volunteers. Furthermore, isoniazid therapy for tuberculosis caused peripheral neuropathies in patients who were sensitive to the neurotoxic effects of the drug. Groundbreaking genetic and biochemical studies by Werner Kalow and others showed that these adverse effects result from polymorphisms in genes encoding the drug metabolising enzymes serum cholinesterase (Kalow and Staren, 1957), cytochrome P–450 (Schmid et al., 1985) and N-acetyltransferase (Evans et al., 1960). These observations laid the foundation for pharmacogenetics.

Functional analysis

Today, many examples of genetic variability in drug response and toxicity are known. In a few cases, genetic tests are beginning to find their way into clinical practice. In cancer chemotherapy with tioguanine, severe toxicity or even death can result if a patient is unable to inactivate the drug. Functional assays of thiopurine methyltransferase in red blood cells or genotyping can identify those patients who are at risk and must be given a much lower dose of tioguanine (Tai et al., 1996; Weinshilboum and Sladek, 1980). This is particularly critical for the 1 in 300 patients who is homozygous for null alleles (non-functional) of the gene encoding thiopurine methyltransferase which converts the drug to its inactive methylated form.

Cytochrome P–450

The large family of cytochrome P–450 genes has been most intensely studied because it contains the main drug-metabolizing enzymes encoded by numerous genes (Weber, 1997). Among the cytochrome P–450 subtypes, CYP2D6 and CYP2C19 play a critical part in determining the response to several drugs. This is particularly important for lipophilic drugs – such as drugs that act on the central nervous system and penetrate the lipophilic blood-brain barrier – because renal excretion is minimal and cytochrome P–450 metabolism provides the only means of effective drug elimination. Thus, homozygous carriers of CYP2D6 null alleles cannot readily degrade and excrete many drugs, including debrisoquine, metoprolol, nortriptyline, and propafenone (Broly et al., 1991). These patients are termed 'poor metabolizers' for CYP2D6 selective drugs. Because of this they are exquisitely sensitive to these drugs. The incidence of 'poor metabolizers' varies greatly among ethnic groups, ranging from 1 per cent in Japanese people to 15 per cent in Nigerians. Similarly, patients with defective CYP2C19 subtypes are highly sensitive to methoin (mephenytoin), hexobarbital (hexobarbitone), and other drugs selectively metabolized by this P–450 isoform.

The principal molecular defect in poor metabolizers is a single base pair mutation (A–G) in exon 5 of CYP2C19 (De Morais et al., 1994). Gene chips designed to test for polymorphisms of the main subtypes of cytochrome P–450 are now commercially available, but not yet in general clinical use. Cytochrome P–450 polymorphisms also affect the inactivation or, in some cases, activation or toxification of xenobiotics, and thus affect an individual's susceptibility to environmental toxins. This is studied in a field of research called toxicogenetics. Launched recently by the US National Institute of Environmental Health Sciences, the environmental genome project aims at understanding genetic factors in individual responses to the environment and parallels the study of genetic variability in drug response (Guengerich, 1998).

PHARMACOGENOMICS

As a scientific discipline, pharmacogenetics has made steady progress, but the human genome project has shattered any complacency as it has revealed profound gaps in our knowledge. By broadening the search for genetic polymorphisms that determine drug responses, the new field of pharmacogenomics begins to supersede the candidate gene approach typical of earlier pharmacogenetic studies. Initially hailed by pharmaceutical biotechnology as the latest trend in biotechnology, pharmacogenomics is now taken seriously everywhere. While genomic techniques serve to identify new gene targets for drug research, and some might refer to this as pharmacogenomics, the broader consensus is that pharmacogenomics deals specifically with genetic variability in drug response. The distinction between pharmacogenetics and pharmacogenomics remains blurred, but here are some of the new ideas typical of pharmacogenomics.

Searching for responsible genes

Each drug is likely to interact in the body with numerous proteins, such as carrier proteins, transporters, metabolizing enzymes, and multiple types of receptors (Sadée, 1998). These proteins determine the absorption, distribution, excretion, targeting to the site of action, and pharmacological response of drugs. As a result, multiple polymorphisms in many genes could affect the drug response, requiring a genome-wide search for the responsible genes. We now know that that there are thousands of receptor genes in the human genome, many of which are closely related to each other because they have evolved by gene duplications. Therefore, we must anticipate that a drug rarely binds just to a single receptor but rather interacts promiscuously with several receptor types. Chlorpromazine, for example, is known to engage several dopaminergic, adrenergic and serotonergic receptors. As a result, polymorphisms in multiple genes can affect the drug response.

Polymorphisms

Polymorphisms are generally defined as variations of DNA sequence that are present in more than 1 per cent of the population. Most polymorphisms are single nucleotide polymorphisms (referred to as 'snips'). As the human genome contains 3 billion nucleotides, and variations between individuals occur in ~1/300 base pairs, around 10 million single nucleotide polymorphisms probably exist. Only 1 per cent of these may have any functional consequence at all, and thus individuals differ from each other genetically by roughly 100,000 polymorphic sites, providing for near infinite variety. As only a small fraction of these single nucleotide polymorphisms will prove relevant to drug response, our goal will be to identify the most important variants.

Microarray gene chips

Novel technology in the form of microarray chips enables us to scan the entire human genome for relevant polymorphisms (Service, 1999; Sinclair, 1999). We can determine simultaneously many thousands of polymorphisms in a patient. At present, these single nucleotide polymorphisms are selected merely as markers evenly distributed throughout the genome, in the hope that functionally relevant polymorphisms can be associated with specific markers by virtue of their proximity on the chromosome. Such genome-wide association studies are already being used in the discovery of susceptibility genes for diseases such as asthma and prostate cancer, but they are equally suitable for determining the genes involved in drug response. Genome-wide scanning can identify these genes even if we do not know the mechanisms by which the drug acts in the body. The French genomics company, Genset, currently uses gene chips with 60,000 single nucleotide polymorphism markers – sufficient for a complete genomic scan – applied to clinical drug trials in partnership with major pharmaceutical companies. Expanding the number of single nucleotide polymorphisms and selecting functionally relevant single nucleotide polymorphisms in coding or promoter/enhancer regions of genes is quite feasible with current technology and would greatly enhance the power of genome-wide scanning. Herein lies the main incentive for the current rush in the pharmaceutical industry to patent single nucleotide polymorphism markers. It might also be possible to salvage useful experimental drugs that would have failed with standard clinical trials, because of an unacceptable incidence of toxicity in a poorly defined patient population. Stratifying patient populations in relation to genetic criteria emerges as a major challenge to the pharmaceutical industry. Undoubtedly, the insights expected to emerge from such an approach are staggering, but they cannot be gauged accurately at present.

Chip technology

Microarrays can further serve to determine the expression pattern of genes in a target tissue. This shows the mechanisms of drug action in a genomic context. It can also clarify interindividual differences in drug response that are downstream of immediate drug effects in the body by sheer force of the massive amount of information emanating from chip technology. Analysing the entire transcriptional programme of a tissue – for example, fibroblasts in response to serum stimulation (Iyer et al., 1999) – provides unprecedented details of a complex system and leads to new insights in pathophysiology and biological drug response. Tissue transcript profiling is especially appropriate in cancers because mRNA can be extracted from biopsy specimens or surgical samples. Altered gene expression in the tumour can serve as a guide for selecting effective drug therapy or avoiding unnecessary exposure to toxic but ineffective drugs – for example, the overexpression of drug resistance genes encoding transporters.

PROMISE OF PHARMACOGENOMICS

These advances are the harbinger of profound changes in treatment. What then do we expect to gain from pharmacogenomics? In the near future, genotyping can help avert severe drug toxicity that is genetically determined but occurs only rarely. Alternatively, drugs may be designed a priori so that they are not subject to extreme variations that result from a few well defined polymorphisms. Drug structures under development are already being selected so that they do not interact with cytochrome P-450 subtype CYP2D6 to avoid unwarranted toxicity in people who metabolize this poorly.

Predicting drug efficacy

Looking further ahead, and on a much broader scale, we could improve drug efficacy by distinguishing between people who respond well to a drug and those who respond poorly. Often, an effective drug response is found in a few patients treated, while most benefit little or not at all. Much could be gained if we could select the optimal drug for the individual patient before treatment begins. Perhaps a gene chip that establishes a single nucleotide polymorphism signature involving multiple genes relevant to therapeutic outcome for each individual will be developed. This signature could offer insights into an individual's susceptibility to disease and responsiveness to drugs, enabling optimal drug selection by genetic criteria. For example, cure rates with combined surgical and drug treatment of advanced colorectal carcinoma range from 20 to 40 per cent, while the remainder of the patients experience little gain or even severe toxicity from chemotherapy. If we could predict which patients will respond best to a particular drug – or better, which drug will yield optimal effects for a given patient – much will be gained. The success of this approach will depend critically on the selection of single nucleotide polymorphisms tested by the gene chip. Single nucleotide polymorphisms must be informative and many must be tested to scan the entire genome. This task is by no means complete and constitutes a major goal of those companies which are focusing on genomics.

LIMITATIONS

There are also formidable obstacles that we are unlikely to overcome in the near future. The dynamic complexity of the human genome, involvement of multiple genes in drug responses, and racial differences in the prevalence of gene variants impede effective genome-wide scanning and progress towards practical clinical applications. Furthermore, the drug response is probably affected by multiple genes, each gene with multiple polymorphisms distributed in the general population. For example, the anticancer drug 5–fluorouracil used in the treatment of colorectal cancer is activated and inactivated by nearly 40 different enzymes. Each of these is currently being scanned for relevant polymorphisms at the biotech company Variagenics. Dihydropyrimidine dehydrogenase is a likely candidate in 5–fluorouracil inactivation. However, whether extensive genotyping will provide useful predictors of clinical response remains to be seen.

Racial differences add further confounding factors. Drug response might be predicted from a certain pattern of polymorphisms rather than only a single polymorphism, yet these patterns probably differ between ethnic groups. This could prevent us from making predictions about drug responses across the general patient population, and it emphasizes the need to stratify clinical pharmacogenomics studies.

Genomic technologies are still evolving rapidly, at an exponential pace similar to the development of computer technology over the past 20 years. We are not certain where genomic technologies will be 10 years from now.

Ethical issues also need to be resolved. Holding sensitive information on someone's genetic make-up raises questions of privacy and security and ethical dilemmas in disease prognosis and treatment choices. After all, polymorphisms relevant to drug response may overlap with disease susceptibility, and divulging such information could jeopardize an individual. On the other hand, legal issues may force the inclusion of pharmacogenomics into clinical practice. Once the genetic component of a severe adverse drug effect is documented, doctors may be obliged to order the genetic test to avoid malpractice litigation.

IMPACT OF PHARMACOGENOMICS

Pharmacogenomics will have a profound impact on the way drug treatment is conducted. We can include here bioengineered proteins as drugs, or even gene therapy designed to deliver proteins to target tissues. These treatments are also subject to constraints and complexities engendered by individual variability. A case in point is the treatment of breast cancer with trastuzumab (Herceptin; Genentech, USA) a humanized monoclonal antibody against the HER2 receptor. Overexpression of HER2 may occur as a somatic genetic change in breast cancer and other tumours. This correlates with poor clinical prognosis and serves as a marker for effective therapy with trastuzumab, either alone or in combination with chemotherapy (Golderberg, 1999; Baselga et al., 1998).

Whether we will see broad use of gene chips in clinical practice within 10 years is questionable, but the mere knowledge of the principles underlying genetic variability will prove valuable in optimizing drug therapy. Pharmacogenomics will lead us towards individualized therapy, but it will also help us understand limitations inherent in treating disease in a broad patient population.

REFERENCES

Baselga, J., Norton, L., Albanell, J., Kim, Y.M. and Mendelsohn, J. (1998) 'Recombinant humanized anti-HER2 antibody (Herceptin) enhances the antitumor activity of paclitaxel and doxorubicin against HER2/neu overexpressing human breast cancer xenografts', *Cancer Res*, 58: 2825–31.

Broly, F., Gaedigk, A. Heim, M., Eichelbaum, M., Mariko, K. and Meyer, U.A. (1991) 'Debrisoquine hydroxylase genotype and phenotype', *DNA Cell Biol*, 10: 545–58 [*Medline*].

De Morais, S.M., Wilkinson, G.R., Blaisdell, J., Nakamura, K., Meyer U.A. and Goldstein, J.A. (1994) 'The major genetic defect responsible for the polymorphism of S-mephenytoin metabolism in humans', *J Biol Chem*, 269: 19–22 [*Abstract*].

Evans, D.A.P., Manley, K.A. and McKusick, V.A. (1960) 'Genetic control of isoniazid metabolism in man', *British Medical Journal*, 2: 485–91.

Goldenberg, M.M. (1999) 'Trastuzumab, a recombinant DNA-derived humanized monoclonal antibody, a novel agent for the treatment of metastatic breast cancer', *Clin Ther*, 21: 309–18 [*Medline*].

Guengerich, F.P. (1998) 'The environmental genome project: functional analysis of polymorphisms', *Environ Health Perspect*, 106: 365–8 [*Medline*].

Iyer, V.R., Eisen, M.B., Ross, D.T., Schuler, G., Moore, T., Lee, J.C.F., et al. (1999) 'The transcriptional program in the response of human fibroblasts to serum', *Science*, 283: 83–7 [*Abstract/Full Text*].

Kalow, W. and Staron, N. (1957) 'On distribution and inheritance of atypical forms of human serum cholinesterase, as indicated by dibucaine number', *Can J Biochem*, 35: 1306–17.

Kleyn, P.W. and Vesell E.S. (1998) 'Genetic variation as a guide to drug development', *Science*, 281: 1820–1 [*Full Text*].

Sadée, W. (1998) 'Genomics and drugs: finding the optimal drug for the right patient,' *Pharm Res*, 15: 959–63 [*Medline*].

Schmid, B., Bircher J, Preisig, R. and Kupfer, A. (1985) 'Polymorphic dextromethorphan metabolism: co-segregation of oxidative O-demethylation with debrisoquin hydroxylation', *Clin Pharmacol Ther*, 38: 618–24 [*Medline*].

Service, R.F. (1998) 'Microchip arrays put DNA on the spot', *Science*, 282: 396–9 [*Full Text*].

Sinclair, B. (1999) 'Everything's great when it sits on a chip: a bright future for DNA arrays', *Scientist*, 13: 18–20.

Tai, H.L., Krynetski, E.Y., Yates, C.R., Loennechen, T., Fessing, M.Y., Krynetskaia, N.F., and Evans, W.E. (1996) 'Thiopurine S-methyltransferase deficiency: two nucleotide transitions define the most prevalent mutant allele associated with loss of catalytic activity in caucasians', *Am J Hum Genet* 58: 694–702 [*Medline*].

Weber, W.W. (1997) *Pharmacogenetics*. New York: Oxford University Press.

Weinshilboum, R.M. and Sladek, S.L. (1980) 'Mercaptopurine pharmacogenetics: monogenic inheritance of erythrocyte thiopurine methyltransferase activity', *Am J Hum Genet* 32: 651–62 [*Medline*].

35

Towards the Millennium of Cybermedicine

Gunther Eysenbach, Eun Ryoung Sa and Thomas I. Diepgen

The world wide web is the universe of network-accessible information, the embodiment of human knowledge. (World Wide Web Consortium)

The evolution of the 'information age' in medicine is mirrored in the exponential growth of medical web pages, increasing numbers of databases accessible on line, and expanding services and publications available on the internet. The handful of computers linked by the predecessor of the internet in 1969 has grown to more than 5 million web sites today. In Spring 1998, the world wide web had at least 320 million web pages of general content (Lawrence and Giles, 1998). In addition, there are countless conversational areas on the internet, like chat rooms and newsgroups, where people exchange messages on tens of thousands of subjects. Somewhere more than 150 million people currently communicate over the internet (8th Computer Industry Almanac, 1998). According to the World Wide Web Consortium (W3C), however, the rapid 'hyper-growth' of the web from 1992 to mid-1995 has now somewhat slowed to roughly gaining an order of magnitude 'only' every 30 months (Pitkow et al., 1999).

Medical information is often said to be one of the most often retrieved types of information on the web. In fact, according to a survey of October 1998, 27 per cent of female and 15 per cent of male internet users say that they access medical information weekly or daily (GVU, 1998). An interesting observation from this and other surveys (Reents and Miller, 1998) is that health and medical content seems to be one of only a few categories on line that women are more likely to use than men.

SUMMARY POINTS

- more than 100,000 medical web sites exist, and their number is still growing rapidly.
- 'Cybermedicine' is a new academic speciality at the crossroads of medical informatics and public health, studying applications of the internet and global networking technologies to medicine and public health, examining the impact and implications of the internet, and evaluating opportunities and the challenges for health care.

- The internet revolution in health care is largely driven by a massive consumer demand for online health resources.
- The fact that patients have access to the same databases as clinicians leads to increased consumer knowledge, which is pushing clinicians to higher quality standards and evidence-based medicine.
- Patient to patient interchanges are becoming an important part of health care and redefine the traditional model of preventive medicine and health promotion.
- Problems of cybermedicine include the quality of online information, lack of standards, and lack of social equity.

No one knows the exact number of medical (including health and 'wellness') web sites, but the frequently cited figure of 15,000 health sites (Reents and Miller 1998) is probably an underestimate, given that Yahoo USA alone lists more than 19,000 web sites under the topic 'health' (Yahoo, 1999) and other international Yahoo catalogues together add roughly another 15,000 sites. Assuming conservatively that a maximum of 30 per cent of all sites are registered in Yahoo (Lawrence and Giles, 1998), we can estimate that there are a minimum of 100,000 health-related web sites available. Health information providers on the web include mostly private companies offering medical products or medical information (news services, electronic journals, databases), individual patients and health professionals, self-support groups for patients, and professional associations, non-governmental organizations, universities, research institutes and governmental agencies.

CYBERMEDICINE: A DEFINITION

The developments outlined above probably have a considerable impact on efficiency and quality of future health care, consumer empowerment, public health, medical education, and several other issues. At the crossroads of medical informatics and public health a new academic speciality is emerging–'cybermedicine', 'medicine in cyberspace,' where 'cyberspace' denotes the internet.

An arbitrary definition of this discipline could be 'the science of applying internet and global networking technologies to medicine and public health, of studying the impact and implications of the internet, and of evaluating opportunities and the challenges for health care'. Of particular interest in our unit for cybermedicine at the Department of Clinical Social Medicine in the University of Heidelberg is the exploration and exploitation of the internet for consumer health education, patient self-support, professional medical education and research, the evaluation of the quality of medical information on the internet, the impact of the internet on the patient–physician relationship and quality of health care, and the use of global networking for evidence-based medicine.

Cybermedicine is distinct from telemedicine, although there are over-lapping issues, especially as the internet can also be used as a medium for telemedical applications. While telemedicine focuses primarily on a restricted exchange of clinical, confidential data with a limited number of participants, for the most part between patient and physician or between physician and physician, in cybermedicine there is a global exchange of open, non-clinical information, mostly between patient and patient, sometimes between patient and physician, and between physician and physician. Telemedicine for the most part is applied to diagnostic and curative medicine, while cybermedicine is applied to preventive medicine and public health. The term 'prevention' in this context covers not only measures to prevent the occurrence of disease (primary prevention), for example by health education on web sites set up by professionals or consumers, but also a reduction in the consequences of disease (tertiary prevention), for example by information exchange among patients through newsgroups, web sites, or via e-mail, leading to improved self-management of disease. In cybermedicine the new role of the consumer redefines the traditional concept of 'prevention' and 'health promotion' (that is, the process of enabling people to increase control over the determinants of health and thereby prevent disease or reduce the impact of disease), which traditionally implied a formal communication process between the health professional as sender and the consumer as receiver, whereas on the internet, health promotion and prevention become largely a process between consumer and consumer.

Other people may have other definitions of cybermedicine. In his book *Cybermedicine: How Computing Empowers Doctors and Patients for Better Health Care*, Warner Slack uses this term in a much broader sense, not only focusing on the internet but referring to the use of computers in medicine in general (Slack, 1997). Another article, entitled 'Cybermedicine' in the *New England Journal of Medicine* (Pies, 1998), merely referred to medical advice services on the internet and thus to only one aspect of what we think constitutes cybermedicine.

THE ROLE OF CONSUMERS

While most physicians still lag behind other professions in their use of modern information technology (Anon, 1997) in many parts of the industrialized world consumers have taken the lead in adopting new media for retrieving and exchanging health information. While tele-medicine is often driven by a 'technological push', cybermedicine is characterized by a remarkable 'consumer pull'.

We would argue that consumers and patients will have a crucial role as a major driving force for clinicians to 'go on line' as consumers accessing electronic information will inevitably increase the pressure on caregivers to use timely evidence and will force them to become acquainted with information technology. The internet is therefore a motor for evidence-based medicine, not only because it provides an infrastructure for health professionals to access resources and databases (Hersh, 1996) but also because it allows consumers to draw from the same knowledge base, thereby increasing consumer involvement in health care decision-making and increasing the pressure on caregivers to deliver high quality health services (Silagy, 1999). It is mainly the latter aspect that is the true revolution (at the same time a challenge) (Coiera, 1996) for health care. While it is still a matter of debate whether the typical patient can translate these possibilities directly into better health (rather than simply getting lost in a stew of information or becoming a 'cyberhypochondriac'), many patients will use this information at least to challenge the evidence base of physicians by confronting them with 'anecdotes' from the internet. This is often referred to as one of the negative sides of medical information on the internet as it puts new strains on the patient–physician relationship, but we can also regard it as a positive incentive for doctors to learn how to use electronic evidence-based resources. As physicians follow consumers into the information age this will further increase the demand and the provision of information on the internet, leading to even more consumer empowerment and patient-centred and evidence-based medicine – a positive feedback loop.

At this point it should be emphasized that according to our own experiences (Eysenbach and Diepgen, 1999a) considerable differences from country to country exist in the ratio of consumers to physicians shopping for medical information, indicating that data from the United States (which are predominant in the literature) must not necessarily be generalized to other countries.

QUALITY ISSUES

The quality of information is a critical factor in the use of cybermedicine for consumer empowerment, patient support, health education, and evidence-based medicine. Pioneering studies that assessed the quality of web sites (Impicciatore et al., 1997) and newsgroups (Culver et al., 1997) or evaluated interactive venues by posing as a fictitious patient (Eysenbach and Diepgen, 1998a, 1998b) all showed that important aspects of quality such as reliability, accessibility, and completeness of information and advice found on the internet are extremely variable, ranging from the useful to the dangerous. While a similar problem is also known from traditional media such as magazines, newspapers and television, the internet adds a new dimension because, first, everybody can be a publisher (often without any quality or editorial control at the stage of production), secondly, originators of messages and their credibility are difficult for readers to assess; and, thirdly, the line between editorial content and advertisements is often blurred. Organizations such as the Federal Trade Commission (FTC, 1999) or the US Science Panel on Interactive Health Communication (Gustafson et al., 1999) have repeatedly warned that much information on the web is misleading or positively harmful. Surveys also show that most internet users would like to be able to identify and filter potentially harmful information more easily (HON, 1999). At the same time, it has been pointed out that many rating systems on the web are 'incompletely developed instruments' (Jadad and Gagliardi, 1998).

But quality issues are not the only problems that have to be solved. Lack of standards is another concern. While internet protocols led to a global standardization of how computers talk to each other, standardization on many higher levels (such as medical applications) still has to be achieved to reach inter-operability of medical internet resources.

The third major challenge is less a technical but more a social issue: how can we avoid global health staying limited to the industrialized world and not reaching the populations and areas that are most in need of improved health? This problem is not confined to developing countries, but even if we look at users of the internet in the 'developed world', where the internet is well established, ethnic minorities are under-represented and low income as well as poor education remain real barriers to accessing health and medical content on line.

The internet will change radically in the coming millennium. One major revolution on the web will be a 'quantity leap', freeing today's internet from some of its technical limitations. The next generation internet will operate at speeds up to 1,000 times faster than today. Sight, sound, and even touch will be integrated through powerful computers, displays and networks. Patients will be able to videoconference with their health care providers, security problems will be resolved, and the internet will increasingly be used for transmitting clinical data, linked with and integrated into educational resources.

The second revolution will lead to a 'quality leap'. Up to now, the web has been used primarily for human to human communication. The vision of the web, however, goes beyond this. The second side to the web, yet to emerge, is that of 'machine understandable information' (Berners-Lee, 1997). If this vision becomes reality in medicine, a part of the web would evolve into a global medical knowledge base that is browsable and searchable across languages and continents. Key to this development is the widespread use of metadata (medPICS/XML/RDF), which means linking human readable content with standard nomenclature such as the UMLS (Unified Medical Language System) and other descriptive and evaluative meta-information, either by authors themselves or by third parties (Eysenbach Diepgen, 1998c, 1999b). In such a global medical knowledge base, diverse medical internet applications and resources such as text, images and retrieval systems of databases would then be interconnected beyond manual 'linking', glued together by middleware and intelligent software agents, helping internet medical users to navigate an unbounded information space. Together, these developments will once again revolutionize discovery and dissemination of knowledge in medicine.

REFERENCES

Anonymous (1997) 'Doctors lag behind executives in using e-mail and the internet', *Telemed Virtual Real*, 2: 135.

Berners-Lee, T. (1997) 'Realising the full potential of the web'. Talk presented at the W3C meeting, London, 3 December.

Coiera, E. (1996) 'The internet's challenge to health care provision', *British Medical Journal*, 312: 3–4.

Culver, J.D., Gerr, F. and Frumkin, H. (1997) 'Medical information on the internet: a study of an electronic bulletin board', *J Gen Intern Med*, 12: 466–70.

8th Computer Industry Almanac (accessed 20 March 1998).

Eysenbach, G. and Diepgen, T.L. (1998a) 'Responses to unsolicited patient e-mail requests for medical advice on the world wide web', *Journal of the American Medical Association*, 280: 1333–5.

Eysenbach, G. and Diepgen, T.L. (1998b) 'Evaluation of cyberdocs', *Lancet*, 352: 1526.

Eysenbach, G. and Diepgen, T.L. (1998c) 'Towards quality management of medical information on the internet: evaluation, labelling, and filtering of information', *British Medical Journal*, 317: 1496–1500.

Eysenbach, G. and Diepgen, T.L. (1999a) *Informations system Dermatologie (dermis.net). Abschlussbericht eines BMBF/DFN geförderten Forschungsprojekts an der Universitätshauklinik Erlangen.* Heidelberg: University of Erlangen and Nuremberg (accessed 28 June 1999).

Eysenbach, G. and Diepgen, T.J. (1999b) 'Labelling and filtering of medical information on the internet', *Meth Inf Med*, 38: 80–8.

FTC: Federal Trade Commission (1999) *Consumer Alert Virtual 'Treatments' Can Be Real World Deceptions*, Washington, DC: Federal Trade Commission, June (accessed 29 June 1999).

Gustafson, D.H., Robinson, T.N., Ansley, D., Adler, L. and Brennan, P.F. for the Science Panel on Interactive Communication and Health (1999) 'Consumers and evaluation of interactive health communication applications', *Am J Prev Med*, 16: 23–9.

GVU (1998) 10th WWW user survey of October 1998 (accessed 28 June 1999).

Hersh, W.R. (1996) 'Evidence-based medicine and the internet' (Editorial), *ACP Journal Club*, 5: A14–A16.

HON (1999) Fourth Survey on the Use of the Internet for Medical and Health Purposes (accessed 28 June 1999).

Impicciatore, P., Pandolfini, C., Casella, N. and Bonati, M. (1997) 'Reliability of health information for the public on the world wide web: systematic survey of advice on managing fever in children at home', *British Medical Journal*, 314: 1875–81.

Jadad, A.R. and Gagliardi, A. (1998) 'Rating health information on the internet. Navigating to knowledge or to Babel? *Journal of the American Medical Association*, 279: 611–14.

Lawrence, S. and Giles, C.L. (1998) 'Searching the world wide web', *Science*, 280: 98–100.

Pies, R. (1998) 'Cybermedicine', *New England Journal of Medicine*, 339: 638.

Pitkow, L., Hjelm, J. and Frystyk Nielsen, H. (1999) Web characterization: from working group to activity. W3C Note, 19 March (accessed 28 June 1999).

Reents, S. and Miller, T.E. (1998) *The Health Care Industry in Transition. The Online Mandate to Change.* Cyber dialogue (accessed 28 June 1999).

Silagy, C. (1999) 'Introduction to the new edition: the post-Cochrane agenda: consumers and evidence', in A. Cochrane (ed.), *Effectiveness and Efficiency*. London: Royal Society of Medicine Press.

Slack, W.V. (1997) *Cybermedicine: How Computing Empowers Doctors and Patients for Better Health Care.* San Francisco: Jossey-Bass/Simon & Schuster.

Yahoo Health Directory (accessed 28 June 1999).

36

Working Whole Systems

Julian Pratt, Pat Gordon and Diane Plamping

Whole System Working is a radical way of thinking about change in complex situations; a combination of theory and practical methods of working across boundaries.

A WAY OF THINKING

From the parts to the whole

Complex social issues such as urban regeneration, teenage pregnancy, or the quality of life of older people are influenced by the actions of many individuals, groups and organizations. They are beyond the ability of any one agency or individual to 'fix'. In trying to tackle them the tendency is to break them into actionable parts. Yet despite the hard work of policy-makers and good people 'on the ground', many of these problems prove insoluble by traditional problem-solving methodologies.

We reasoned that it might be more fruitful to think of them as issues for an interconnected system to tackle together. We use the word 'system' to refer to a network of people and organizations which share a particular purpose – improving the quality of life of older people in a town, for example. We chose to shift our attention from parts to the whole and thus to the connections between parts – how the whole system fits together.

One group of 10–20 got together because they wanted to do something about improving transport for older people. There was a strong nucleus of elders, people from the voluntary sector, the police and a transport company. Initially, the struggle was to find a way of using the strengths of this unusual membership. The group first tried to act as if it were able to represent older people and hold those in the formal system to account. We encouraged them to identify something they could all work on together and they decided on bus services. Recognizing that bus drivers had a shared interest in this they focused on the question, 'How can we enable bus drivers to provide the service that older people want?'

Several older people, with experience of getting things done by campaigning, wanted the group to campaign to persuade the bus company to schedule longer journey times, to allow more time for passengers to sit down, to go back to two-man bus operations and to extend the hours of the concessionary bus pass.

However, by retaining the identity of a system containing many perspectives, the group discovered that what they could productively do together was for older people and managers from the bus companies to travel together on the buses and share their experiences. This led to improved understanding of the bus operators by the older people. It also led to recognition by the managers that older people are a resource with useful things to say about bus design and operation. As a result, they immediately put into effect some inexpensive but significant modifications to the buses; took the comments of the older people into the driver-training programme; and invited older people to view and assess new buses the bus operators were thinking of buying.

Organizations as designed systems

As a means of illuminating whole system thinking we use the contrasting metaphors of organizations as designed systems and as living systems (Morgan, 1986). Some management thinking and practice uses the metaphors of designed and mechanical systems (like computers or telephone exchanges). We can recognize this approach by its language – cogs and leverage, redesign, re-engineering and so on. It is based on scientific ideas that have increased our understanding of the world by analysing wholes into their component parts. In organizational life the 'messes' and complexity are broken down into a series of manageable problems and tackled separately.

In a designed system of this sort behaviour is sequential – analysis, planning, action and review that occur one after another, feeding into further cycles. Policy and strategy are separated from implementation. The parts of a designed system can be separated, standardized, optimized and reassembled to improve the efficiency of the whole.

This approach in organizations is particularly appropriate when you know the desired future and how to achieve it. It helps ensure that people make decisions with transparency, create audit trails and avoid fraud. Structures based on hierarchies provide effective ways of preventing individuals or organizations from doing their worst.

Organizations as living systems

We find it fruitful to use metaphors derived from living systems, or ecosystems, which lead us to think of individuals, teams, departments and organizations as purposeful entities linked in a web of interdependence. We think they can interact intelligently, autonomously and through a process of constantly adapting with each other. They are not limited to behaving in ways predetermined by a designer, planner or chief executive.

We find this metaphor more sympathetic to the individual creativity of conscious human beings and the familiar patterns of behaviour structured by social context. Many different sorts of people co-create their shared future, in more equal relationships.

This approach in organizations is particularly appropriate when it is not possible to know in detail what actions will be needed in the future, not least because part of the solution is to trigger behaviour change in others. Structures based on peer relationships provide effective ways of enabling individuals and organizations to do their best.

The behaviour of the whole

We distinguish between the concepts of 'control' and 'order'. Control is about 'checking and controlling action'. Order is about 'the condition in which everything is in its proper place, and performs its proper functions'. Order is about pattern, not about having to control each detail. Order is about the characteristic shape of a tree, not where a particular leaf or branch is.

In complex adaptive systems, such as living systems, order is an emergent property of the system as a whole. In all its rich particular detail, order can arise from the repeated application of quite a small number of guiding principles.

If you think of organizations as living systems you pay attention to certain features such as connections, meaning and relationships. If you think of organizations as designed systems you pay attention to improving the parts and to controlling how they fit together.

A WAY OF WORKING

What's involved

Whole system working is a way of seeing the world that leads you to do work in different ways. It is not a single methodology but an overall approach with a set of distinct characteristics. We have identified nine principles, or characteristics. We use the traditional device of a wheel to allow us to keep an awareness of the whole set of ideas while giving attention to the component parts (Figure 36.1).

Meaning Spend enough time talking together about what you want to do (purpose) and why you want to do it (meaning) before rushing into fix-it mode. Particularly when there are differing perspectives it helps to include lay people and people who use services from the start, as their views often provide the basis for recognizing common ground.

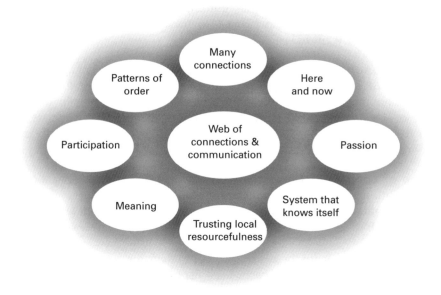

Figure 36.1 *Characteristics of whole system working*

Trusting local resourcefulness Permit trust to grow that there are appropriate solutions already within the system. Enable people to recognize capacities and assets.

System that knows itself Shared purpose enables people to recognize that 'we're in this together' and that their futures are linked. Find ways to reveal the way the system works as a whole.

Passion Living systems have the capacity to fuel themselves. The renewable fuel in human systems is passion. Give people the freedom to engage with the purpose they feel passionate about.

Here and now Practise these conversations while doing real system work rather than talking about the way systems work. Spend the valuable time you have together exploring purpose and meaning – if you can reach understanding about this you will know what you need to go away and do on your own.

Many connections Find ways to have conversations with unusual mixes of people – diversity is an asset, not a problem. Ensure there are enough perspectives to grow a more complete (i.e. whole) system picture.

Patterns of order   Seek out the 'guiding principles' that people actually use in their day-to-day work. Do these give rise to the sort of behaviour you want to see?

Participation   Use processes that allow everyone to engage as an expert individual. This means redefining our understanding of expertise as synonymous with certification. It means enabling people to use personal experience and stories, and inviting people to participate in their own right rather than as representatives. Focus on co-producing solutions.

Web of connections and communication   Grow new connections. Information is about the transfer of data (through reports, lectures and presentations). But real communication, which co-ordinates behaviour, involves sharing of understanding (through conversation and dialogue).

These principles are the nearest we get to devising a sort of algorithm to describe the overall approach. Each aspect is important, but none is sufficient on its own. Bringing together people with many perspectives but no shared commitment, for example, may end up as a shouting match. Encouraging people to follow their passion without a sense of shared meaning may lead just to performance and posture.

Putting it into practice

Whole system working is designed to help people make connections that enable them to find sustainable solutions to complex organizational problems. It is an approach that aims to deal with 'the whole' and not just 'the parts'. In putting it into practice we are looking for ways in which people recognize they have to seek solutions at a system-wide level. For this to happen our experience is that we must give attention to three essentials: language, people and design.

Language – what is the system-wide issue?   Most problems, most of the time, are dealt with entirely appropriately by an individual, a team or an organization – they are not issues that require the attention of a wider system. It is therefore important to be clear whether there is an issue that a system wants to tackle together. In whole system working, crafting the question that brings people together is critically important. Formulating the content and the wording is part of the change process. It is about shared purpose and meaning and therefore careful phrasing is vital.

The way we ask questions often reflects beliefs about 'whose problem' it is and 'whose responsibility' it is to solve. For example, whose problem is it if there are long waits in casualty departments? Are the solutions about reorganizing the department or are they to do with clinical practice elsewhere in the hospital, in general practice, the availability of district nurses, the local authority's community care policy, or all of the above?

Working to identify a system-wide issue, something that only the whole system can address, is crucial.

If we form questions around deficits we exclude groups whose involvement is critical to new solutions, and so perpetuate shifting the blame. We know of a multiple-stakeholder conference where the invitation was to 'tackle the problem of youth crime'. Framing the issue in this way did not draw in young people. They continued to be seen as the problem, and the conference did not produce any new energy to make a difference.

This contrasts with an approach where the original concern was teenage truancy from school but became 'How do we make this a good place to grow up in?' This question mobilized a very different system, which extended far beyond the formal education and policing networks. Re-articulating the problem, in ways that tap into people's passion *for* something, can release different forms of energy. 'How do we make this a good place to grow up in?' bounds the issue in important ways. Its clarity ensures that any person knows whether this is an issue they want to contribute to; but its openness allows them to contribute to building the agenda. It is an invitation to share responsibility to co-produce solutions, not just react to pre-formed problems. Language is critical.

People – who is the system? We use the word 'system' to describe something that assembles itself around a shared purpose, the system-wide issue we discuss above. The next step is to identify who are the right people and in this context 'right' is about getting a sufficient mix of people working together to support new connections, new information flows and new possibilities. For this to happen you need unusual mixes of people from all levels within an organization and across organizations. You need citizens and service users and individuals who know 'how to connect', as well as those with formal power. The work is about co-producing solutions – identifying what we each have to do 'to make things work differently around here'. Those with formal power must be prepared to trust that between them local people can come up with locally sustainable solutions.

Living systems are made up of continuing relationships. This shared future is essential for sustainable change in a system's behaviour. In human terms it is tempting to think that if sufficient representatives of organizations are brought together then somehow 'the system is in the room'. But if there is no commitment to future action then what you have is a sample of each kind – an ark, not a system.

So in taking this approach you are always looking for a rich mix of individuals who are prepared to take responsibility for participating and *continuing* to make a difference.

Design – getting the system's attention This is about designing meetings and choosing methods of working that enable local people and organizations *to work constructively together* to uncover new possibilities for action. These methods can be designed for use in large or small meetings. They are about participative ways of working that help people get clear about their purpose and release the sort of creativity that fuels new working practices.

Since a lot of organizational work is done in meetings, when you begin to take a whole system approach this leads you to redesign meetings. You invest time 'up front' in conversations to establish purpose and a shared sense of being 'in this together'. You look for ways to enable people to identify what it is they feel passionate about, and want to take responsibility for doing together. Meetings become more creative – fun, even. This is an approach that is worth taking when you realize that more-of-the-same just won't produce new solutions, no matter how hard people try. It is about looking for possibilities. It is not a substitute for the committee-style meetings and planning processes which organizations also need, but for different purposes.

Your aim in 'getting the system's attention' is to enable people and organizations to recognize that actions taken by one will have often unpredictable consequences for the others, and that because their futures are linked they can trigger reciprocal changes in the behaviour of others; to recognize, in other words, that they are functioning as a living system. If your aim is to change the system's behaviour then the big question becomes: how to work effectively with the great diversity in a complex system? Sometimes this requires large numbers of people to work together in the same room at the same time (Bunker and Alban, 1997), but the guiding principle is about engaging multiple perspectives, not about size (Plamping et al., 1999). The attraction of working simultaneously with large numbers of local people is that their time and energy are focused on a shared concern in a very public and energizing way. However, this is no more than a broadening out of a way of working to include a greater number of people in the building of networks, sharing of purpose and exploration of possibilities.

The whole of a system is not in the usual sense controlled; rather it is 'self-ordered'. Any living system is probably perfectly formed to achieve its current purpose. If you don't like the way it is behaving you have to design ways of getting its attention to help it reconsider its purpose and choose new principles to guide behaviour. Our experience is that if the right mix of people is brought together and meetings are designed according to the principles we have outlined, then you can trust their judgement and the system can alter its behaviour.

WHAT HAPPENS

Different sorts of things begin to happen in different situations. It's the process of uncovering rather than importing or inventing solutions that generates the possibility for change that is not only locally appropriate but sustainable:

> At a meeting of the older people's JPT (joint planning team) two of the older people's representatives were noticeably upset. Their distress was caused by their personal situations and concern about the circumstances of other older people known to them. At first it seemed that the meeting would (briefly) sympathetically listen to these personal anecdotes – but regard them as having no general relevance, certainly not to admit them as evidence of more widespread system failures – and then carry on with its business. But Mr K. from the Health Authority stepped in and supported the older people. He agreed to their suggestion that time should be given at each meeting for airing of personal stories – from anyone. This was quite a dramatic intervention. There was nearly dissension in the statutory ranks. But others rallied to support Mr K., and it was widely discussed and agreed. This was a critical point where something suddenly shifted. (Local authority manager)

> Service planners and providers always find it very difficult to hear these stories. They don't want to hear them. They have to deny them or rule them out of order as mere anecdotes, not hard evidence. For to accept the elders' stories as true would mean having to confront and admit that things are not as they – the funders and providers – present them. This is very threatening. So to get stories allowed is a small triumph. But the crunch has to come in what happens as a result of what people say. (Voluntary agency director)

> There are already small changes in services as a result of elders' stories. For example there will be changes to security in sheltered housing as a result of an anecdote described at a planning meeting. The manager came along to the next meeting and we all discussed it. (Voluntary sector worker)

As people recognize their part in a wider system they begin to go beyond simply 'doing their own bit':

> One of the 'classic' boundary issues in the health service is when people get admitted to hospital, and when they leave hospital to return home. Communication between GPs and hospitals is crucial. In one of the places we worked, a group of GPs knew the importance of a really good 'admission letter' to ensure that their local hospital got all the information it needed when a patient was admitted, and they had worked hard to produce a good format. During the course of a whole system event they realized that, no matter how good the letter was, the hospital was not able 'to hear' what they were communicating because of the way junior hospital doctors rotate between departments. In other words, they realized that if they wanted to get their message across, and to influence what the hospital actually did, they would have to become involved in the hospital's induction programme for doctors. And this they set about doing. (Pratt et al., 1999, p. 54)

There are more examples in our book (Pratt et al., 1999), and in the independent evaluation of the action research programme in which the approach was developed (Jee et al., 1999).

Probably the most powerful thing that happens, yet the most difficult to pin down, is the emergence of a new willingness to collaborate and a new energy to re-engage with long-standing issues. People who see their world in this way find lots of ways of doing their work differently, of allowing good practice to emerge locally.

Sometimes the tangible results don't seem to be very dramatic. But in a living system, small changes in the fundamental 'code' may lead to major differences in the behaviour of the system. We are encouraged by remembering that humans have 98 per cent of their genes in common with orang-utans – 2 per cent can make a big difference!

REFERENCES

Bunker, B.B. and Alban, B.T. (1997) *Large Group Interventions – Engaging the Whole System for Rapid Change*. San Francisco: Jossey-Bass.

Jee, M., Popay, J., Everitt, A. and Eversley, J. (1999) *Developing Urban Primary Care: Evaluating the London & Northern Health Partnership's 'Whole System Approach'*. London: King's Fund.

Morgan, G. (1986) *Images of Organization*. Newbury Park, CA: Sage Publications.

Plamping, D., Gordon, P. and Pratt, J. (1999) *Action Zones and Large Numbers*. London: King's Fund.

Pratt, J., Gordon, P. and Plamping, D. (1999) *Working Whole Systems: Putting Theory into Practice in Organisations*. London: King's Fund. See also www.wholesystems.co.uk

37

Future Health Scenarios and Public Policy

Michael Peckham

The clinical 'present' benefits from some of the most exciting examples of twentieth-century creativity and ingenuity. By contrast, many aspects of the organization and structure of health care are historical and struggling to contain a revolution in science, technology and social development. Manifestations of this are the tentative and often ineffectual approaches to chronic illness and preventable disease as well as variations in standards and methods of treating acute problems.

The clinical future can be thought of in two ways: the future of clinical practice and the broader future of which clinical practice forms part. Either way it is clear that the clinical future is necessarily bound up with the future of society. In terms of financing and style it will be influenced by the efforts of governments to balance social development, political freedom and industrial competitiveness. At present the achievements are uneven. Even in rich countries individuals or even segments of cities are disadvantaged and excluded from many of the health and other benefits enjoyed by the rest of society.

Despite the spectacular advances of medicine and the general improvement in health statistics across the world, the gap between our technological sophistication and social primitiveness is stark. Thus, as mankind enters the third millennium, it is capable not only of etching nanocircuits with electrons or of performing microsurgery on neonates, but also of engaging in ethnic cleansing and the widespread violation of human rights. This discordance is not new but it is more stark.

GENOME

Genomic and genetic research coupled with informatics is today's equivalent of the discovery of X-rays a century ago and the future consequences are as unforeseeable as were the implications of Röntgen's finding. The DNA revolution has had a fairly protracted gestation since the double helix structure of DNA was described in 1953, but all is now

Edited from a chapter in M. Marinker and M. Peckham (eds), *Clinical Futures*. London: BMJ Books, 1998.

rapidly changing, ushering in a new era for diagnosis, treatment and disease prevention.

In the 1990s it was shown for the first time in sheep that nuclear material from an adult mature cell fused with the enucleated ovum could form an embryo which after implantation in a surrogate mother could go on to produce a normal lamb. The first successful experiment used cells from the udder of a living ewe, but subsequently a lamb has been produced from fused cells cultured in the laboratory. The technology of nuclear transfer demonstrates that mature cells can be persuaded to revert to an embyronic form. Foetal cells have been implanted with some success into the brain of patients with Parkinson's disease. One possibility is for brain cells from individual patients to be dedifferentiated using nuclear transfer methods and implanted back into the donors. Other anticipated applications of nuclear transfer include the production in pigs of organs that are tolerated as xenotransplants in human recipients, also the preparation of cattle, sheep and pigs with the human genetic material for producing human proteins that can be harvested and used to treat patients.

From genetic research we can anticipate novel molecule and protein therapies, the targeting of existing therapies, and the genetic dissection of diagnostic disease categories. Knowledge of genetic risk will influence personal behaviour, including eating habits and other behavioural patterns. Population genetic testing will reveal the anatomy of hidden disease and pre-disease states necessitating a redefinition of 'health needs'.

The genomic revolution will be driven by advances in silicon microchip technology and robotics, allowing molecules generated by computer to rapidly be tested in multiple simultaneous experiments. The results will aid drug discovery, elucidate the role of genes in health and disease and lead to the development of new diagnostic methods. Home-based kits will become available, allowing for example self-testing for pregnancy and self-monitoring for drug therapy. These new technologies raise the prospect of home-based blood sampling and automated drug prescription.

Knowledge of the genome of pathogenic micro-organisms will yield new methods of disease prevention. A recent report on complete genome sequence of the tuberculosis bacillus noted that 'the combination of genomics and bio-informatics has the potential to generate the information of new therapies and interventions needed to treat this airborne disease and to elucidate the unusual biology of its aetiological agent, *Mycobacterium tuberculosis*'. Vaccine development based on well-characterized antigens, an understanding of antigenic variation, and knowledge of the molecular basis of virulence will lead to new prophylactic and therapeutic interventions as well as to an epidemiological understanding of the spread of disease based on genetic subtyping.

Population genetic testing, new methods of genetic diagnosis and the subclassification of disease categories on the basis of genotype will be short- to medium-term developments. Novel therapeutics and the routine use of therapies involving the transfer of genes into either somatic cells or germ cells of recipients are likely to be further away.

There are consequences for governments in the large scale and rapid industrial developments in genetics and health. Industry invests massively in genetic and genome R&D, as well as in the information systems needed to handle the outputs. Know-how, data, diagnostic tests and therapies will encourage the move into health care offering testing, screening, treatment, counselling and population monitoring. Unchallenged this will result in a huge disparity between the commercial and public sectors in terms of knowledge, expertise and technology, with implications for costs and equity. Policies will be needed to ensure that genetic information is available to and used appropriately by the public sector.

The genomic era will also lead to a reappraisal of what constitutes individual identity. DNA fingerprinting already provides a precise method of identification. Genes and external features such as iris pigmentation patterns and facial contours, and the dissection of 'normality' in terms of the relationships between genes, behaviour and personality, will extend concepts of individual identity.

THE INDIVIDUAL IN AN INTERCONNECTED SOCIETY

In the interconnected society the individual is subsumed into a global milieu. However, other trends will give emphasis to individuality. Genetic 'uniqueness' will acquire a new dimension as it becomes possible to describe the genes along an individual's genome. Individualization of therapies will become a reality and genetic contributions to development and behaviour will be elucidated, with educational interventions and childbearing tailored to the individual. The use of molecular genetic methods in archaeology and anthropology will transform our knowledge of population movements and cultural origins and challenge preconceived notions of ethnicity and origin.

At the same time, and in response to a technology-dominated world, people will seek 'whole person' forms of health care. Already more than 5 million people in the UK each year seek complementary and alternative medicine and doubtless more would if they could afford it. Similar trends are seen in other countries and many of those who go to non-orthodox practitioners are young, without known physical symptoms or disability. This quest for holistic care to complement orthodox medicine may reflect the attraction of a one-to-one relationship between patient and the practitioner which used to be a feature of orthodox health care but which is being compromised by rapid throughput, larger primary care groups, and other trends.

DEFINING THE HEALTH 'PROBLEMATIQUE'

For any given society, defining what constitutes the set of problems under the label 'health' should be a prerequisite for developing and applying appropriate correctives. Currently health problems are articulated from viewpoints that are either too narrowly focused or impossibly diffuse. Over the next two decades there will be a shift away from the economic objectives that dominated the twentieth century. Health will become a central concern of governments based on a concept of health that emphasizes individual creativity. Purposeful living, protection from physical and mental injury and prevention and treatment of disease and disability will be integrated and form the basis for policy decisions.

HEALTH SERVICES AS OBSTACLES TO HEALTH

Health services in the form in which we know them today will evolve into new structures in the first decades of the twenty-first century. The change will be driven by the need to deliver a pan-governmental multisector commitment to health development as well as the treatment of disease and disability.

In the case of the British National Health Service, its political profile, media worthiness and public standing tend to place it beyond open debate. However, to disregard the possibility that the health service as presently constructed may become an obstacle to health development will be seen to run counter to the spirit of enlightened thinking that led to its creation in the first place.

A number of trends will allow future change to be presented and accepted as a positive and innovative development. The concept of a national service will be increasingly difficult to sustain with devolution and regionalization in the UK and common health interests coming to the fore in an enlarged European Union. It will prove frustratingly difficult to tackle many of the broader health and social problems through a service that needs to maintain a capacity for providing high-quality specialized medical care. By attempting to face in two directions at once, towards public health as well as towards high technology health care, the NHS will be seen to underexploit technology-driven medicine while failing to make a significant impact on societal health problems. Excessive expectations will lead to a growing disillusionment with orthodox medicine, as reflected in popular demand for complementary and alternative forms of health care. The result of these trends will be a waning of public support for the NHS in its current form which will be seen as overloaded and unable to fulfil its commitments.

A further disturbing trend will be the apportionment of blame to lower socioeconomic and other disadvantaged groups for their ill health. This will be ascribed to self-inflicted damage caused by adverse behaviour, poor eating habits and other factors that are judged to be within the power of individuals to change. There will be a discernible shift of opinion favouring safety-net health care provision for poorer people, with the more affluent covered by insurance or self-payment. Such arguments will be countered by a better understanding of the NHS contribution to the social fabric as well as to health. The emergence of two-tier health care and the threat to social cohesion will be an added stimulus to the creation of an alternative system.

At the time of the change a retrospective analysis of health and social problems will illustrate the mismatch between what the NHS provided and the real-life problems it sought to address. Of particular concern will be the growing inadequacy of provision for isolated, frail elderly people and the limited success in identifying and dealing with potentially preventable health problems.

The new system will include a well-researched and tested incentives framework for attainable disease prevention and the maintenance of health. Research funds will be invested in the elucidation of relationships between social structures and health. The antenatal and early childhood determinants of adult health will become a central issue in public health and health care.

The evolution and outline above will reflect the fact that, despite policy changes and reforms, old health service structures that are ill adapted to change will be seen to linger on: the distinctive architecture and ambience of the 'historical' hospital; old-fashioned communications systems; inertia in documenting the products of health care.

In future it will be unthinkable not to apply the best that can be achieved with current knowledge, skills and resources with a reasonable level of uniformity in health care. Professional leaders and their constituencies will refocus UK health on outcomes rather than on content. If this task is neglected and if the gap between the effort devoted to research and technological development on the one hand and practical application to produce measurable health benefits on the other is not closed, it will increase regulation, weaken professional commitment and cast doubts on the value of research.

Health systems will be obliged to demonstrate that they meet the needs of their users. Looking back it will seem an extraordinary aberration that variations in standards of care were allowed to persist in a technologically sophisticated era dominated in other sectors by consumer choice. In the twenty-first century, we will be astounded at the permissiveness of late twentieth-century health care, with wide variation in hospital referral rates and the rates at which different procedures are performed; for example the fourfold difference in the rates of performing coronary artery revascularization procedures between different health authorities, with the highest rates in those areas with the least need.

At present it is uncertain whether the concept of the 'customer' is relevant to the NHS and if so who the customers are: the government which pays for the service from general taxation; or the consumer as a co-payer and taxpayer; or local payers – health authorities and primary care groups. Criteria and mechanisms for establishing consumer needs will be introduced together with clearly defined and workable account-ability arrangements to the public and to government. In addressing customer needs it will be necessary to clarify what kind of intervention is most appropriate to meet those needs. This may be a social rather than a health intervention. 'Total problem' strategies will be devised to avoid problems, such as obesity, becoming medicalized. As John Vaisey observed: 'ill health could be defined as what the doctor decides: it is created or accepted in a medical consultation, thereafter the medical machinery starts up and whatever the problem a medical solution is looked for'. Since the potential for increasing technological complexity is practically unlimited, judging the right level of technical sophistication in health care will be crucially important. In the absence of any agreed criteria the pursuit of quality could also be taken to extreme lengths, with concomitant demands on resources.

Innovation, through finding new ways of using old techniques or through the invention of new technologies, changes the way medicine is practised and this in turn feeds back into the type of facilities needed, the manpower required, the flow of patients, and other modifications to existing services. At the origin of policies formed centrally are changes that have already started to happen at grassroots level. A good example is the development of endoscopy, leading to minimally invasive surgery, the emergence of day surgery, and new hospital requirements.

Despite the fact that health care, perhaps more than any other sector, is presented with a profusion and great diversity of new methods and is subject to constant change, development and innovation are concepts and functions that have had a remarkably low profile in the NHS. Yet the affordable exploitation of new opportunities should have the highest priority. Currently the NHS as an organization is slow to respond to new challenges. Innovation is often seen as a threat. It is difficult to know how to gain entry to the system in order to interest senior decision-makers in potentially valuable new developments. A good current example is telemedicine.

The coming decades will see the concept of growth and productivity introduced into health care, drawing on and adapting industrial models to the specific purposes of a public service. 'Growth' in health care will be thought of in two ways. First, the extent to which public health and health services are able to accommodate and absorb the increasing number of new technologies. Secondly, the extent to which these are deployed in an expanding pool of 'consumers', for example elderly people or those who have intractable conditions, for whom treatment will become available. Statements of productivity will be based on what is achieved with constrained resources in terms of cures, preventive interventions, changes in health status and quality of life, new developments and exploited intellectual property.

The notion of competitiveness also has relevance to the health service but in a different context to that of industry. Publicly funded health care competes with other government departments for resources as well as with the demands of other sectors for public funds. Health services contribute to national competitiveness by improving the health of the workforce and the population, through social advancement, through efficient and effective handling of resources, and through exportable innovation.

At present there is no well-defined mechanism for incorporating new technologies in a systematic way to further the development of health care provision. New medical and other interventions together with the analyses of clinical trials and systematic reviews form, as it were, a predevelopmental depository without there being any clear-cut procedures for drawing upon and exploiting the contents. In particular there is no dedicated development and innovation capacity underpinning the design and implementation of policies that make use of new opportunities to address the priorities of government.

To address the deficiencies a 'technology gateway' will be introduced into health care. Its functions will be based on pre-set criteria and serve to screen entry into the health care system of new forms of practice and to provide an exit mechanism for those that have been superseded or found to be unnecessary or ineffective. The technology gateway will be the means by which the relationship between R&D, policy formation and health care is formalized. The criteria by which decisions are reached will be drawn up with input from the range of interests involved in health care, including contributions from professional and lay people. They will be based on economic measures and health outcomes – including changes in health status as perceived by patients – and take into account other factors such as emergent developments and the envisaged level of technological complexity to be sustained by the NHS.

THE FUTURE OF MEDICINE

Medicine is in a quandary. Is its prime function to care for the sick? Is it to prevent ill health? Or should it do both? Where does 'medical' responsibility for caring for the sick begin and end? Prevention of sickness extends from medical interventions such as vaccination through to ways of tackling social and economic causes of ill health, and wider global influences such as environmental damage. Where in this spectrum is the physician to play a part? At present the answers to these questions are not clear cut and there is a degree of polarization between the 'biomedical' doctor and the 'public health' doctor, as there is between medical and non-medical professionals.

Overall the public continues to hold doctors in high esteem. If difficult resource decisions and choices have to be made the public overwhelmingly feels that these should be made by doctors and not governments or managers. However, this could change. The medical profession needs urgently to contribute to a clarification of its future role because far-reaching decisions will be taken in the next few decades. There are a number of pointers to future change. The first is the trend towards complementary and alternative methods of health care. Another is for nurses to assume greater responsibility for patient care. Other professional staff such as pharmacists are also extending their remit, managers have become firmly established in health care and many would argue that the public health function could be discharged perfectly well by non-medical personnel. At the same time, the trend in medicine is towards increasing specialization with the creation of larger groups of primary care physicians. Both trends risk distancing patients from doctors in terms of total care. Also lay people are becoming more informed, making use of their access to information including the internet and coming to consultations better armed with knowledge.

These trends could point to a largely technical role for doctors confined to the 'high tech' end of health care with other functions performed by non-medical staff. Patient contacts would be predominantly with non-medical personnel with tele-linkages to the specialist. The doctor would then become as remote from his or her patients as the airline pilot is from passengers.

If this scenario is to be substantially different, education, training and attitudes must be transformed. Medicine has fought a defensive position over health reforms and many other matters. Today it is not clear where the thinking presence of medicine resides or whether any of the colleges and associations are free enough from their historical interests to examine 'clinical futures' with sufficient detachment.

CONCLUSION

Franz Vranitsky, a former Austrian Chancellor, is said to have commented that 'anyone with visions needs to see a doctor'. It is true he was referring to Europe rather than health. However if the past is anything to go by, attempts to predict changes in medicine are generally wildly inaccurate.

Nevertheless, looking at the future may have some merits. It may alert us to opportunities which would otherwise be downplayed or missed, or prevent us taking steps that inadvertently block fruitful lines of action or inquiry. A view of the future may help shape society and prepare individuals to live with and master new technologies. Finally, by detaching ourselves, if only transiently, from daily routine in order to reflect on what might come, we may be able to see contemporary problems and potential solutions more clearly.

Conversely, forecasting could delude us into making unwise decisions, having unreasonable expectations, or it might even provide an excuse for inaction; on balance, however, the benefits outweigh the disadvantages.

Rather than a futuristic exploration, the emphasis here has been on problems that need to be solved and some of the opportunities for change. In particular the future must see an integration of scientific medicine within a broader framework that tackles social and other determinants of health. This is not an 'either/or' choice but an absolute requirement if there is to be a balanced approach to health development.

Index

abortion, 89, 294, 296
accountability in NHS, 198
acupuncture, 315
acute care provision, 331–2
adolescents
  and economic hardship, 231–2
  see also young people
advocacy
  role of GPs, 296–7, 298
  role of international organizations, 131
  see also public health advocacy
aetiology, and 'black box' epidemiology,
  170–2
agency *see* self-determination
aid for health development, 125
AIDS/HIV, 8, 39, 119
Amick, B.C., 46
anatomical atlas, 17
Anderson, R., 255
art *see* arts initiatives; body art
arts initiatives
  economic impact of, 154, 157–8
  principles of, 158–9
  social impact of, 153, 154–7, 158, 159–60
  and social policy, 153–4, 158
Assey, J.L., 288–9
asthma, 166, 209
autonomic nervous system, 246

balancing strategy and chronic illness, 263
Balarajan, R., 171
basic needs, women's campaigns for, 92–4
Baudrillard, Jean, 36
Baumol, William, 49
beauty, and cosmetic surgery, 188–9, 191,
  192
Beeson, P.B., 44
behavioural modification, 48
behavioural problems of children, 231, 232
biomedical model
  limitations of, 245
  separation of disease and self, 258
birth *see* childbirth
birth control
  campaigns about, 88–9
  see also abortion

'black box' epidemiology, 170–2
Black Reports, 48, 65
Blainey, D., 166
Blake, William, 14
Blaxter, M., 259
body
  disciplining, 22–3
  power exercised over, 17
  sexuality and care of *see* nursing
  technology and status of, 187–8
body art (Orlan's), 186–90
  audience responses to, 185, 187, 194
  and 'real life' cosmetic surgery, 190–2
Bond, S., 271
Bourne, C., 303
breast milk substitutes, 108
Bristol Cancer Help Centre, 313
Brown, L., 274
budgets *see* health care resources
BUGAUP (Billboard Utilizing Graffitists
  Against Unhealthy Promotions), 108
burnout and uncaring, 275
Bury, M., 255, 256, 258, 261, 262, 263
bus services for older people, 358–9
Butler, P., 104
Byteheway, B., 320

caesarian sections, 209–10
Caldwell, J.C., 63
cancer
  genetics and drug responses, 344
  lung cancer and smoking, 5
  mythologies about, 3
  prevention and cure of, 165–6
  research on Bristol Cancer Help Centre,
    313
  research on ethnicity and, 171
cardiovascular disease
  cost of preventing, 164
  see also coronary heart disease
care settings, 271–2
CARE-Q, 273–4, 275
caring
  balancing curing and, 272
  burnout and uncaring, 275
  concept of care and, 268–70